# Stress and Pheromonatherapy
## in Small Animal Clinical Behaviour

# Stress and Pheromonatherapy
## in Small Animal Clinical Behaviour

Daniel Mills, Maya Braem Dube and Helen Zulch

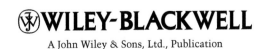

A John Wiley & Sons, Ltd., Publication

*Registered Office*
John Wiley & Sons, Ltd, The Atrium, Southern Gate, Chichester, West Sussex, PO19 8SQ, UK

*Editorial Offices*
9600 Garsington Road, Oxford, OX4 2DQ, UK
The Atrium, Southern Gate, Chichester, West Sussex, PO19 8SQ, UK
2121 State Avenue, Ames, Iowa 50014-8300, USA

For details of our global editorial offices, for customer services and for information about how to apply for permission to reuse the copyright material in this book please see our website at www.wiley.com/wiley-blackwell.

*Library of Congress Cataloging-in-Publication Data*

Mills, D. S.
Stress and pheromonatherapy in small animal clinical behaviour / Daniel Mills, Maya Braem Dube, Helen Zulch.
    p. ; cm.
  Includes bibliographical references and index.
    ISBN 978-0-470-67118-4 (pbk. : alk. paper) – ISBN 978-1-118-45881-5 (ePDF/ebook) –
ISBN 978-1-118-45880-8 (emobi) – ISBN 978-1-118-45865-5 (epub)   1. Pets–Behavior.
2. Pets–Effect of stress on.   3. Pets–Psychology.   4. Animal behavior.   5. Animal psychology.
I. Braem, Maya.   II. Zulch, Helen.   III. Title.
    [DNLM:   1. Behavior, Animal.   2. Pets–psychology.   3. Pheromones–therapeutic use.
4. Stress, Psychological.   SF 412.5]
  SF412.5.M55 2013
  636.088'7–dc23
                                        2012024774

A catalogue record for this book is available from the British Library.

Top cover image: Dog looking out from underneath a fence, contributed by tjhunt, iStockphoto.com; Bottom cover image: Portrait of Russian Blue cat, Copyright Nailia Schwarz, by licence from Shutterstock Images LLC.
Cover design by Garth Stewart

Set in 10/12pt Palatino by SPi Publisher Services, Pondicherry, India

1  2013

# Contents

# Preface

This book is the culmination of many years of research and experience, and we are grateful to colleagues, friends and students (too many to mention) who have helped us develop our ideas on these topics over this time. We appreciate your generosity, openness and constructive criticism in equal measure. Science makes progress through discussion, sharing and a willingness to change ideas as new knowledge and opinion becomes available; and it is in this spirit that we have written this text. We have tried to address several emerging issues within the field of clinical animal behaviour, some more controversial than others. But this controversy makes them academically interesting, since at times we have to resort to the basic principles of biology and scientific philosophy to make a judgement about what we consider to be the most appropriate interpretation of what we perceive. It is fair to say that differences of opinion have been a feature of pheromonatherapy from the outset, ever since Patrick Pageat appeared on the world stage at the World Small Animal Veterinary Association (WSAVA) in 1996 and suggested that the facial secretions of the cat consisted of five pheromone fractions, one of which appeared to inhibit urine spraying.

For some, there was concern over the use of the term 'pheromone' in this context, especially when it became apparent that the fraction was in fact a mixture of chemicals rather than a single substance, since this did not fit with the common view of a pheromone. Another issue was that this mixture seemed to consist of relatively common fatty acids. How could these have such powerful effects? Pheromones were largely considered to be specific chemicals that triggered the release of behaviour (recent work shows that ants can use some of these chemicals in a much more flexible way than was previously appreciated, but their role in mammals, who have more flexible behaviour patterns, is more questionable), although a possible exception related to sexual attractants and chemicals that caused sexual arousal in males (what some might call our 'base urges' – reflecting a highly cultural perspective on behavioural control). So what was this French vet doing using the term 'pheromone' in relation to chemicals which seemed to have broader effects on behaviour? Some suggested the term 'social odour' or simply 'semiochemical' should be used instead. However, as we will argue later, this perhaps ignores some of these chemicals' special properties relating to the control of emotional processes, and we should not be distracted by semantics, but instead focus on the claims being made.

The inclusion of *Valeriana* extract in the early commercial formulations raised further concerns among sceptics: they suggested that the fatty acid element was just a placebo and that the effect (if there was one) was due to the psychoactive properties of this herbal extract. However, this herbal fraction has only ever been included in the commercial sprays and never the diffusers, which have been shown to have a similar level of efficacy. The use of this fraction for the management of spraying was also recently subjected to the most rigorous form of assessment in medical treatment evaluation (meta-analysis) and found to be significantly better than placebo, but even so sceptics remain. Healthy scepticism is good for science, but evangelical preaching of opinion against scientific evidence, like blind acceptance, is not. We hope this book will help the reader to distinguish between these extremes and contribute to the debate on either side in a more informed way. What is important is that we make rational and consistent judgments when faced with uncertainty and are prepared to change our opinion as new evidence comes to light. Otherwise it is a matter of faith, not science.

The use of feline facial and other supposed 'pheromone' fractions extracted from a wider range of anatomical sites and species in the control of behaviour has also been quite an alien concept to many within the veterinary profession (who were the original target of the marketing of these products). So it is not surprising that there has been much confusion and some misunderstanding. It is perhaps for this reason that Ceva Animal Health, the commercial producer of the main products currently available, has invested in a sustained programme of research into their application and use, seeing education as key to acceptance. This includes a lot of research by the first author of this text, much of which was directly supported by Ceva, but only ever with a view to obtaining independent opinion and evaluation. Unlike some of the horror reports which are heard about in the human medical field, Ceva has never sought a spin on our interpretation of results. Rather, it has sought to learn alongside us, and it is fair to say our opinions have changed over time. Also, as data have accumulated and our understanding has increased, the use of pheromonatherapy has been more broadly embraced by both the veterinary profession and nonveterinary behaviourists alike. However, much remains to be learned about their specific mechanism of action, and so this text is a starting point.

In the beginning, many vets were also unclear about how relevant this emerging field of clinical animal behaviour was to them. We hope, as guardians of animal welfare, with a special legal obligation in many countries to this effect, that it is now much clearer, despite the fact that at the time of writing, in the UK, only the treatment of behaviour problems with drugs is considered to be a veterinary act subject to any specific legal regulation. All other aspects of treatment are subject to no such regulation, although attempts are being made to develop benchmark standards for the recognition of professional competence by the Animal Behaviour and Training Council (www.abtcouncil.org.uk).

It is not just the veterinary profession that has been confused. Even within the broader field of clinical behaviour practitioners there is no widely accepted paradigm for the discipline, with some advocating a more medical approach, akin to that used in human psychiatry, and others emphasising the importance of psychology and ethology to the understanding of these problems. Our approach is unashamedly broadly biological, since it is this which underpins all life sciences. However, even within this academic field there remains much debate on many relevant topics, including the regulation of behaviour. Animal behaviorism, in an effort to reduce subjective bias, has focused on the observable – stimuli and responses – with what happens between these being largely ignored or avoided for fear of being unscientific. As a result, the importance of normal affective systems (emotional reactions, moods and temperament) in regulating behaviour has perhaps not been fully appreciated, and it has lacked much consistency in its application in practice. It is our contention that a deeper understanding of these affective systems is what distinguishes a behaviour counsellor from an animal trainer. Our focus is on creating a happy and well-behaved animal, rather than simply an obedient one. Fitting in with others involves adjusting one's behaviour in anticipation of events, rather than just attending to cues for instruction.

A lot has happened in the last 15 years or so to address many of the issues mentioned in this introduction, which is why we feel this book is timely. It represents a synthesis of ideas, offering not only a framework for understanding how pheromonatherapy can be used to encourage desirable behaviour (when there is still much to learn) but also a fresh approach to understanding the nature of clinical animal behaviour problems. This, we believe, allows for more precise treatment and a deeper understanding, especially of those cases that do not seem to fit the typical presentation. Science is by its very nature imperfect, since it progresses by falsifying what we previously believed to be true, but that does not mean we should be afraid to propose ideas to explain our observations. While we have tried to develop our ideas logically on the basis of sound science, we have also tried to produce a readily accessible text for those who want to learn more about the subject. Over time, we hope to produce more academic publications expanding on the details of some of the underpinning concepts presented here; but for now we wish to present an initial framework, which we believe will help to move things on, since it allows us to generate testable hypotheses.

We do not want arguments over the meaning of words to get in the way of the overall message, nor do we want to invent a totally new language. Instead, and especially with a view to a readership beyond the academic, we have tried to accept 'the diversity of language' as a starting point. In order to do this, we feel it is important to define how *we* are using certain terms, in order to try to avoid confusion. In time it may be that a new language is necessary, but we will leave that for another day. Thus we continue to use the word 'pheromone' in places where some might prefer 'semiochemical', 'social odour' or some other term, largely out of recognition that 'pheromonatherapy' appears to have entered the English language as a word used to describe the deliberate application of these chemicals to affect the behaviour of captive animals. But in using the word 'pheromone' thus, we think it is important to highlight at the outset that the reader should be careful about making assumptions as to how the clinically used chemicals work or exactly what can be generalised on the basis of our knowledge of pheromones in a broader academic setting.

At many points in the book, we try to clarify other potential inconsistencies in scientific language in a similar way. Indeed, we also devote a considerable amount of text to the other keyword in the title of this volume: 'stress'. We argue that the concept is of very limited value without an appreciation of its qualitative property in a given context if we wish to manage it effectively. The limitations of previous thinking only become more fully appreciated in light of an understanding of the role of affective systems in the control of behaviour, a topic which has often been ignored, but which we also try to address at some length in Part I. Although Part I deals with some fundamental concepts, it only focuses on those areas which are likely to be less familiar to the typical reader. It does not deal with those which we believe are well covered in other clinical animal behaviour texts, such as pure and applied learning theory, history-taking and counselling skills, so the less experienced reader should reference such other texts as appropriate.

In Part II we illustrate the application of these concepts to a range of specific situations. This is not intended to be an exhaustive list of common conditions encountered, or even of those in which pheromonatherapy may be applied, but rather covers those situations in which there has been the most research to support pheromonatherapy's efficacy. Thus we do not deal with aggressive behaviour, despite its obvious prevalence in clinical-behaviour case loads. The research is not finished and clearly no trial is definitive, but we try to explain why we favour a particular interpretation of the uncertainty that remains. Recently, Ceva Animal Health has produced a freely available text summarising each published trial to date. We have therefore not repeated the details here; rather, the reader can obtain this supplementary text from Ceva if interested.

In conclusion, it is our genuine hope that this book will be useful to both academics and practitioners alike in the field of clinical animal behaviour and will stimulate further positive and constructive debate, not just about the use of pheromonatherapy but also about other important concepts relevant to animal welfare. We do not wish you to blindly believe everything, nor do we want you to dismiss things out of hand, but rather we hope to make you think and reflect, and perhaps to make new discoveries as a consequence. It is in this way that we can genuinely hope to do all that is in our power for the ultimate benefit of our patients.

# PART I

Principles and Concepts
Underpinning the Management
of Stress-related Behaviour
Problems

# Chapter 1

# How Animals Respond to Change

## 1.1 UNDERPINNING PRINCIPLES RELATING TO STRESS IN COMPANION ANIMALS

### 1.1.1 *STRESS AND CHANGE*

It has been said that the only constant in life is change, and it seems that some of us cope better with this than others. In this chapter we will explore why this might be. We will focus on factors that not only affect humans but are also relevant to nonhuman animals. Attempting to adapt to change is an intrinsic part of being alive. As a feature of any living system, the environment changes around us all the time, and we have a number of mechanisms for dealing with this. Two obvious ones that are commonly described in the literature are:

- *Physiological processes*: Pure changes in physiology are often thought of as being relatively simple (metabolic changes), for example a change in sweating when the body's temperature starts to rise. These changes may be mediated by either the nervous or the endocrine system, or a combination of both. Often changes in simple physiology are relatively inexpensive, energetically speaking, for an animal to implement.
- *Behavioural processes*: Behaviour responses, for example an animal panting when it is hot (Figure 1.1), involve much greater use of resources and energy, and so are perhaps better considered as the second line of response in the majority of cases. However, physiological processes are at the root of changes in behaviour too: it is just that behaviour changes are more obvious and involve a shift in the animal's posture or position.

Sometimes an animal adapts to a stressor by making a mental adjustment (cognitive change), for example accepting something novel in the environment as nonthreatening, and this too is ultimately a reflection of physiological changes in the brain, even though we might focus on the cognitive outcome.

*Stress and Pheromonatherapy in Small Animal Clinical Behaviour*, First Edition.
Daniel Mills, Maya Braem Dube and Helen Zulch.
© 2013 John Wiley & Sons, Ltd. Published 2013 by John Wiley & Sons, Ltd.

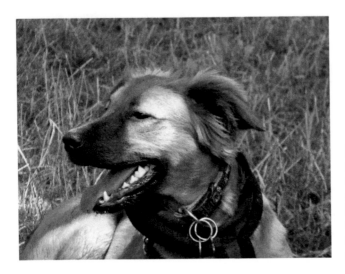

Fig. 1.1 Panting is a response to thermal stress. Animals encounter stressors all the time, but their behavioural flexibility means they can usually cope without significant distress.

Thus, in response to stress, we can recognise three types of change in the body:

- A metabolic shift.
- A change in behaviour.
- A psychological adjustment.

These are not independent, but rather are usually closely related, though perhaps with one being more obvious than another at a given time, depending on the demands being made or anticipated given the circumstances. Overt changes in behaviour are typically more demanding and are therefore often a secondary line of defence when metabolic shifts are not possible or do not work.

## 1.1.2   HOMEOSTASIS AND ALLOSTASIS

The concept of homeostasis has dominated thinking about how animals adapt to change for a long time, but in its purest form it has the potential to limit our understanding in some important ways, as we will see. *Homeostasis* basically means that an animal's body works to restore an optimal state whenever this is disturbed (stressed). So if blood sugar goes up, the body will try to bring it down again, since high blood sugar can be harmful. An immediate response might be to increase production of insulin in order to increase the uptake of glucose by cells in the body. At a behavioural level, an animal may stop feeding in these circumstances, and at a cognitive level it may no longer show positive interest in cues suggesting food. The concept of homeostasis can be applied not only to stressors associated with internal changes, such as changes in blood sugar, but also to external changes such as unpleasant and dangerous environments or situations that are confusing to the animal: thus, if something scares the animal it may run away in order to restore the preferred state of relaxation in a safe and secure environment. Sometimes an animal must work very hard to restore balance, or it

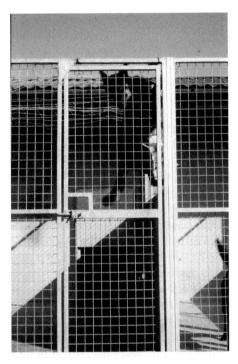

Fig. 1.2 A dog trying to escape from its kennel. Successful escape would restore homeostasis, but this is not possible because of the height of the pen walls. It is better to see the walls as a barrier which gives rise to frustration to the animal's attempts at escape than to simply consider the animal bored, since this focuses attention on the types of intervention which might be most effective. If we consider the animal to be bored, we are using a vague concept and our recommendations for intervention may be equally vague – such as unspecified 'environmental enrichment'. As we will see later in the text, if we recognise that the animal is frustrated by a specific stimulus, we can ask the question: what action is being frustrated and why? The answer in this case is that there are things outside it wants to gain access to. So treatment should focus on not only removing this frustrated desire by ensuring the stimuli outside are less interesting, but also, and more importantly, making the inside more engaging for the animal. This means enrichment needs to be applied that is dynamic and interesting. A few toys will not be enough.

may be frustrated in its efforts by an inescapable situation, such as when a dog wants to get out of a kennel (Figure 1.2).

From these examples, it should be apparent that although responses may share some common features, such as an increase in arousal, stress responses vary according to the nature of the trigger. Thus the specific response is quite different when the trigger is a rise in blood sugar than when it is frustration at a barrier.

The key feature of homeostasis that we will now consider more closely is that the body tries to minimise the impact of stressors (things that disturb us from an optimal set point in some way) by *responding* to changes. The word 'responding' is emphasised as it suggests that it is the disturbance which drives the process.

A concern with this idea is that if we provide an animal with a balanced diet, fresh water, an optimal temperature and so on in a nonthreatening environment, we might be tempted to think that the animal should not be stressed. This was one of the errors which led to the belief that factory farming would be good for animals. We now recognise that because animals have evolved in environments in which change inevitably exists, their bodies have come to expect change and so they are driven to do things even when everything seems optimal. This is probably because such a state is never very long-lasting in nature, so there is no evolved mechanism to simply accept that life is good and will remain as such.

An outcome of the evolutionary expectation that life exists within an ever-changing environment is the development of an anticipation of change within the core processes governing the regulation of the body's metabolism. The body therefore changes in anticipation of change. This is what is meant by the term *allostasis*, which provides a better model than homeostasis for many physiological processes. The key difference between allostasis and homeostasis is that in allostasis responses are driven by the *anticipation of change* as well as by actual change. So if an animal is always fed at the same time each day, insulin will eventually be produced at a certain time, even if there is no food available and even if this leads to a significant lowering of blood sugar which the animal then has to counter by producing the antagonistic (opposing) hormone glucagon.

From the preceding example, it might be tempting to think of allostasis as simply a training of the homeostatic response, but it is much more than that, as it helps to explain why animals have natural rhythms to their metabolism and activity even in the absence of cues. It also helps us to understand the wider and changeable psychological needs of animals, which we discuss in the next section.

### 1.1.3   *PSYCHOLOGICAL NEEDS*

One of the things which many animals do when they have all their fundamental physiological needs met is seek information. There are several reasons why this is useful if there is an inbuilt expectation of change. For example, it allows them potentially to exploit resources more effectively in future (e.g. by knowing where the next meal could come from if the current supply were to dry up) and it might reduce the risk of future harm (e.g. by knowing how strong different potential competitors are). Therefore, when times are good we will often see animals investigate and play much more. Object play allows animals to learn about the physical properties of things, while social play can help them learn about the characteristics of other individuals, including their strengths and weaknesses. An important implication of this is that, in such circumstances, providing for some of these activities should not be considered a luxury, but rather essential for an animal's well-being. In humans, a hierarchy of needs has been described in the literature by Maslow (1943), which indicates what individuals seek as different needs are met. While some of the higher levels originally described may not be directly applicable to nonhuman animals, this hierarchy can be adapted to give a guide as to animals' priorities in different circumstances (Figure 1.3).

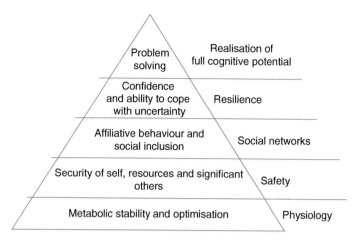

Fig. 1.3 A hierarchy of needs for animals, adapted from Maslow's hierarchy of needs for humans. The labels to the right indicate the type of need, with those at the bottom being initially most important. As the lower-level needs are increasingly met, the higher-level needs become increasingly important. Thus if an animal's physiological needs are being met, the need for safety and security is more pressing, so it can be expected that the animal will become less willing to take high risks to obtain its food and so on. All of the needs depend on the acquisition of information in order to be met efficiently, but the type of information changes with ascending levels.

Another use of this hierarchy is to help us appreciate why an animal is not performing particularly well in a given aspect of its life and what needs to be done to help resolve the issue. For example, an owner might complain that their pet lacks confidence, and this might be at least partly due to unstable social relationships at home, which mean that the animal is focusing resources on social networks as a priority. Without addressing this lower-level need, it may be difficult for the animal to grow in confidence, as its priorities are elsewhere.

This hierarchy indicates that safety or a sense of safety is a big priority for animals after their physiological needs have been met. Most pets are well fed and watered, and so the issue of safety deserves further consideration. *Safety* broadly means knowing that you can escape potential harm, and so requires that the animal has some freedom to withdraw from situations that it finds unpleasant. In the home, this means the animal has a safe haven, or some other secure attachment. We will return frequently to the importance of providing coping strategies when we discuss the use of pheromones in a clinical context to help animals cope in a variety of settings. The need for safety also helps us to understand why the inappropriate use of punishment, especially by an owner, can be so disruptive to an animal's well-being. Quite apart from being ineffective in altering the underlying motivation for the unwanted behavioural response and disrupting the bond between the owner and their pet, the inconsistent use of aversive methods leads to the animal's lacking a sense of safety. Thus common basic requirements for managing almost any behaviour problem are that all punishment should cease and that a healthy relationship between the owner and their pet should be established. Only with these foundations in place can we expect the animal to have the confidence to change inappropriate emotional responses. Once again, pheromones can be useful in this process, as we shall see. However, there are also important constraints on what can be achieved, which are considered in the next section.

### 1.1.4   THE GENOME LAG AND EVOLUTIONARY CONSTRAINTS

Companion animals evolved in a particular environment over centuries and today often live in a very different one. The modern environment can be very stressful for both humans and their companion animals. The fact that evolution may not have equipped them with the mechanisms to deal with the sorts of stress or that they face in the domestic home can pose a problem. Let us look at the dog as an example: it is a social animal and is adapted to live in close social groups. Hence, being left alone can be very stressful for a dog and it will use the mechanisms that it has received through evolution to cope with this situation, such as howling in order to try to reestablish contact with the members of its group. Other possible behaviours it might attempt include trying to escape from the environment in which it is isolated, which can result in considerable property damage (Figure 1.4). We might think that a dog should know it can't break through a wall, but solid, all-enclosing walls are not something it has evolved to deal with. An important thing to appreciate here is that although a behaviour may not be very effective (i.e. maladaptive), that does not mean the underlying behavioural control

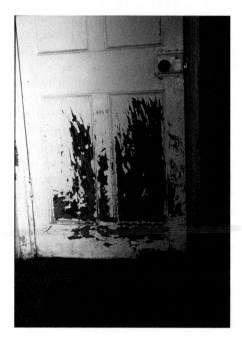

Fig. 1.4  A dog may try to escape even if it cannot succeed. The lack of success can simply lead to persistent behaviour, as seen in the damage to this door.

systems are broken (i.e. malfunctional). There is sometimes a tendency to think that a behaviour must be pathological if it does not bring an obvious benefit, but this is not always the case; an animal may simply be using its evolutionary rules of thumb in an inappropriate context because of the artificiality of the environment. This has important implications as it means we should not be looking for treatments to correct a supposed malfunction, but rather we should be looking at the environmental contingencies and perceptions of the animal that are leading it to perform in this way. However, although the response may be a functional one, that is not to say it cannot be problematic or give rise to pathological processes as a result of its inappropriate deployment in given circumstances (we will return to this in Section 1.2).

Most stress responses have evolved in order to help animals cope with acute (short-term) crises, for example 'There is a predator and I need to escape', 'I am alone and I need my friends' and so on. Unfortunately, the stresses that we tend to face in modern living are often much more prolonged (possibly going on for years), and even a mild stress can end up having quite an impact, as an animal's coping mechanisms are not developed to deal with prolonged challenge. By way of example, imagine you are required to hold up a cup of water. It is not a big problem and you should be able to do it easily. But if you have to hold it up for hours it becomes a much more significant issue. In the same way, the odd stressor may be fine on its own, but when it goes on for months or years we can see wider effects on the functioning of an animal and the system it lives in. We will return to this later when we talk about factors affecting the impact of a stressor. At this point it is simply important to appreciate that animals are often not well adapted to deal with stressors that go on for a long time, even if they are small, because in nature stressors are typically resolved quite quickly one way or another. This is one reason why a thorough history of any animal presented for problem behaviour is important. For example, two cats may have never got on very well together but have tolerated each other. Over time this can lead to more substantial changes such as certain recurring health problems, an increased risk of diabetes and perhaps more overt aggressive behaviour problems.

Another important evolutionary constraint on adaptation relates to the type of response elicited. Different species have evolved in different niches and have different lifestyles. Accordingly, they may use different rules of thumb to resolve an issue. Thus cats and dogs differ in the typical behaviours that they can offer in order to help them adapt:

- Dogs are a social species that use a well-developed communication system to cooperate and to coordinate their behaviour with other group members.
- Cats are more independent but are generally capable of living in groups. Their social communication skills are not so refined, as living alone is their evolutionary inheritance given the type of prey they feed upon, which does not require pack hunting.

Thus a dog, when faced with a problem, will be much more likely to look for social support for help (which might involve trying to engage the owner in the issue) than a cat, which would be more likely to try to resolve things itself. In either case, this can involve the animal changing the chemical environment around itself in order to cope. Alarm pheromones can help an animal avoid a dangerous area and so remain safe, but there are also pheromones that signal safety, which allow the animal to focus less energy on environmental monitoring and more on other things. We will discuss these pheromones in detail later, but first we need to consider the concept of safety in more detail.

## 1.1.5   *SAFETY AND ITS ROLE IN LIFE*

We have already mentioned that safety is an important need for animals, but it is worth considering in more detail what it means to be safe and the consequences of this.

A safe place is somewhere that is associated with the absence of harm and the absence of signs of harm. It is therefore a place in which an animal can relax and explore with confidence. This has many important implications for animal management and welfare. A *safe haven* is somewhere that an animal feels in control of events. One of the most common misunderstandings that we encounter is confusion between a 'safe haven' and a 'bolt hole'. A *bolt hole* is somewhere that an animal runs to in order to hide or to watch and hope that whatever is bothering it will pass. A *safe haven* is somewhere that an animal goes where it feels safe and in control of events. It is quite difficult to convert a bolt hole into a safe haven; to create a safe haven we need to create a place where the animal is not disturbed and where it can choose to go if it does not want to interact with us. If we really want to give the pet a place where it is truly in control, we must not impose ourselves or our interests on it in this area. It is obviously important for all who come into contact with the animal to appreciate and respect this.

Young animals frequently use an attachment figure (typically the mother) as a secure base from which to explore the world. This can be transferred to other individuals, but such individuals must be supportive of the animal, recognising and respecting its communication and responding appropriately (e.g. not forcing it into situations with which it expresses discomfort). Pheromones, like dog-appeasing pheromone (DAP), which is produced by bitches shortly after whelping, appear to be particularly important in this process. As we will see later, these chemicals seem to have an intrinsically reassuring effect through the limbic system, which helps provide the pup with a secure base from which to explore and learn about the world.

As a simple rule, it is important for social individuals to have at least two points of safety in their lives:

• A physical place (safe haven).
• A social companion (secure base).

The importance of a social companion may be lower for a more independent individual, but recent work suggests that this should not be generalised to species; that is, while cats in the wild may be quite independent, in the home they can form strong attachments and dependencies. If an animal has no need for a social companion, the physical safe haven may be especially important.

## 1.1.6   *STRESSORS AND THE STRESS RESPONSE*

The term 'stress' is often used in a very confusing way to refer to both an animal's response to something and the cause of that response. In this book, we will use the term *stress response* to describe an animal's behavioural and physiological reactions to a threat and the term *stressor* to describe the trigger of these: that is, the stimulus.

The *stress response* can be defined as the physiological, behavioural and psychological response to a challenge to an individual's optimal state of well-being. As we have already seen, this is not a simply defined fixed point, as might be thought from a homeostatic perspective, but will vary with numerous factors. When trying to assess the stress response, it is important to distinguish the measures we can assess objectively from our interpretation of them. For example, a dog may run away in response to a loud noise, which is something we can measure objectively (e.g. the time it takes to respond (*latency*), its speed, the distance it travels, changes in its heart rate). But if we say 'The dog is scared', that is an interpretation, which may be much more difficult to quantify and objectify. There is room for debate when it comes to interpretations; for example, some dogs that run up to their owner when they hear a loud noise are not actually scared but are just seeking the owner's attention or have found that the noise is a good way of getting the owner to give them more attention – this has been referred to as a *pseudofear*. In these cases it is important to examine what the owner does in response to the pet coming up to them and to determine whether they function as the previously mentioned secure base or whether they are reinforcing the dog's attention-seeking behaviour, as these outcomes will require different types of intervention to resolve. Owners will typically report interpretations and one of our jobs as clinicians is to sensitively and objectively assess these, rather than accept them as fact.

If we consider a *stressor* as anything which moves an animal out of its normal optimal range, this means there are many different types of stressor and that not all stressors are bad. It further means that there are likely to be many forms of *stress response*, as different responses are required to cope with different types of stressor. An animal can be moved out of its normal optimal range by something unpleasant: for example, a pet running away from a loud noise or a cat hiding from a chasing dog. Both of these responses lead to increased arousal. On the other hand, increased arousal is also required for essential activities like reproduction and play that are generally considered to be more pleasurable. Hence, we should be careful not to interpret all stressors or the resulting changes elicited as indisputable evidence of poor welfare. The determination of an animal's well-being is an inference which should be drawn from multiple pieces of evidence (a process sometimes referred to as *triangulation*).

There are many features which relate to a stressor's impact on an individual, such as:

- *The type and number of stressors*: Some animals may find auditory stressors, such as the level of noise, more stressful than visual ones. Similarly, if certain stressors are combined, this may be much more stressful for some individuals and not for others. For example, in the case of fireworks, some animals are able to cope with the noise or with a flash of light on its own, but when the noise and the visual stressor occur simultaneously, the animal perceives the situation as much more threatening.

- *The intensity of the stressor*: Some animals may be able to cope with softer noises, for example, but find it difficult when the volume increases beyond a certain level.
- *The duration of the stressor*: As already discussed, a stressor might be quite mild, but if it goes on for a long period of time it can be difficult for an animal to cope with it. It is therefore important to evaluate how long a particular stressful situation has been going on.
- *The predictability of the stressor*: The concept of predictability can be very important for an animal's welfare. If something is very predictable, it can make it easier for the animal to prepare its defences and to cope as a result. For example, an animal might habituate to certain stressors that have been going on for a long time (e.g. road work in front of the house) but react strongly to rarely and unpredictably occurring stressors (e.g. a thunderstorm). If the animal cannot predict the situation, it cannot divert resources in order to cope, as it does not know when the problem is going to arise. For a given individual, the optimal level of predictability of a stressor varies enormously: something that is too predictable can actually also be stressful, as we do seek some change in our environment. We often interpret it as 'boring' if something is extremely predictable. We know it is going to happen and so we do not pay much attention to it. If something that the animal knows it can't cope with is predictable, this increases arousal in advance without an expectation of being able to cope.
- *The level of control an animal has over a stressor*: If an animal has control over its environment, it is easier for it to cope and to take appropriate measures. If we return to the example of sound sensitivities, things like fireworks and thunderstorms are often very difficult for an animal, because it has very little control over when the sound will happen (in this example, predictability and control are linked, but this is not always the case). This is made worse if it has no safe haven. Noises like thunderstorms can be particularly problematic, because the sound seems to move around in an uncontrollable way and cannot be clearly located – the stressor is both unpredictable and uncontrollable. Having no way of removing itself from the situation because it is locked in the house and/or being on its own may be additional stressors that an animal has to cope with at such times. Hence, it is not surprising that problems such as noise fears and separation distress often occur together. When a case is referred for one of these conditions, it is very important to check that the other is not present as well, as they may be linked.
- *The previous consequences of the potential stressor – what the animal learns*: Has the animal been able to cope in the past? If it has then even quite severe situations may be tolerated. But if an animal has had other unpleasant experiences associated with a potential stressor, something that might seem relatively mild to us may actually become very severe for it. For example, if a dog starts to show mild signs of anxiety in response to a noise and the owner tells it off, the mild noise now becomes a predictor of punishment from the owner and so can actually

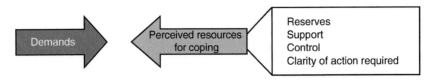

Fig. 1.5 Stressors give rise to concern over an animal's welfare when the demands they impose exceed the animal's perceived resources for coping. There are therefore many features outside the properties of the stressor which affect its potential impact. Resources for coping include not only the physical reserves of the animal but also aspects which are often influenced by the handler, such as the level of perceived support the animal has, the level of perceived control the animal has over the situation and the clarity of action required to deal with the problem. The fact that this process depends on a perception of the animal's means there are few hard and fast rules about whether a given stressor is necessarily harmful to a given individual.

become much more stressful, and the animal is likely to react even more strongly the next time it faces the stressor or predictors of the stressor.

When we think about the impact of a stressor, we often tend to focus on its physical properties, such as its intensity, duration, frequency, predictability and so on, but as the last few examples show, a central principle underpinning how much impact a stressor will have relates to the animal's interpretation of whether and how it can cope (Figure 1.5). An animal may face quite a big challenge, but if it predicts (and has learned) it can cope with change (i.e. it is resilient), the impact of the stressor may be rather small, including that on the animal's welfare. On the other hand, a phobic animal may not be able to cope with a relatively minor and – to bystanders – obviously harmless stressor, such as a fly. Coping with it seems like an insurmountable challenge and the animal's welfare is therefore seriously impacted.

## 1.1.7   *SELYE AND THE GENERAL ADAPTATION SYNDROME*

By now it should be apparent that stress responses are quite varied; nonetheless, there is still a tendency to refer to a general stress response. This idea is particularly associated with Hans Selye (1907–1982) and what he termed the *General Adaptation Syndrome (GAS)*. This basically describes the most common form of arousal, resulting from a range of stressors. It describes three phases of response to a stressor and has greatly influenced our understanding of how stress can be harmful to the body, and so deserves some attention.

Selye's three phases of the GAS consist of:

- *The alarm phase*: Selye termed the immediate response the *alarm phase* or the *alarm reaction*, with the following reactions within the body:
  - *An increase in both epinephrine (adrenaline) and norepinephrine (noradrenaline)*: These are hormones from the centre of the adrenal gland, the *adrenal medulla*,

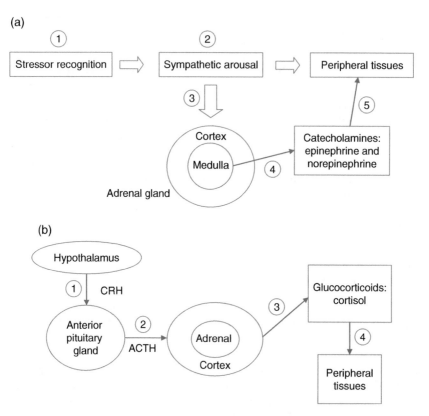

**Fig. 1.6** Schematic of the sympathetico-adrenal (a) and hypothalamic–pituitary–adrenal (b) axes and general physiological and behavioural changes. (a) (1) the stressor is recognised, which leads to (2) changes in the sympathetic nervous system, which is the fight/flight system; (3) nerves associated with the sympathetic nervous system travel to the core of the adrenal: the medulla; (4) the medulla releases epinephrine and norepinephrine, otherwise known as *catecholamines*; (5) the nervous system also directly impacts on specific tissues – both the catecholamines and the direct nervous input result in a variety of changes in these peripheral tissues, which prepare them for action. (b) (1) the impact of a potential stressor is registered within the hypothalamus of the brain, which results in a release of *corticotrophin releasing hormone* (CRH); (2) CRH is transported to the anterior pituitary gland, which sits at the base of the brain and results in the release of *adrenocorticotrophic hormone* (ACTH), another releasing hormone that affects the adrenal cortex – this response requires a cascade of hormones in order to take effect and so is a slower response than that from the adrenal medulla; (3) this cascade of hormones results in the release of glucocorticoids, which include the hormone *cortisol*; (4) the glucocorticoids in turn have a variety of effects on peripheral tissues.

which are released as a result of increased activity in the sympathetic nervous system (Figure 1.6). Their production is closely associated with the fight, flight, freeze and fidget (or fiddling about/flirting) strategies, which are aimed at repelling, running away from, cautiously tolerating and redirecting attention away from the stressor, respectively.

○ *An increase in corticosteroids (the hormones cortisol or corticosterone, depending on the species) from the cortex of the adrenal gland*: This is a result of activation of the hypothalamic–pituitary–adrenal (HPA) axis (Figure 1.6).

○ *An increase in blood sugar*: Epinephrine, norepinephrine and corticosteroids all raise blood sugar and so help mobilise energy reserves. Another hormone change that we see in this immediate reaction is a drop in hormones such as insulin, whose role is to lower blood glucose. So, overall there is a rise in blood glucose in anticipation of having to take action, such as running away from a predator or a serious threat.

○ *Diversion of reserves within the body to support immediate survival*: The body diverts its reserves towards taking immediate action in response to the potential threat and away from longer-term activities. So, in the alarm phase, the hormone changes also result in a suppression of the immune system and a reduction of the hormones that help increase productivity. Obviously, if you are faced with a predator, functions like reproduction and fighting off disease are relatively unimportant compared to staying alive in the immediate future. There is no point being very healthy but dead!

- *The period of resistance*: After the immediate alarm phase, Selye described what he termed a *period of resistance*, which has the following characteristics:
  ○ The levels of adrenal hormones (epinephrine, norepinephrine, corticosteroids) all remain quite high.
  ○ The levels of the *anabolics* (i.e. molecules that help build up reserves in the body, such as the blood glucose-lowering hormone insulin) return back to normal.
  ○ Raised blood glucose levels are maintained, in order to sustain and prepare for further activity as might be necessary.

- *Adaptation or exhaustion phase*: It may be that the previously mentioned response is sufficient for the animal to be able to cope, in which case the animal *adapts* successfully. However, if the response persists for a long period of time, *exhaustion* may occur, with a risk of a whole range of pathological processes as a result. It is important to appreciate that the balance between adaptation and exhaustion can be a fine one and that animals may appear to adapt for a reasonable period of time but ultimately become exhausted, which can lead to serious health and welfare problems (consider the example of holding up the cup of water). Even if an animal appears to be adapting, it may be making an enormous effort to do so and that too is a cause for concern.

Although Selye proposed that the GAS was the general way in which animals responded to stressful situations, it was soon recognised that it was not perhaps quite as general as he initially thought. There is a whole range of specific responses that animals may employ when faced with unpleasant situations. For example, many species respond to a rise in the environmental temperature with a drop in corticosteroid levels, rather than an increase. Similarly, when sheep are dehydrated, there may be no perceptible adrenal response at all. This makes sense from an adaptive biological perspective, because raising blood glucose when you are hyperthermic or dehydrated will actually tend to increase activity within the body and so increase demand for water, as well as raise body temperature further as a result – not to mention that the water may be more useful in aiding cooling through panting or sweating. It makes a lot of sense not to produce a response which is likely to make matters worse.

Animals vary enormously in how they cope with a given stressor, not just between species but also between individuals of the same species. For example, an increase in temperature may be far more difficult for one animal to cope with than another (consider the short-nosed – *brachycephalic* – breeds of dog in this context, which can have difficulty panting efficiently). If we think about changes in the social environment, we will also see enormous individual differences, with some animals showing behavioural problems and others seeming to cope fine.

Another concern over the common interpretation of the GAS is the emphasis it puts on *cortisol*. It is easy to see why this happens as there seems to be an ever-growing list of known effects of cortisol on the body. Not only does it have the physiological effects discussed, it also produces behavioural changes and biases. For example, as part of its effect in helping to maintain blood sugar, it actually stimulates appetite. This is why you might feel the need to eat lots of chocolate when you are chronically stressed. This may seem strange, considering that we would expect an animal's priority to be escape, but it is important to note that we are now talking about longer-term stressors. The role of cortisol in this context is to help the animal cope with these longer-term impacts of stress; for example, after the stress is over, the raised cortisol will stimulate the animal to eat and, thereby, to replenish its reserves – this helps to explain why physiological arousal lasts longer than the stimulus causing it (a characteristic of emotional reactions). Cortisol also produces quite important cognitive changes. It biases an animal's attention towards negative events, which means that the animal may view otherwise neutral stimuli as potentially threatening. This is not just of academic interest, but also of clinical importance, because in clinical practice synthetic and much more powerful versions of the glucocorticoids are used to control a whole range of medical conditions. One must keep in mind that treating an animal with these medical drugs may actually induce concerning changes in the animal's behaviour as a result. An increase in appetite is a commonly recognised side effect of the use of glucocorticoids, but less attention has been paid to their cognitive effects, and so some behavioural advice – aimed at reducing the impact of an increased sensitivity to aversive events – may be useful when dispensing these drugs.

Prolonged or excessive cortisol can be quite toxic to parts of the brain involved in memory, like the hippocampus, with obvious and immediately apparent effects. For example, as a result of chronic exposure an animal may forget things that it has previously learned. In the human literature, *stress-induced dishabituation*, which is when a person forgets things that they have previously learned as a result of chronic stress, is well documented, and we are increasingly recognising it in companion animals too. This can result in the appearance of a number of behavioural problems, including noise fears. If a problem appears at an unusual age, it is important to check whether or not the animal appears to have been under chronic stress recently, particularly if the behaviour in question is one which the animal had learned not to show: this might be a strong indicator of stress-induced dishabituation. In such cases, the focus of treatment must be not just to correct the behaviour problem but to look at general stress management for the animal so that the problem goes and stays away.

We may also see changes in the reactivity of the adrenal cortex, particularly in the case of long-term or repeated stimulation. These changes, however, can be difficult to predict, as the adrenal cortex may become less responsive or exhausted, or it may become sensitised. This is clearly an area in need of further research. The relatively routine *ACTH stimulation test* can be useful in some cases when we see a marked change, in the sense of either an over- or an underreaction, in the adrenal response. Changes in response can indicate that an animal has been subject to long-term stress, but the fact that individuals vary enormously in their normal response to the test often makes interpretation difficult. The test would really be most useful if we could assay an animal before it underwent a stressful experience as well as after, in order to assess the stressor's impact. If we were to perform the test before an owner moved house and again afterwards, we might see marked changes in the responsiveness. We mention this here simply because it is something that we might want to make better use of in future.

Undoubtedly cortisol is very important, but it is just one of many hormones which are involved in how animals cope with environmental changes (i.e. stressors in the environment). Cortisol is produced as a result of ACTH release from the anterior part of the pituitary gland in the brain. This structure also produces a whole range of reproductively important hormones: notably *prolactin* (Prl), most widely known for its role in milk production in females, but with other effects not associated with reproduction; and *luteinising hormone* (LH) and *follicle stimulating hormone* (FSH), which occur in both males and females and are associated with the production of the gametes. All of these hormones rise after initial stress and can stay elevated for several hours after the stress has disappeared. However, in response to chronic stress, levels will fall, and so we may see knock-on effects of stress with respect to reproduction.

Prolactin is of particular and growing interest within the field of veterinary behavioural medicine in that it is regulated by inhibition rather than stimulation. The removal of inhibition results in its release. Dopamine, a neurotransmitter generally involved in the activation of goal-directedness of a wide range of behaviours, seems to be one of the main factors that inhibits the release of prolactin. A high release of prolactin suggests that there is very little dopamine coming from the hypothalamus to control it; that is, the animal is not seeking out the good things in life. This may explain a whole range of behavioural changes that can be seen in relation to stress. Dopamine is associated with behavioural activation; that is, the approach an animal takes towards potential signs of reward or potential rewards. If an animal has low levels of dopamine, it may become more apathetic and less responsive towards rewards, which is reflected in its behaviours. It makes sense that an animal becomes less sensitive to rewards in times of stress, because it is probably focusing on escaping from an unpleasant situation.

In France there has been an effort to try to validate a system for both scoring and monitoring animals' responses to chronic stress, which has resulted in the production of the *Evaluation of a Dog's Emotional Disorder (EDED)* scale (see Appendix A).

Interestingly, recent work has suggested that the scoring used in this system might correlate quite well with prolactin levels.

The relationship between dopamine and prolactin and our ability to indirectly infer the level of dopamine activity from prolactin screening might also have implications for the choice of drugs used to treat particular disorders. In treating behaviour problems, it has been noted that not all patients respond in the same manner to the same medication. The postulated explanation for this is the involvement of different neurotransmitters in the same superficial behaviour presentation in different patients. If one can assess which neurotransmitters are involved in a patient's behaviour, a more targeted use of medication can be implemented. For example, if an animal is showing changes in behaviour that seem to be associated with a reduction in dopamine levels, it makes sense to use drugs, such as selegiline, that are likely to act on the dopamine system. In support of this, data are emerging to show that where anxiety is associated with a change in prolactin level, drugs like selegiline may be more effective than drugs like fluoxetine. Fluoxetine might also be indicated for the presenting complaint, but it works on the serotonin neurotransmitter system, indicating that often more than one neurotransmitter system is involved in behaviour and in behavioural changes.

There are a number of other hormonal changes in the pituitary gland that occur in response to stress, particularly changes in *oxytocin*, which is associated with bonding behaviour, and the endogenous *opiates* (*endorphins*, *enkephalins* and *dynorphins*), which are also associated with bonding but in addition also with *analgesia* (pain-killing). Both of these groups of chemicals also have effects on memory that should not be underestimated.

The domestic environment is very complex and individual animals will vary in how they perceive different changes in this environment according not just to genetic differences but also to their developmental history. Developmental history is referred to as *ontogeny* within the scientific literature. Individual differences are very important for a number of reasons. First of all, they remind us that it is actually the animal's perception of the stressor rather than its physical nature that is important. What is too loud for one dog or cat may be fine for another. It is important when working with cases that we appreciate that all animals are individuals. In behaviour therapy, it is particularly important to pay attention to individual differences, because when it comes to finding solutions, they have to be tailored to the individual animal, its circumstances and the resources of the system in which it lives. We should avoid the temptation of thinking one solution fits all.

Finally, contrary to its common representation, the GAS is not very specific to unpleasant situations. In fact, the changes in cortisol seem to be a reaction to any change that requires increased arousal, whether it is pleasurable or aversive. Based on this, some people have proposed using two different terms to distinguish between stressful situations that are harmful and those that are not:

- *Distress*: Responses associated with unpleasant events, such as punishment or fear.
- *Eustress*: Stressful situations which an animal may find pleasurable, such as reproduction or play. *Eu* is the Greek word for 'well'.

## 1.1.8   *MOBERG'S MODEL OF STRESS*

A lot of recent work on stress physiology has emphasised both the importance of individual differences in perception on the outcome of stress and the potentially detrimental effects of excessive activation of the stress-response system. This is well described by Gary Moberg's model of stress (Figure 1.7).

As a result of the stress response, animals change what they would normally do, which can put them at risk of a range of behavioural, psychological and medical problems.

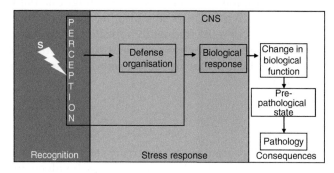

**Fig. 1.7** Moberg's model of stress.

## 1.1.9   *RESILIENCE*

We mentioned the concept of *resilience* earlier in relation to an animal's ability to cope with stress. Resilience incorporates at least four important capacities:

- The ability to minimise the impact of a stressor on normal functioning.
- The ability to retain competence even when normal functioning is disturbed.
- The ability to recover very quickly when there is an impact.
- The ability to increase coping potential in future as a result of exposure to stressors.

One approach to animal welfare is to try to minimise exposure to stressors, but the reality is that some exposure is inevitable. Unfortunately, if an animal has been largely protected from stress, it may have less ability to cope and so be at greater risk of suffering even in the face of relatively minor threat. We started this chapter by saying that the only constant in life is change, and so a sensible strategy is to try to ensure that animals have the capacity to cope with changes. There are many ways of doing this, which we will discuss later in the text, but a general rule is to ensure that an animal is exposed to stressors that are within its coping capacity. This might mean gradually building up the intensity of the stressors it is likely to face in later life, which is the main goal of a lot of habituation and socialisation practices for young animals. But there is a lot more that can be done, such as ensuring that the animal has some control over its environment, including possible stressors, and a secure base from which to explore stressors, so that it learns that it can cope, as well as teaching it acceptable and transferable coping strategies. Pheromones may be important in this regard as they can potentially help to reassure an animal that it can cope and can increase its coping capacity and thus increase resilience.

## 1.2   THE EFFECTS OF PERSISTENT STRESS, OR 'WHY STRESS CAN BE SO STRESSFUL'

We have already explained that the stress response has largely evolved to deal with acute problems and that when an animal is placed in a situation where there is a persistent stressor, an initially functional system might actually turn into a harmful one. In this section we consider this in more detail by first considering two types of persistent stressor – the frequently repeated stressor and the chronic stressor – before examining the impact of persistent stress more generally on the body. We finish the section by introducing the concept of stress auditing in clinical behaviour management.

### 1.2.1   TWO TYPES OF PERSISTENT STRESS

First we will consider the frequently recurring stressor. The *sympathetico-adrenomedullary (SAM) system* is the dominant process involved in making the adjustments necessary to respond to an unexpected event (surprise). Its function is to increase arousal and prepare the animal for possible further action. Although both epinephrine and norepinephrine are produced as a result of this process, it is thought that there is a bias depending on the type of stressor involved, with epinephrine more closely associated with psychological stressors and norepinephrine with physiological stressors. Repeat activation of these systems typically results in one of two changes: either the animal *habituates* to the stimulus (i.e. learns to ignore it as an irrelevance and stops responding to it both physiologically and behaviourally) or it becomes *sensitised* to it (in which case the physiological and behavioural response may become heightened). Behavioural and physiological responses do not necessarily occupy the same time period. This is important because an animal may appear to have adjusted behaviourally to an initial startle but still be quite highly aroused physiologically. This may be one of the factors that increase the chances of sensitisation in the longer term, if the process is repeated. Unfortunately, there is still a lot we do not know about why an animal may sensitise, and so it can be hard to predict. Even if we do not see sensitisation of the immediate response, we may see more general changes in an animal's behaviour if it is in an environment where this system is frequently activated. With frequently recurring stressors, we will typically see one or more of the following signs:

- Hypervigilance (scanning etc.).
- Hyperreactivity (jumpiness).
- Anxiety.
- Irritability.
- Recurrent anxious conflict behaviours, such as shoulder-licking or hair-pulling in cats (Figure 1.8) or hollow barking in dogs.

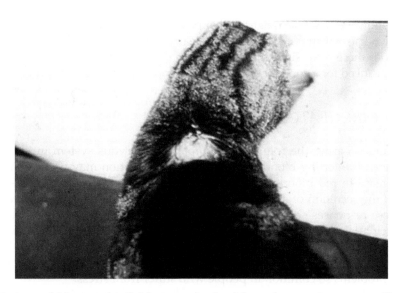

Fig. 1.8 A cat which started to lick between its shoulders whenever it unexpectedly encountered the new puppy that had moved into its home. An important differential in this case is a skin tumour or vaccine reaction.

By contrast, we see quite a different profile in the face of chronically enduring stressors, because these lead to an exaggerated influence from the *HPA system*. In the previous section we mentioned the importance of the glucocorticoids in raising metabolic rate and suppressing the immune system, as well as of reductions in dopamine production. If we understand these changes, the effects of chronic activation of the HPA axis become easier to comprehend. Typical changes are as follows:

- A higher metabolic rate means that the risk of damage resulting from the previously mentioned processes is increased and so we may see an acceleration of age-related problems, including cognitive dysfunction.
- Reduced dopamine activity means that there is less behavioural activation and so the animal may be behaviourally depressed.
- Stress-induced dishabituation may be observed in these circumstances as the animal learns that previous stimuli to which it has habituated may no longer be irrelevant.
- Finally we are more likely to see a whole range of stress-related illnesses, which are explained further in the subsequent sections. Since cortisol suppresses the immune system, the animal may also be vulnerable to a whole range of infections, such as chronic or mild recurrent skin conditions, gastrointestinal disturbance (vomiting or diarrhoea) and/or urinary tract problems (especially in cats) with associated behavioural changes. If animals frequently experience these problems, the significance of chronic stress in their aetiology needs to be considered.

There are, however, a whole range of other physical diseases which are more directly caused by persistent stress, although less clearly linked to one pattern or the other. We consider these next, since their occurrence in a patient should be a prompt to consider the need for a combined medical–behavioural management programme.

## 1.2.1.1   *CIRCULATORY DISEASE*

We mentioned earlier the role of the sympathetic nervous system in increasing heart rate and diverting blood supply. Splenic contraction may occur and result in an increase in red blood cells released into the system. There may also be a change in the secretion of antidiuretic hormone, which increases water retention. All of these responses serve to increase blood pressure and in the short term to improve circulation. However, if this short-term response is prolonged, we may see the chronic effects of increased blood pressure. This transition from the body's short- to long-term coping attempt is one of the factors which makes blood-pressure problems so common in people who suffer from stress.

## 1.2.1.2   *METABOLIC DISEASE*

In the initial stress-response phase, several processes are triggered in order to help the animal to be ready for action:

- Mobilisation of blood glucose, which involves a shift within the autonomic nervous system towards increased sympathetic activity and reduced parasympathetic activity.
- Reduction in insulin and increase in the glucocorticoids, such as cortisol.
- Changes in glucagon, epinephrine and norepinephrine, all of which serve to raise blood glucose.

However, the long-term effects of these changes in blood glucose can be quite problematic. In people, we recognise diabetes mellitus as a problem resulting from high levels of stress over a long period of time, and we are becoming increasingly interested in this from a veterinary point of view as well: that is, the role of the environment in diseases like diabetes mellitus in both cats and dogs.

## 1.2.1.3   *ENTERIC DISEASE*

If an animal is going to engage in flight, it wants to get away as efficiently as possible. Hence it makes sense to have as little food in its gastrointestinal tract as possible, as too much would slow it down. There is also not a lot of point in diverting energy reserves to digesting the food because it may not be alive to digest it if it does not manage to get away from the situation! Consequently, it is not surprising that we see a change in activity in the gastrointestinal system in stressful situations: the stomach and the small intestine slow down and there is a reduction of blood flow to these areas. In some animals, we may actually see vomiting, because this helps to eject food and reduces the bulk carried. At the other end of the gastrointestinal system, the large bowel might actually speed up in order to eject food for the same reasons, which helps explain why we will often see diarrhoea and colitis as a result of persistent stress.

## 1.2.1.4   GASTRIC CHANGES

The association between gastric ulcers and chronic stress is well known. In the short term, the responses which ultimately give rise to an increased risk of ulcers make sense biologically speaking; the problem arises because the animal fails to adapt to the persistent (perceived) threat of harm. Escaping the perceived threat is of highest priority, and so the body does not prioritise digestion and as a result the blood flow to the stomach is reduced. The inside of the stomach is a very hostile environment: the acid can potentially do a lot of damage to the stomach if its lining is not properly protected and the cells are not regularly replaced. The reduction of blood flow to the stomach is not a problem in the short term, but in the longer term it might result in an increased rate of cell death, which in turn can lead to gastric ulcers. This is not, however, the only stress-related risk factor for gastric ulceration.

During stress, the pattern of the stomach's muscle contraction also changes: contractions become slower and more sustained, which means that less blood actually reaches the stomach efficiently. This results in further compromise of the blood flow and an increased risk of damage to the lining. Prostaglandin production is also reduced during stress. Prostaglandins are important factors in tissue repair. A reduction therefore leads to a decrease in the stomach's ability to repair itself. Psychological changes happening in the body more generally may also result in an increased production of hydrogen ions, and there is an increase in acid production by the stomach in order to try to eliminate these from the body. In addition, in chronic stress, the activity of the immune system is also reduced. Bacterial infection may be an important factor in the occurrence of gastric ulcers, which means that stress-induced immunosuppression can contribute to increase the risk of gastric ulcers. It is easy to see how in combination with the stomach becoming less able to protect itself and producing more acid, this further increases the risk of ulcers.

Finally, if the stress eventually stops there may also be a big outsurge of acid, known as *acid rebound*, which alone can result in the burning of holes within the lining of the stomach. There are therefore lots of factors to explain the relationship between stress and gastric ulcers. Very little attention has been paid to this in cats and dogs but it is of growing interest, particularly in race horses, and is a known problem in pigs.

## 1.2.1.5   APPETITE CHANGES

Animals may increase or decrease their appetite when 'stressed'. The reasons for these apparently contradictory effects can however be understood and predicted. The effect of stress on appetite relates to both the effect of the glucocorticoids on appetite and the effect of their releasing factor, 'CRH' (corticotrophin-releasing hormone or corticotrophin-releasing factor), in the brain, which strongly suppresses appetite. CRH has a very short half-life – that is, it does not exist very long in the body – but even during its short existence it is very effective at reducing appetite, which is obviously desirable in the immediate crisis of a potential threat. However, after CRH has been through the system, the effects of the glucocorticoids become more apparent. These compounds increase appetite and encourage the animal to replenish its reserves. Glucocorticoids survive a lot longer in the circulation than CRH: they have a longer half-life. In a situation in which an animal is under chronic stress, a lot of CRH is continuously released and, as result of this, a lot of glucocorticoids are released as well. However, the effects of CRH are much stronger than the effects of the glucocorticoids. This means that we see a reduction in appetite. If the animal experiences a series of small stressors, rather than one continuous one, we will get pulses of CRH being released, followed by pulses of glucocorticoids, which survive in the circulation for longer. So, while we see an initial period of loss of appetite, this state is very rapidly replaced by a period of increased appetite and so overall the animal will be eating more. The important difference here is that in chronic stress there is no relief, whereas in a series of multiple stresses we have periods of stress, periods of relief and periods of stress again.

## 1.2.1.6   *REPRODUCTIVE DISTURBANCE*

It is well recognised that chronic stress suppresses reproductive activity. In males, the release of endorphins and enkephalins inhibits the production of luteinising hormone-releasing hormone (LHRH), which is important in sperm production. The change in the autonomic nervous system also means that sexual arousal becomes more difficult, which can result in impotence. Increases in prolactin levels not only increase the production of milk but also suppress reproductive cycling in females. There can also be a change in the metabolism of fat cells, which are important for removing androgens. As a result, females can become more masculinised. Both of these factors combined lead to females becoming less efficient at the reproductive level. In some cases, this can be very important when trying to manage the behaviour of breeding animals.

When evaluating a patient, we need to be aware of any history of chronic or intermittent gastrointestinal disturbance, marked changes in appetite, whether or not the animal has diabetes and any history of reproductive problems if it is entire. If any of these features are present in the history, it may indicate that persistent stress might be involved, and this needs to be addressed even if the stressors are not the specific triggers of the presenting problem. Most behaviour problems do not arise because of a single cause but occur as a result of a range of risk factors coming together in a particular individual at a particular point in time, which pushes it over an acceptable threshold of behaviour. Hence, chronic stress may result in its own specific problems but may also contribute to the production of a whole range of other, less-specific problems.

## 1.2.2   *OTHER BEHAVIOURAL EFFECTS OF PERSISTENT STRESS*

So far we have emphasised the importance of a failure to manage or accommodate some form of change as a cause of stress-related problems and focused on the impact of this on the body due to the maladaptive effect of a functional system. However, at a cognitive and behavioural level there will be other changes, as the animal tries different strategies to help it cope. As we mentioned earlier, a change in behaviour is often a relatively energetically expensive way of trying to adapt, which will feature if simpler physiological changes do not succeed. We can therefore expect major changes in behaviour in cases where the animal is faced with persistent stressors. Its initial response will typically be based on the evolutionary rules of thumb that it has inherited and on developmental experience, which will depend very much on the initial cues and signals in the environment. However, the fact that the stressor is persistent means that it is highly likely that the animal will perceive that the strategy has not worked. In this case it has a limited number of choices:

- *Continuation of the original response*: One option is to continue the original behavioural response, which may be some form of the fight, flight, freeze or fidget response. These behaviours may become more intense with repetition as the animal tries harder to succeed with the same strategy. The frustration which can arise at the lack of success also means that the animal may become more irritable in general or intensively aggressive in the given context, or may run away, take flight, freeze or fiddle about (i.e. seem hyper) more readily.
- *Alternative strategy*: The second option is to develop an alternative strategy: the animal might for example shift from running away (flight) to becoming aggressive (fight).
- *Give up*: A third possibility is for the animal to give up, which is manifested as behavioural and possibly affective (emotional) depression. If an animal learns it has no control over its environment, a condition known as *learned helplessness* may result, which has been used as a model of depression in many studies.

In any case, we need to appreciate that if an animal continues to try to solve a problem unsuccessfully, we are likely to see both behavioural and emotional changes associated with frustration. In the case of persistent stress, these responses may themselves become quite persistent or repetitive. Although frustration is a commonly described outcome, it is important to appreciate that it arises from many different contexts, and it is useful to distinguish these from both a diagnostic and a therapeutic perspective. For example:

- Frustration may occur because an animal is denied access to something that it wants and so is thwarted in its efforts to obtain that resource: e.g. a dog pulling on a lead in order to interact with another dog
- It may arise because an animal gets less than it was expecting from a given situation. This might be conceptualised as a form of disappointment: e.g. a dog

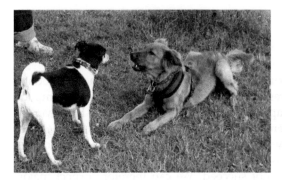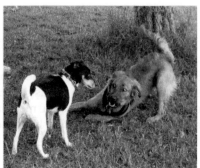

Fig. 1.9 Notice the behaviour in these still images taken of one dog trying to get another to play. The dog on the right shows elements of approach and avoidance, and while in this context it is not a problem, this sort of ambivalent behaviour is indicative of frustration.

who gets given a dog biscuit when it was expecting a piece of chicken may ignore the reward, which would have been acceptable if it had not expected something better. In some situations the dog's behaviour might become aggressive.
- It may arise because an animal is uncertain about what it should do. In this case the animal is in a state of anxious conflict: e.g. a dog who is told to 'come here' by an angry owner.

Depending on the circumstances, the animal may respond passively, for example with behavioural depression, or actively with a more vigorous response. The latter seems particularly likely if the animal is highly aroused and/or predicts it has control over the situation and can alter the outcome. However, in some circumstances the animal's response may be quite measured. Some responses may simply reflect confusion and the trialling of different potential solutions based on previous experience because the animal cannot solve the problem, or an attempt to lower its arousal in order to accept the situation and settle itself emotionally so that it can move on to other projects. Therefore the behavioural manifestations of frustration are quite complex, and several categories are recognised; unfortunately, these do not precisely map on to the forms of frustration described earlier, but some may be more likely in certain contexts than others.

- *Ambivalent behaviour*: This involves doing a little bit of one behaviour and a little bit of another. Often this consists of a mixture of approach- and avoidance-type actions, as the animal is in conflict. So an animal may step forward and then step back: this is especially common when one animal is trying to invite another to play but is uncertain about how its overtures might be accepted (Figure 1.9). In this example, the frustration is unlikely to become persistent (although it may become quite ritualised) as the conflict is not chronic and can be resolved simply by walking away, but a failure to respond clearly may increase frustration further and increase arousal: for example, the dog may bark and become even more animated.

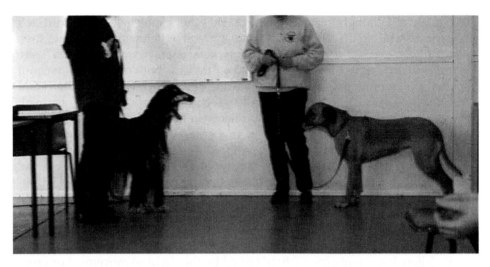

Fig. 1.10 A dog showing displacement behaviour in a stressful situation. The Afghan hound on the left yawns in response to a direct stare from the Rhodesian ridgeback.

- *Displacement behaviour*: This consists of simple behaviours which seem completely irrelevant to solving the problem. When an animal is in a state of conflict, different behavioural programmes may compete for expression with no single one being clearly optimal, which can result in an excessive information load for the animal as it struggles to make a decision. It is thought that in these circumstances the brain may evoke simple behavioural patterns which allow it to refocus and then potentially return to this attentional dilemma, by which time the preferred choice may be more obvious. In cats, a common displacement behaviour is turning round and licking between the shoulder blades (Figure 1.8); this does not solve many problems but it does focus the animal on something else for a short period. The behaviours expressed in these circumstances are typically quite fixed motor patterns; that is, self-contained sequences of behaviour that can be easily executed (we will return to this in Chapter 2). In dogs, common displacement behaviours include circling, yawning (Figure 1.10), cocking the leg and sniffing around. Sometimes these behaviours can seem very bizarre: a dog that just snaps its jaws (fly snapping), for example. Because the behaviour does not resolve the actual problem, it can end up being repeated over and over again if the conflict persists, and it can become compulsive and stereotypic with time.
- *Redirection of the behaviour*: This means the animal attempts to perform the behaviour aimed at resolving the problem towards something other than the cause of the problem. In this case, the frustration is not focused on a conflict between competing behaviours but rather on the thwarting of a behaviour. Typically the behaviour is associated with high arousal and so may be more difficult to inhibit once this level of arousal has occurred. By expressing the behaviour in a redirected form, it is thought that the animal can move on from

the situation, although this may have created other problems for it. Redirected behaviours are often seen in relation to aggressive behaviour, which is then referred to as *redirected aggression*. Dog owners often recount that they were bitten by their dog (who is known to have problems with other dogs) when it spotted another dog passing on the other side of the road while on the lead and they tried to intervene to calm it down or refocus its attention. As it is on a lead, the dog is unable to get to its target and hence in its excitement it turns around and bites the nearest thing, which in this case is the owner's hand or leg. Redirected aggression is not uncommon in multi-cat households. A typical story might be that an owner has two indoor-only cats. Another cat enters the garden, which the indoor cats can see through the window. One of the cats in the household is very highly aroused by the presence of the stranger. If it were outside, it would probably threaten and swipe out if the other cat did not retreat. However, a pane of glass stops it, and so it becomes frustrated. Unfortunately, the second resident cat happens to walk by at this point and so the highly aroused cat turns on its fellow housemate (possibly triggered by the slightest movement or proximity). Such events can lead to longer-term problems, which may be the presenting complaint expressed by the owner; for example, a fear of the dog's apparent aggression to the owner and the associated disruption of the relationship between the owner and the dog in the first instance, and inter-cat conflict between housemates, leading to communication problems, possible avoidance of one another and more aggression, in the second. Only a thorough history will reveal the situational origin of these problems.

It is thought that some of these conflict behaviours may acquire ritual significance in some contexts, for example when an individual is unsure about the intent of another, and in such situations they may help to reduce tension between individuals, as they indicate that the sender does not intend to be a threat. In this context, many conflict behaviours are popularly referred to as 'calming signals'.

In conclusion, some animals seem to be more active copers, who often seek to take control of a situation and so might tend to become more aggressive and to take the initiative when frustrated, whereas other animals are more passive in their coping style and so may become more withdrawn. If we see one of these behavioural changes, it indicates that the animal is having difficulty in coping with its environment and that there may be a need for therapy to help the animal deal with stress. This is one of the important roles of pheromonatherapy. If the cause of any frustration remains, the behavioural manifestation of the frustration may become quite persistent or recurrent. With time, the repeated or persistent performance of a behaviour makes it easier and more likely that the behaviour will recur in similar circumstances. This may form the basis for a form of compulsive or stereotypic type of behaviour (there are other ways that this can arise, for example from persistent reward-seeking, which is the basis of many pharmacological models of stereotypic and addictive behaviour). With time, and if there is little environmental variation, secondary neurological changes may occur, possibly as a result of mechanisms that have evolved to increase behavioural efficiency in consistent situations. These may make the behaviour less varied and ultimately quite fixed and reduced in its form. At this point, we might refer to the behaviour as a stereotypy. Thus persistent frustration can result in repetitive behaviour, which may be a form of either compulsive behaviour or stereotypy. While superficially similar, these behaviours appear to be associated with different underlying neurological changes and so may be mechanistically different.

## 1.3    OTHER CONSIDERATIONS FOR ASSESSING WELFARE

### 1.3.1    *RECOGNISING SIGNS OF POSITIVE WELL-BEING*

In order to evaluate the well-being of an animal, it is important to consider another perspective on the issue of welfare. Historically, most focus has been on detecting signs of distress and the assessment of welfare has largely been based on the absence of these. But it is just as important to recognise the positive signs that indicate that an animal is coping. The following are characteristics of a 'normal' healthy animal or, perhaps, signs that an animal is enjoying life. However, as with the signs of distress, no one sign alone is sufficient. Our assessment should include the balance of signs of positive and negative well-being:

- Psychologically healthy animals can be expected to show a good variety of behaviours, as they efficiently organise their behaviour to meet competing needs at different times. These behaviours will be very variable in form, adapted to different situations and well matched to the shifting priorities presented by a changing environment. The emotional intensity with which behaviours are performed should be evaluated, with the animal seeming to be in control of its behaviour.
- The animal will typically be alert, curious and wanting to investigate things. As mentioned previously, if it feels secure, it is normal for an animal to engage in more information-gathering behaviour. The environment should be sufficiently complex, variable and changeable to ensure that there is a reason to do more than sleep the whole time, in order to maintain a healthy level of cognitive activity.
- The animal will probably be very playful and will want to interact with other members of its social group. Play takes several forms: it can be solitary, object-directed or social, but it is often informative to the animal and self-rewarding. This is why it is often considered a very useful measure of things being good for the animal.

By contrast, an animal that is struggling will typically not show these signs or will show the opposite. For example:

- A very limited range of behaviours of a very limited type, such as stereotypic behaviours (repetitive behaviours with no obvious function).
- Excessive fear, anxiety or irritability, in which the response is out of all proportion to any threat or frustration.

- Bouts of spontaneous panting, restlessness and/or shivering.
- Depression or social withdrawal.
- Hyperactivity and focal attention problems.

There may be a temptation to label these animals or signs as 'abnormal', but the term 'abnormal', like the term 'stress', is difficult to define clearly as it is commonly used in a very confusing way, with different meanings in different contexts.

## 1.3.2   BEHAVIOURAL ABNORMALITY

The concepts of normality and abnormality are widely used in reference to animal behaviour and its evaluation in terms of animal welfare. However, it is not always clear what they mean in practice. While behaviours vary according to context, animals also have species-specific behaviour patterns with an element of consistency, and abnormal behaviour may be considered anything which deviates from this standard. This poses the problem of recognising what 'normal behaviour' is and what standard should be used: the behavioural measure (pattern of behaviours, individual form, intensity, functionality etc.), its level of deviation and its context must be defined, and sometimes we are left with only our intuitions about some of these features. In many instances the term 'abnormal' is simply used to describe behaviour that is rare (literally away from the statistical norm), but in these circumstances it must be recognised that there is not necessarily a link between the  abnormality (i.e. the frequency of the behaviour in the population studied) of a behaviour and animal suffering. The point of reference may be important in this context. For example, in horses, if the stabled population is considered the reference point, then using a statistical approach it can easily be argued that it is not abnormal for them to show repetitive behaviour, since so many do.

In other instances, the functionality or adaptiveness of the behaviour may be used as the reference for normality, but in this case, the terms 'functional' or 'adaptive' are preferable to 'normal' as they are more precise and less likely to give rise to confused associations with animal welfare. This again raises the question of the context for the definition of the key terms of reference; that is, does functional and adaptive behaviour relate to specific circumstances or the underlying mechanism even if it does not achieve its goal? One possible solution involves seeing whether the behaviour occurs in wild free-roaming animals, but a problem here is that the environment is very different and so the behaviour may be absent because it is not needed. Stereotypic behaviour, for example, might be considered abnormal because it is generally not seen in wild free-roaming animals. It is, however, frequently seen in captivity, and one hypothesis is that it reflects frustrated motivation based on natural behavioural predilections, such as the desire to acquire information when the environment appears to provide little (a barren environment) or to escape from an aversive environment. So large felids in the zoo may walk along specific pathways in their cages, gerbils tend to dig and mice climb up their cage walls and repetitively gnaw.

In psychology, the concept of *social deviance* is sometimes applied to assess the abnormality of a behaviour. This involves assessing other people's impression of the behaviour and the impact that it might have on them. A major problem with this approach is that it depends on the subjective opinion of the person using the term. The philosopher Wittgenstein has argued that many concepts have a similar problem of definition. Things that belong within a given category have certain resemblances without necessarily sharing all of the same features, like members of a family. As with stress, all of the underlying defining features that make up the concept of abnormality need to be identified, and then the problem of simple assumptions about the link between the concept and welfare should be more apparent. Eight criteria that might be used when referring to something as 'abnormal' have been proposed, and they have different relationships with the welfare of the performer. It is worth keeping these criteria in mind (as well as the evidence in support of their use) whenever the term 'abnormal' is being used:

- *Suffering*: Behaviours related to suffering may be divided into those that cause harm to the performer (e.g. self-mutilation) or another, those that are associated with an attempt to adapt or cope with a suboptimal environment and those that are associated with an inadequate or noxious state (e.g. signs of frustration).
- *Maladaptiveness*: This refers to the failure of a behaviour to fulfil its goal at either an appetitive (goal-seeking) or a consummatory (goal-execution) level (e.g. a failure to achieve a desired state). Maladaptiveness may also refer to suboptimal behaviour, such as the ingestion of a non-nutritive foodstuff. As noted earlier, there is a distinction to be made between maladaptiveness and malfunctionality.
- *Malfunctionality*: This means that the underlying mechanism regulating the behaviour is disordered for some reason; that is, there is damage or disruption to the underlying neurological processes, resulting in significant deficits in the ability of the animal to execute behaviour. This might be because of a lesion in the brain or damage to peripheral nerves (neuralgia), as is thought to occur in orofacial pain syndrome in cats. Gathering the evidence for this can be challenging in behavioural medicine, and it is important not to confuse this with maladaptiveness, which arises from the application of evolutionary rules of thumb within unnatural settings. Malfunctional behaviours will typically be maladaptive, but the reverse is not true. The brain often has a large reserve and multiple ways of solving a problem, so if one system is damaged, it may use another to solve a problem, and so only when damage or disruption is quite extensive (e.g. extensive seizure activity) will any malfunction become apparent.
- *Unconventionality*: This refers to the statistical rareness of a behaviour in a given context (see earlier).
- *Unpredictability*: It is often implied that behaviours that cannot be predicted are abnormal because they have no recognised control. However, spontaneous behaviour is a rare occurrence and apparent spontaneity is usually a reflection of the knowledge of the reporter of the behaviour. Once the occurrence of a behaviour can be explained, it may cease to appear abnormal. For example, an owner who cannot predict their dog's aggression might describe it as abnormal, but a clear stimulus may be discerned by a therapist.

- *Incomprehensibility*: Similarly, if the nature (as opposed to the occurrence) of a behaviour cannot be understood, it may be described as abnormal until it is explained.
- *Observer discomfort*: If a behaviour causes concern to its observer for any reason then it may be described as abnormal. For example, some people may consider mounting behaviour directed towards a toy or blanket offensive and so describe the behaviour as abnormal.
- *Violation of standards*: Anthropocentric standards may be set which, if they are not met, result in the classification of a behaviour as abnormal. For example, there may be an expectation that a given behaviour will not occur, such as aggression towards people, so its occurrence is seen as abnormal by definition, even if it can be understood.

Many of these criteria are subjective, but still they encapsulate the essence of how the term 'abnormality' can be used. Any behaviour described as abnormal may meet one or more of these criteria in a given context. It is important that any link to welfare is demonstrated logically and not inferred by virtue of the use of the term 'abnormality' for the behaviour alone. Just because a behaviour fulfils one of these criteria does not imply that it fulfils any other; that is, abnormality is not necessarily a welfare problem.

## 1.4   STRESS AUDITING

So far we have focused on how individuals change, why they might change in a given way and the consequences of this. Later chapters deal with how specific types of stressor might give rise to different behaviour problems. However, in many cases there is also a certain level of background stress, which can increase the risk of a problem being expressed, exacerbate any problem that is being expressed or affect the ability to implement effective change. As with specific stress responses, this background stress has a qualitative feature, which may serve to alter the likelihood of specific emotional reactions, making them more likely when the background environment is congruent with the specific types of stressor encountered (e.g. a lot of background frustration will potentially increase the likelihood of frustration responses) but less likely when they are incongruent (e.g. if the home is relaxed, the animal may be less likely to show specific fear responses, or these responses may be more attenuated). It is therefore important to both recognise and manage this background context to the problem. Temperament and prevailing mood play an important role in the risk of specific reactions in a given context. As we will see, pheromonatherapy may be useful in helping the patient to adapt to this. Before we consider the management aspects though, we present a framework for the systematic evaluation of circumstances potentially requiring intervention. This is what we call *stress auditing* (Table 1.1).

A *stress audit* is a systematic evaluation of the daily management routines and environment of an animal with regards to the demands being placed upon it. There are two elements to the environment – the physical environment and the

Table 1.1 Summary of the stress-auditing process.

| | |
|---|---|
| Examine demands made upon the animal regarding: | • Daily management<br>• Daily routines<br>• General environment |
| Consider demands in terms of: | • Expectancy placed upon the individual<br> ○ Animal's 'role'<br> ○ Clarity and consistency of expectancy<br>• Physical characteristics of the stressor in relation to preparation and available resources to help the animal cope<br> ○ Affective quality (threatening, frustrating, socially depriving etc.)<br> ○ Magnitude<br> ○ Duration<br> ○ Predictability<br>• Situation faced by the animal<br>• Opportunity for control<br> ○ Social contingencies: supportive vs conflictive |
| Consider quality of support | • Communication<br>• Feedback<br>• Consistency |
| Consider where there is change | • Amount of change<br>• Preparation and communication of capacity to cope |

social environment – and it is important to recognise the difference between these, as animals have evolved processes for dealing with the specific challenges associated with social interactions.

## 1.4.1  *DEMANDS PLACED UPON THE ANIMAL*

A *demand* is any requirement for change or adaptation that restricts an animal's autonomy or deprives it of a safe, resource-rich environment which meets its needs; that is, anything with the potential to induce anxiety/fear, frustration or significant social deprivation. Within the context of a stress audit, the first aspect to consider arises from the *expectations* placed on the animal; that is, what role the animal is expected to fulfil by its carers, how these expectations are communicated to the animal and the consistency of these expectations among all those who interact with the animal. For example, an owner may want their dog to alert when there are strangers but not when there are familiar visitors. This variable role can be a difficult task to communicate efficiently. If the owner has never taught the dog to 'shh' and 'settle' on command, they may complain about its 'hysterical behaviour' when visitors arrive. Here the expectation has not been clearly communicated to the animal and may have resulted in a conflict that is in danger of spiralling out of control as the owner tries to suppress the unwanted behaviour with punishment.

Next we consider the *physical characteristics* of any demands or potential stressors and the preparation given and resources available to the animal to help it cope. In this regard, we might want to consider not just the magnitude of the stressor but also its duration and predictability. For example, many owners want to interact with their cats for prolonged periods. This is a normal pattern of behaviour for people who are typically intensive and prolonged interactors. Unfortunately this is not the norm for cats, who are less-frequent and shorter-duration social interactors. Therefore, unless a cat has been trained to accept prolonged petting, this may be stressful (frustrating) and can even result in overt aggression if the owner does not read and respond to the cat's behaviour effectively or prevents it from leaving. If the owner holds on to the cat when it would rather leave, they are, in effect, reducing the cat's control over the situation, and this is another important aspect of the stress audit: how much *control* does the animal have over the stressors/demands it encounters? Control increases the perceived ability to cope and so reduces negative affective tendencies.

## 1.4.2   SUPPORT PROVIDED TO THE ANIMAL

When an animal faces a demand, it will cope best if those around it are supportive rather than indifferent or, as often happens, conflictive. Very often, owners feel the urge to punish their pets when they do not behave as they would like them to when facing some stressor. Not only does this potentially reinforce the animal's anxiety or frustration, it also reduces its perception of its wider coping capacity. It is important to appreciate that in this context, we are not simply referring to any conflict associated with the presenting problem, but conflicts that occur more generally in the animal's day-to-day existence.

There are several other aspects to the quality of support given to a pet which are worth considering. These may relate to the social or physical resources available to help the animal cope: for example, the provision of a safe haven or the expectation that an owner will recognise and intervene to abort a situation in which the animal is expressing discomfort. When support is considered, we need to bear in mind its consistency, how well its availability is communicated and any feedback provided from its provision. Where support is consistently available and the pet is aware of this through communication by the owner, it should be easier for the animal to cope with demands made upon it.

## 1.4.3   ELEMENTS OF CHANGE

In summary, when change is required of an animal we need to consider carefully at least the following elements if we want to assess whether it is reasonable to expect the animal to adapt successfully:

- The amount and type of change required, especially in relation to the emotional processes it is likely to elicit.

- The clarity of communication to the animal that change is happening and that the animal will be able to cope with this (again focussing on each emotional process separately).

For example, if we want a dog to cope with being left alone (social deprivation and potential barrier frustration) while we are at work, we should not expect it simply to be able to accept that we are going to leave it for a prolonged period (amount and type of change required). We should consider getting the dog used to shorter periods apart first (communicate the change in small steps) and perhaps providing it with some signs of reassurance (such as safety signals like the dog-appeasing pheromone) to communicate confidence in its ability to adapt. Indeed, it has been found that working dogs adapt better to being kennelled if they are introduced to the kennels for short periods initially and allowed to habituate to the environment.

## 1.5 CONCLUSION

In conclusion, it is important to recognise that stressors vary both qualitatively (i.e. in the type of psychological impact they have – such as anxiety versus frustration) and quantitatively (i.e. in their intensity, frequency and duration). The response that arises will depend on the coping ability of the animal, which will be affected by whether the animal perceives the event as potentially significant and, if it is significant, by its prediction about its ability to adapt to the change demanded by the event. There is much we can do to help animals, by both downgrading the significance of events that we want them to accept and by increasing their expectation that they can cope. By increasing an animal's resilience, not only is the animal's welfare generally improved, but the risk of specific problems is reduced, and when problems do occur the prognosis for successful treatment is improved. It is therefore essential to take a broad overview of the general demands being placed on any animal presented for clinical behavioural assessment and identify where there are conflicts of interest between the owner and their pet, rather than simply focus on the presenting complaint. Such conflicts then need to be addressed accordingly. This can be done by encouraging the owner to develop a way of being with their animal that meets its needs according to its circumstances, rather than through the prescription of specific behaviour-modifying exercises. This approach also recognises that problems arise not so much because of a specific cause but rather as a result of the accumulation of a number of risk factors, many of which may be relatively minor but nevertheless enduring in the animal's general management. Specific events may result in the animal expressing its difficulty in coping in a specific way (i.e. trigger a specific undesirable response), although the problem may be much more general. It is therefore not surprising that by focusing on the general management alone in the first instance, in some cases the primary presenting complaint may disappear, as the animal is generally better able to cope with the specific event triggering this complaint. This focus on general husbandry and communication is not only conducive to a better quality of life for both owner and pet, but also in many cases much easier to implement than more formal behaviour-modification exercises.

## REVIEW ACTIVITIES

- Compare and contrast the stressors to which different companion animals are exposed in modern life and how their ability to cope may vary according to their species-specific evolutionary tendencies.
- Design practical safe havens for different companion-animal species and create instruction sheets to explain to owners how to install and maintain them.
- Explain the relationships between the various hormones and neurotransmitters which are affected when an animal perceives a stressor in the environment and how these can be used to assist evaluation of the type of stressor being perceived by the animal.
- Draw up a check list of the general physical health and behaviour signs a patient might show which would indicate the need for a more comprehensive stress audit.
- Discuss the relevance of frustration as a component of behaviour problems in animals, as well as how frustration can be minimised or avoided to improve welfare.
- Consider a range of questions that you could ask an owner to assess the positive welfare of a pet.
- Design a practical advice sheet for the owner of a new puppy and one for the owner of a new kitten, describing the philosophy behind helping their pet to become resilient as it matures.

## REFERENCES

Maslow AH (1943) A theory of human motivation. Psychological Review 50: 370–396.
Moberg GP, Mench JA (2000) The Biology of Animal Stress. Wallingford: CABI.

## FURTHER READING

Bassett L, Buchanan-Smith HM (2007) Effects of predictability on the welfare of captive animals. Applied Animal Behaviour Science 102: 223–245.
McEwan BS, Wingfield JC (2003) The concept of allostasis in biology and biomedicine. Hormones and Behavior 43: 2–15.
Pageat P, Lafont C, Falewée C, Bonnafous L, Gaultier E, Silliart B (2007) An evaluation of serum prolactin in anxious dogs and response to treatment with selegiline or fluoxetine. Applied Animal Behaviour Science 105: 342–350.
Panksepp J (2011) The basic emotional circuits of mammalian brains: do animals have affective lives? Neuroscience and Biobehavioral Reviews 35: 1791–1804.
Sapolsky R (2004) Why Zebras Don't Get Ulcers. New York: Holt Paperbacks.

# Chapter 2

# Affective Processes and the Organisation of Behaviour

## 2.1 INTRODUCTION

In this chapter we consider how recent advances in neuroscience give us greater insight into the organisation of behaviour and the implications of this for clinical behaviour management. Particular attention is given to the influence of motivational-emotional processes, since the route to problem behaviour management is often (but not always) through controlling the type and/or level of arousal, which determines the behaviour being exhibited.

We start by considering an important historical influence on our thinking about the control of behaviour: behaviorism. The importance of this approach to the acceptance of psychology as a scientific discipline is difficult to overestimate, but a failure to appreciate its limitations can hinder our thinking in light of the rise of neuroscientific and cognitive biological approaches to the study of behavioural control. There is clearly a need to go beyond thinking about things in terms of stimulus and response, if we are to try to gain a more thorough insight into why a specific individual responds in a given way in a given circumstance.

This requires understanding how the external world is represented internally by a given individual and then how this information is used to inform the behavioural decisions of an individual and his/her style of behaviour. Additionally, we need to recognise that emotional processes are at the heart of the facilitation of the individualisation of behavioural responses to external events (Figure 2.1). We consider the process of individualisation of response by examining the processes involved in subjective appraisal of the environment, especially attention and perception. Perceptions are internal representations of stimuli or events, external or internal, and many are necessarily subjective in order to allow the individualisation of behaviour responses. Part of this subjective appraisal process is the application of personal value qualities to some stimuli and events, which results in an emotional response towards them. In its broadest form, this 'emotionally significant quality' can be considered in terms of its incentive versus aversive value; however, other more specific qualities are also recognised in certain other events and stimuli, for example on the basis of

*Stress and Pheromonatherapy in Small Animal Clinical Behaviour*, First Edition.
Daniel Mills, Maya Braem Dube and Helen Zulch.

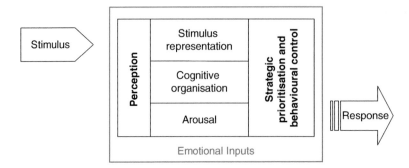

Fig. 2.1 From stimulus to response. Most stimuli have to be processed in order to influence the behaviour of an organism. This processing is subject to cognitive organisation (shown to be at the centre of the process) and potential emotional influence (providing the surrounding context) at all stages.

their social significance to the individual. Motivational–emotional systems serve to integrate subjective and objective information about the significance of a stimulus in relation to the strategic priorities of an individual and regulate the responses that follow as a consequence. These responses must fit within a strategic context and individual behaviours are often neither strategy- nor emotion-specific. However, the emotional content of an action may be evident from the form or style of the behaviour expressed. These features allow these actions to have communicative value, and important clues to both the quality and the intensity of the emotional arousal associated with a given behaviour may be revealed from a careful analysis of its ethological and contextual characteristics. Recognising these features provides greater insight into the goals of a performer, together with their commitment to achieving these goals, and this additional information can help us in our consideration of the most appropriate way to bring about effective behaviour change.

## 2.2   BEYOND BEHAVIORISM

Historically, the science of animal psychology was dominated by a behaviorist perspective, in which the emphasis was on stimuli and responses. This was for sound academic reasons, as there was a need to create a solid scientific basis for psychology that lent itself to objective experimentation. Stimuli and behaviours are observable entities, and associations between them can be carefully measured and recorded. This led to the development of experimental environments in which the contingencies between different events could be carefully controlled, epitomised by the Skinner box (Figure 2.2). It was thus possible to show how different forms of behaviour could be entrained through the careful delivery of reinforcement to shape responses, without necessarily making recourse to the underlying biological mechanistic processes (i.e. the workings of the brain or subjective experience). However, there are several problems with this approach:

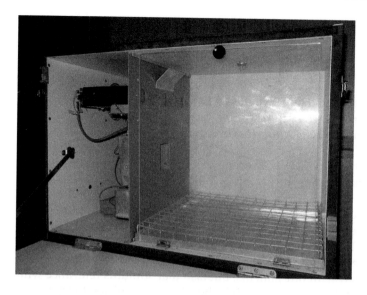

Fig. 2.2 A Skinner box used for animal learning studies.

- First, the absence of a reference to the processes within the central nervous system (CNS) led some to suggest that these were not important to understanding the origins of behaviour within an individual. As a result, 'behaviour' and 'stimuli' became the default organising principles for explanation. However, behaviours are a means to an end, and the CNS processes need to be prioritised before these.
- Second, the environments used for experimental purposes were necessarily sterile and standardised, so that when scientists introduced a change, they could deduce what environmental events were influencing behaviour. However, animals do not live in a sterile environment in nature, and these experiments show what *can* bring about a specific behaviour, but not necessarily what commonly does affect behaviour in the real world.
- Third, the standardisation of the experimental environment means that there has been an emphasis on general effects, and individual variation (i.e. the uniqueness of individuals/personalities or even sex differences) has often either been ignored or considered an inconvenience. This approach is limiting in the clinical setting, since we treat individuals and it is their individuality which determines our treatment recommendations.
- Fourth, a focus on reinforcement to build behaviours which superficially resemble other behaviours led some to suggest that these behaviours were equivalent in motivation. This is an important fallacy: an animal might show a particular (learned) behaviour based on various different motivations. For example, if an animal is reinforced for lying down, this does not necessarily mean it wants to rest. Alternatively, if you reinforce an animal to hold a table tennis bat and hit a ball, this does not mean the animal is *playing* table tennis in the sense in which we talk about *play* from a psychological or biological perspective. However, this was exactly the claim made by leading behaviorists like Skinner.

- Fifth, the emphasis on the externally observable has meant that models of behavioural control have focused on behaviour as the core unit for motivational organisation, rather than some broader and more flexible concept, such as goal orientated strategies (see first point).

The advent of modern brain-imaging methods and other techniques in neuroscience has highlighted the significance of these limitations and, as we will see, helps us understand their relevance when it comes to considering the explanation of clinical behaviour problems.

We now recognise the importance of acknowledging that individuals live in their own personally constructed world, or 'umwelt'. The term *umwelt* refers to the subjectively perceived world of an individual. It differs between individuals because the same stimuli have different relevancies to different individuals as a result of differing species-typical tendencies and individual life histories. Thus we must not only acknowledge that our sensory priorities differ from those of our patients and that different stimuli, or changes in stimuli, may be of greater or lesser relevance to us compared with our patients, but also that stimulus relevance will vary between subjects of the same species. It is the job of the clinician to try to get insight into the perspectives of the patient in order to understand their umwelt as much as possible.

For this reason, we begin with a brief description of perception and how it influences behaviour, before going on to examine the process of behavioural organisation and decision-making.

## 2.3    SELECTIVE ATTENTION AND PERCEPTION: BUILDING A PERSONAL WORLD VIEW

There is an obvious tendency to think of perception as an externally driven activity, in which the brain streams the mass of information coming into it. While this inevitably happens, it is also now recognised that the process has a substantial top-down element to it as well. The reality is that when we consider the range of sensory channels available to us, more impulses from stimuli in the environment are presented to the brain than it can fully process. It is therefore not surprising that mechanisms have evolved, such as sensory bias and selective attention, which enable the brain to create some sort of prioritisation and organisation of the sensory information to be gathered. Indeed, failure of these processes can seriously compromise the ability to function. That is not to say that the senses and brain do not process an enormous amount of information the whole time we are awake, but in humans our conscious sensory world is only a very small part of the total sensory intake. Because this form of representation is a very demanding process, it has a quite limited capacity. What we experience consciously are:

- Our chosen foci of attention.
- Any significant discrepancies from the background monitoring that is going on the whole time.

If we have to learn to do something new, we must concentrate hard initially, but with practice and experience it not only becomes easier but ultimately may be semiautomatic, without the need to attend much to what we are doing. However, if something unusual happens, we suddenly become very aware. Take for example the drive to work. How often do you drive and not give it a second thought? But if a bird were to suddenly fly out in front of your car, you would quickly focus and adjust your behaviour accordingly. Our brain has a working model of how things should proceed under normal circumstances and the subconscious can take control of many of the predictable things that simply require monitoring or have routine solutions. This does not typically require a high level of arousal, although it does require a lot of brain activity. Unexpected events often increase arousal and are brought to the attention of a variety of brain systems that can help the organism cope with this occurrence. It can be argued that consciousness allows information to be accessed simultaneously by many different brain processes and that this facilitates complex problem solving in relation to unexpected or unfamiliar events. The issue of consciousness in nonhuman animals is a controversial subject, but it seems reasonable to suppose that some form of consciousness exists in the species we encounter in a clinical context, even though we cannot know what it must be like to live in their world. Therefore:

- We should not expect animals to normally attend to routine and highly predictable events unless specific training has been given for this. Thus if things are highly predictable, an animal may simply not pay attention to them. Creating notable (but nonthreatening) surprises may be necessary to get an animal to change focus. But by the same measure, if we can bias an animal's attention so it does not rate a given event as significant, the animal will soon learn not to be aroused by this event. Controlling attention, if done correctly, can therefore be a very useful strategy in problem-behaviour management.
- An animal's priorities at any given time will shape what it attends to or notices in the environment and the associated arousal. So if an animal is frightened, it will usually increase arousal and focus on potential signs of danger. This has important clinical implications:
  - Anything even slightly ambiguous is more likely to be interpreted as threatening than it would if the animal were feeling more confident and relaxed about its circumstances.
  - If we try to communicate that all is okay, the animal may simply not notice these efforts and so our efforts are doomed to fail. We need to switch attention and possibly the underlying emotional state (mood) of the animal first. This is where stress auditing (Chapter 1) can be very helpful.

- Different species are likely to have different sensory biases in the way they perceive things and in what things they attend to. We know that cats and dogs have a vastly superior sense of aerial chemical detection compared with humans and might possibly use odour as a primary basis for constructing their umwelt, and this may partly explain the potential power of pheromonatherapy. By the same measure, changes in the olfactory environment, which we humans might be completely unaware of, can have a significant impact on the

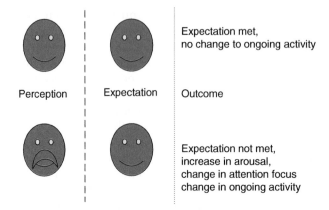

Fig. 2.3 The brain monitors and has expectations of how things should be. If perceptions differ from these expectations, this may serve as a trigger for behaviour change. Thus, if an animal expects to see a clean-shaven face and sees a face with a moustache, there is a mismatch and a consequent increase in arousal, which may lead to a defensive response, such as growling by an anxious dog.

behaviour and attention of cats and dogs. However, alongside this, it has been found that both humans and dogs use their faces a lot to communicate, and many dogs may actually make use of visual facial information in social exchanges with humans and other dogs. Therefore in their social interactions, with people at least, they may depend less on olfactory signals than less socially sophisticated species like the cat.

These points serve to emphasise that perception and attention are active, not passive, processes. The brain has expectations of what the world should be like and monitors for discrepancies in these (Figure 2.3).

An important question which then arises is: how does the brain develop these expectations? The answer lies in certain predisposed tendencies that are shaped by experience. These tendencies relate to the significance attached to the range of qualities perceived in an event or stimulus, which are subsequently stored. In particular, early in life, the brain scans an enormous amount of incoming information for associations and patterns – what goes with what – and then uses these to build up physical and in some instances psychological expectations. For example, a newborn does not innately have the knowledge of who its mother is, but rather acquires this knowledge from its perceptions. It is initially attracted to her because of certain properties she possesses, such as warmth and chemical signals that orientate it towards her. This ultimately leads to suckling and the delivery of milk. The consequences of the newborn's interactions with its mother are that it forms an attachment to her. This means a particular type of emotional significance is given to the features that make up the mother and to the actual individual perceived as the mother. The nature of maternal attachment is such that this quality is not normally applied to anything else (although other forms of attachment do exist). Thus the recognition of a maternal figure is an intrinsically emotional process. As the young grow, they can 'recognise' their mothers through perceptions from a wider range of sensory modalities, such as sight and sound, and their association with features already established. In cats and dogs, the maternal attachment figure does not leave her offspring alone for the first few days, and given her importance to her young it is not surprising that her absence results in a series of distress responses focused on reestablishing contact. This highlights two important features of the young's perception of their mother. First, that they have developed an expectancy of their mother's presence; that is, they not only expect their mother to have certain physical characteristics, but also that she will be close by. Second, these expectations and their fulfilment (or not) are closely associated with certain strategic responses, and these responses are very emotional.

Thus, emotional processes involve personal appraisals relating to the significance of stimuli and events, and the associated behaviour they elicit. Emotion is therefore intrinsically linked to both cognitive processing and behavioural control systems.

Before we discuss these other aspects of emotion, it is worth considering other factors which contribute to individual differences in perception and expectation. The previous example illustrated some strong intrinsic biases to perception, but other biases and abilities arise as a result of our experience. The brain is an extraordinary pattern recogniser and organiser, and the types of association we are exposed to during development appear to affect the types of pattern it can detect later in life. To illustrate this, let us consider a couple of human examples. Some individuals who have been brought up in East Asia may confuse their 'r' and their 'l' sounds. These letter sounds (phonemes) do not exist in their native language and so their brain has never needed to distinguish between them. As a result, the brain is unable to distinguish between them without a lot of training later in life, and until such training is received the two phonemes are perceived as the same. The error that is made in speaking may seem strange to Europeans, because their brains are able to make the distinction and so have an expectation associated with words containing these phonemes. Simply pointing out the error does not resolve the problem; rather, it depends on appropriate exposure. This is not a unique phenomenon, since we often fail to recognise the subtleties of sound in a new language until we have had a lot of practice and experience.

The second example refers to a phenomenon known as the 'other race effect'. We are generally poorer at distinguishing between and remembering the faces of individuals from ethnic groups that we have not had a lot of exposure to during our childhood. The explanation is similar to that in the previous example, in that the lack of experience means we lack the ability to perceive the relevant features to allow discrimination. This developmental phenomenon has important implications when considering the behaviour of nonhuman animals. For example, animals may perform poorly in certain discrimination tasks due to perceptual (rather than sensory) deficits arising from limited exposure to the necessary conditions during development. It is also one of the reasons why limited socialisation and habituation can be so harmful later in life. With limited experience, when something new is encountered which is aversive, the brain fails to discriminate much about this aversive experience and so the problem immediately becomes more general. The brain simply does not have the relevant connections to allow it to perceive differences that would help to limit the effects. By the same measure, if only one person ever gives instructions to a dog, the dog may have difficulty perceiving the same instructions from another individual, at least initially. However, we can also use this knowledge to help prevent problems and set things up to enable animals to achieve their potential. If we want to develop an animal's ability with respect to a particular capacity, we should perhaps immerse it (especially during the relevant developmental phase – sensitive period) in experientially rich and diverse environments associated with that capacity. The brain will then often automatically establish and strengthen connections between reliable associations and so develop the ability to perceive potentially significant patterns, even in very complex settings. Thus a diversity of social experiences should result in a more socially competent individual. This is one way in which cognitive flexibility can develop, leading to greater adaptability and potentially problem-solving ability.

An exciting recent example of this concerns the use of human language by dogs. It has been shown that some dogs have a remarkable ability to learn relatively large vocabularies, while others do not. A common feature of the high-performing dogs seems to be that they are immersed in language directed towards them from an early age, similar to the chat between a mother and her child (what has been termed 'motherese'). It seems reasonable to suppose that this experience results in a brain that is better able to pick out the relationships between words, and in one documented case it has been suggested it may even allow a basic understanding of some form of syntax. However, by the same measure, if we keep an animal in a very simple and unchanging environment, we can predict that it will become very habitual in its behaviour and lack cognitive flexibility. This may help to explain why animals kept in barren enclosures are predisposed to stereotypic behaviour associated with their monitoring behaviour.

Although the potential ability (hardware in the brain) to encode certain features may be common between members of the same species, it is the developmental experience which is key to the actual development of both individual perceptual abilities and expectancies of the world. When an animal is born, there are many more connections between cells in the brain than it needs or are useful. As a result of experience, connections are maintained and strengthened between reliable patterns and are broken between those that are not detected.

Some of the patterns that are perceived are highly complex and depend on the existence of more general internal constructs within the brain for reference, against which multiple features of a stimulus can be checked (Figure 2.4). This allows the filling in of missing information, in order to create more general expectations. This has been studied quite extensively with regards to certain aspects of vision.

In the case of visual information, it seems there is an inherent ability to process contrasts in shading as boundaries and to use this information to break complex shapes down into more simple ones, known as 'geons' (Figure 2.5). These geons form the basis of the three-dimensional construction and recognition of the world; that is, the ability to recognise familiar objects from unfamiliar angles. But there are many visual other aspects of an object to process too, and these aspects tend to

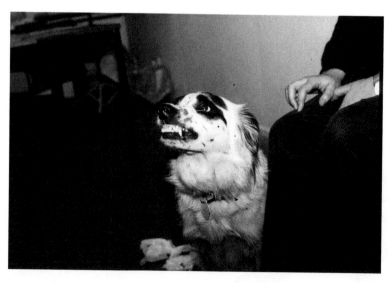

Fig. 2.4 Expectation can be built on direct mapping of a stimulus or on mapping of a range of features against a more complex construct. For example, the mapping of an individual's identity from its odour may be a relatively straightforward process, in that this combination of chemicals is uniquely associated with this individual. However, in the case of perceiving a threat, we cannot directly map the visual features of each encounter to a matching memory; rather, we must map more general salient features against a flexible model. In this way we can expect to be bitten by this dog, if we are not careful, even if it is the first time we have met him.

be processed separately. Colour is processed independently of form, as is movement, and the significance of these qualities varies from species to species and perhaps even within species.

Expectations relating to general constructs may also develop in relation to behaviour. Thus when almost any object is dropped, our brain will expect it to fall to the ground. We may not even attend to such events as they are so predictable, unless our attention is specifically drawn to one (perhaps by a child holding a ball and saying 'Look!' before dropping it). These types of general expectancy in effect become general rules for physical cognition, which can be used by the brain to help with problem solving: 'Drop something heavy and it will fall down.' The extent to which similar expectancies develop in relation to social cognition is less clear, but it seems emotions may have a role to play in this context. As we have seen, the perception of the mother is associated with certain expectancies, and there are other useful individualised social distinctions that can be made which may have beneficial general effects on behavioural efficiency. For example, a given individual might be another's mother, daughter, sexual partner, friend or enemy, and we would expect her to elicit a different type of emotional response and type of interaction in the other accordingly. Thus emotional processes may be used to give a particular quality to certain stimuli, and to develop certain expectancies as a result, which if not met may attract attention. This 'emotional quality' of a stimulus

(a)

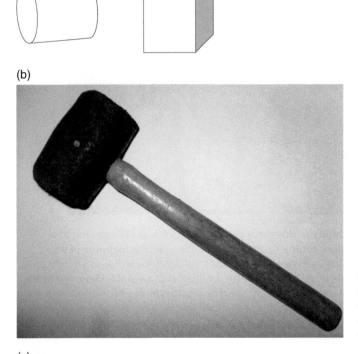

(b)

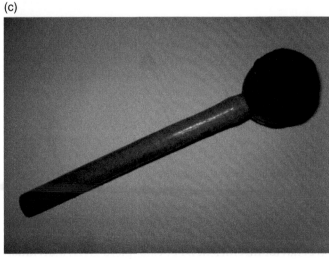

(c)

Fig. 2.5 (a) Examples of two geons: a cylinder and a cube. By detecting the edges of a complex object from changes in colour, texture and brightness, it can be broken down into standard, simpler, three-dimensional units such as these, with known properties. This allows the brain to create expectations about the object, such as what it should look like from another angle. Thus the image of the mallet (b) can be broken down into a couple of cylinder geons, which allows it to be recognised from a different angle (c).

may be as much a part of its definition as its more objective features and, as we will see later, has an important role in setting behavioural priorities at any given time.

Finally, we should not forget that in some cases perceptual abilities are limited by sensory capacity. An interesting potential example of this has been found in dogs. It seems that the longer a dog's nose, the wider the visual focal area for visual discrimination in the eye (the fovea); that is, the more it becomes a visual streak rather than a focal spot. This means that short-nosed dogs (such as many lapdogs) may have a fovea like that of a human, which might be good for face reading, whereas the fovea of a long-nosed breed (such as many sight hounds) is more like that of a horse, which is good for horizon scanning.

Pheromones may be particularly important in some of these perceptual processes, including the emotional appraisal and organisation of stimuli. What makes them different to other semiochemicals is they are not simply odours with which arbitrary associations are learned. Rather, they are chemicals that are biologically predisposed to affect behaviour, through general perceptual effects. So a chemical which increases the likelihood of a fear response is a pheromone (alarm pheromone), whereas a chemical which identifies a specific individual of whom I am afraid is not. This is not to say learning cannot occur in association with pheromones – far from it – but rather that learning is not necessary for them to have their effect. Thus a sexual pheromone will cause sexual arousal, and if it is reliably paired with another stimulus it may be possible over time to produce sexual arousal in association with that stimulus even in the absence of the pheromone, as a result of classical conditioning. So pheromones are unconditional stimuli which signal the intrinsic relevance of something. This relevance may result in high levels of arousal, as in the case of sex or alarm pheromones, but may also encourage reduced arousal, in the case of 'safety signals', which allow an animal to prioritise or explore other nonthreatening stimuli in the environment. This is particularly important when we consider how pheromonatherapy works in problem-behaviour management.

In this section we have considered how the brain organises the information it receives in order to minimise the processing demands associated with environmental monitoring. Some of this organisation relates to identifying general properties of stimuli, such as their physical characteristics; other aspects relate to properties of more individual relevance, such as the social relationship between the stimulus and the appraiser. Events which do not meet expectations may attract particular attention, with a view to changing behavioural priorities. In the next section we expand on the idea of individual relevance and the role of emotions in this regard.

## 2.4   INCENTIVES AND AVERSIVES

It is worth pointing out that a consensus has not been reached by scientists on exactly what aspects of personal relevance are encoded by the brain in relation to the external world, so what follows is partly a personal interpretation of current neuroscience. Nonetheless, as we will see later, it is a paradigm that works well in clinical animal behaviour problem management and is grounded in a solid biological foundation.

Broadly speaking, things which are of importance to an individual can be divided into the objects or events which it desires to have (*incentives*) and those which it hopes to avoid (*aversives*). However, even if something generally engenders desire or avoidance within an individual, its immediate impact on the individual's behaviour (i.e. its immediate relevance to the individual) might vary depending on other priorities. The form and type of emotional arousal that is elicited in these situations may be an important aspect of the behavioural decision-making process, and the consequences of the animal's decision provide an opportunity for learning.

## 2.4.1  REWARDS, PUNISHMENTS AND BEHAVIOURAL CHANGE

In some cases, what is desired relates to the presence of something, such as food or companionship; in other cases, it is relief from something, such as the ending of excessive noise or a painful experience. In either case, an individual might work to achieve these ends and the control of the situation that results might reinforce this behaviour; that is, make it more likely when similar circumstances arise. When the probability of a behaviour recurring in similar circumstances has increased as a result of the acquisition of an incentive, *positive reinforcement* of the behaviour is said to have occurred. When the probability of a behaviour recurring in similar circumstances has increased as a result of escape from an aversive, *negative reinforcement* of the behaviour is said to have occurred. It might be argued that both of these situations relate to the acquisition of some form of incentive, but the incentives are qualitatively different, and so the two processes are not the same. In one situation the incentive is typically an additional resource, in the other it is a form of comfort or safety. Similarly, the things an animal wants to avoid might relate to the presence of certain stimuli, such as things, which can directly cause harm or are otherwise aversive, or on the other hand to the loss of things that are valued – in other words, incentives. In either case, the occurrence of these events might cause an animal to change what it is doing and make it less likely to perform the preceding behaviour in similar circumstances. In this case, the event has been an effective *punishment*. As with reinforcement, punishment can be *positive* when it involves the application of a stimulus (in this case an aversive) or *negative* when it involves the elimination or loss of a stimulus (in this case an incentive). Thus positive and negative punishment are qualitatively different events. It is worth emphasising that within the terms 'positive and negative reinforcement' and 'positive and negative punishment', the terms 'positive' and 'negative' refer to the acquisition or loss of a stimulus (incentive or aversive) to achieve a given effect (reinforcement or punishment) and not to the subjective quality of the event, which can be more specifically defined (Table 2.1).

These four types of event are associated with the information required for success in different aspects of survival and optimality. Positive reinforcement is associated with the acquisition and exploitation of resources, negative reinforcement with finding comfort and safety, positive punishment with harm and negative punishment with the loss of resources. Therefore it is not surprising that the behaviours performed in relation to these events can result in qualitatively different experiences: the acquisition of an incentive is associated with satisfaction, the

Table 2.1 Representation of different forms of reward and punishment in terms of the acquisition or loss of a given stimulus, in relation to attempting to get a dog to be quiet when another dog passes.

|  | Positive = adding something: incentive or aversive | Negative = taking away something: incentive or aversive |
| --- | --- | --- |
| **Reinforcement**<br>• The behaviour is shown more frequently | **Positive reinforcement** of being quiet when another dog passes, e.g.<br>• Attention: verbal praise, looking at the dog…<br>• Tactile: petting…<br>• Food: giving a treat…<br>…when it shows the desired behaviour | **Negative reinforcement** of being quiet when another dog passes, e.g.<br>• Tactile: releasing the tension on the collar…<br>…when the dog stops barking at another dog |
| *Example and qualitative process* | • *Acquisition and exploitation of resources*<br>• *Satisfaction* | • *Finding comfort or safety from harm*<br>• *Relief* |
| **Punishment**<br>• The behaviour is shown less frequently | **Positive punishment** of being quiet when another dog passes, e.g.<br>• Attention: telling the dog off in a loud, harsh voice…<br>• Tactile: tugging on the lead, hitting the dog…<br>…when the dog barks at another dog | **Negative punishment** of being quiet when another dog passes, e.g.<br>• Attention: isolating the dog…<br>• Tactile: stopping petting…<br>…when the dog barks at another dog |
| *Example and qualitative process* | • *Harm*<br>• *Fear or pain* | • *Loss of resources*<br>• *Disappointment or frustration* |

elimination of an aversive with relief, the arrival of an aversive with fear or pain and the loss of an incentive with disappointment or frustration.

When working with reinforcement and punishment in practical situations, the two will appear to go hand in hand; that is, positive reinforcement with negative punishment (e.g. the dog receives a treat when it shows the desired behaviour, such as a 'down' (= positive reinforcement), but does not receive a treat when it does not show the desired behaviour (= negative punishment)) and positive punishment with negative reinforcement (e.g. the owner jerks on the lead to stop the dog forging ahead (positive punishment) but stops jerking when it stays at his side (= negative reinforcement)). However, it may be that one of these is much more salient to the animal and so of more relevance in bringing about behavioural change. Which has greater salience is likely to be a feature of the individual circumstances and this needs to be evaluated by the clinician as it has

Table 2.2 Emotional quality of actions associated with different types of event related to incentives and aversives. Terms in *italics* are derived from the typical human feeling in each circumstance, which is used as a shorthand to describe the underlying emotional expression in a nonhuman animal (accepting that the subjective experience is likely to be different). The anticipated potential loss of an incentive may result in *Anger* if the subject attempts to resist it or in *Depression* if the subject does not (loss of control). Likewise, it might be suggested that *Terror* is associated with the uncontrollable but anticipated gain of an aversive.

| | Comparable human feeling | Comparable human feeling |
| --- | --- | --- |
| Contingency | Incentive | Aversive |
| Gain | *Happiness* | *Fear* |
| Anticipation of potential gain | *Desire* | *Anxiety* |
| Loss | *Sadness* | *Relief* |
| Anticipation of potential loss | *Anger* | *Hope* |

implications for the emotional states involved in a behaviour as currently manifested and its alteration.

It is not just the behaviours associated with the immediate delivery of reinforcement and punishment which have an emotional quality, but also their antecedents: that is, behaviours expressed in anticipation of the reward or punishment. These anticipatory states have a different emotional quality. By way of shorthand, we can give these contingencies a label comparable to a possible human feeling in such a circumstance, while accepting that we are not implying that animals necessarily share the same experience. For this reason we have put the terms in *italics* in Table 2.2. In the case of potential incentives, the contingent events serve to invigorate behaviour and maximise the chance of gaining the desired outcome, whereas in the case of aversives, they aim to minimise the risks associated with its arrival. In the case of anxiety, inhibiting ongoing behaviour allows the exploration of alternatives, while in the case of anger, mobilising reserves helps resist the potential loss.

The important point to appreciate here is not that the animals we encounter have qualitatively different feelings in relation to different events (we cannot know the subjective feelings of others, including our fellow humans) but rather that events which are of specific importance to an animal are associated with different emotional responses that inform the behavioural priorities of the individual.

## 2.4.2   GENERAL BIOLOGICAL AND BEHAVIOURAL PRIORITIES ASSOCIATED WITH INCENTIVES AND AVERSIVES

One potential outcome of the ability to anticipate is preparation and therefore the potential to maximise one's interests. We can expect animals to be capable of and

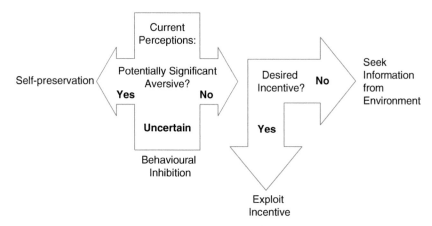

Fig. 2.6 Schema indicating the initial decision-making process in relation to operational priorities. Behavioural activity directed towards maximising the acquisition of incentives is the norm; in the absence of a specific incentive, this will be expressed in the form of general exploratory behaviour. The perception of a significant aversive always has the potential to intrude into ongoing activity.

efficient at undertaking this task. In order to operate efficiently, the importance of strategies directed towards gaining something potentially valuable needs to be evaluated against other competing options, even in the absence of an immediate reward. Otherwise, animals would always prioritise immediately available incentives over less accessible but potentially more valuable ones. Similarly, the avoidance of a minor immediate aversive would take priority over longer-term safety strategies. A key requirement for the efficient execution of strategic or planned behaviour is therefore the ability to prioritise the relative significance of different events in order to effectively inhibit potentially competing activities. This inhibitory control in relation to strategic planning is an important function of the prefrontal cortex.

The brain is an active information-seeking machine and so individuals normally seek information from the environment in order to learn about it and potentially exploit it more effectively at some future date. Thus, exploratory activity is the default mode of operation when awake, in the absence of specific demands associated with potentially significant incentives or aversives in the environment. However, if exploiting a specific incentive (including the opportunity to mate) is advantageous at any given time, behaviour will be directed towards achieving this. Intrusion by a potentially significant aversive may occur at any time, in order to minimise the risk of harm. This top-level decision-making process is represented in Figure 2.6.

Uncertainty about the aversive nature of something perceived as potentially significant can result in behavioural inhibition while it is being reevaluated. Further indecision may result in conflict activities, such as displacement behaviour (see Chapter 1). It may be that these help the animal break out of the conflict before undertaking a renewed appraisal of the current circumstances. Ambivalent behaviours might also occur in this circumstance, as monitoring the consequences of its own approach–avoidance behaviour may result in the acquisition of information that helps the animal decide about its significance.

A prerequisite for this model is the existence of a neuroanatomical comparator of incentives and aversives, and this seems to exist within the septohippocampal system. This system stops ongoing behaviour when there is a discrepancy between stored information and what is detected in the environment. In this way it can respond to both unexpected events and unfamiliar events in a similar manner. In the former situation there is a mismatch with predictions, whereas in the latter there is no match. When reading the literature, confusion can arise because the emotion associated with activity within this 'behavioural inhibition system' is often referred to as 'anxiety', but this is not the same as the *anxiety* that arises from the prediction of an aversive (i.e. anticipation of a fearful event). Behavioural inhibition system anxiety relates to uncertainty and an unresolved approach–avoidance conflict, and so we will use the term *conflict* to refer to this state. Gamma amino butyric acid (GABA) and benzodiazepine receptors appear to play a particularly important role in the regulation of this system and it is therefore not surprising that drugs acting on these receptors can be particularly useful in the management of behaviour problems associated with this type of circumstance.

At a higher level, there appears to be a degree of hemispherical specialisation in the processing of information leading to behaviour associated with aversives and incentives. The right hemisphere is typically more active in aversive or avoidance situations and the left in incentive or approach situations.

## 2.5   MOTIVATIONAL–EMOTIONAL PREDISPOSITIONS AND BEHAVIOURAL CONTROL

### 2.5.1   *MOTIVATIONAL–EMOTIONAL SYSTEMS AND INDIVIDUAL PRIORITIES*

In the previous section we saw how a top-level appraisal of the incentive and aversive value of externally and internally perceived events can determine the broad mode of operation of an animal. These are a self-preservation mode versus an incentive-exploitation mode, with behavioural inhibition occurring when a personally significant but unexpected or uncertain event occurs. Within both of the affirmative-action modes there are several biologically distinct priorities (motivational–emotional predispositions). These predispositions reflect the personal needs of the animal, and have to be monitored, evaluated and acted upon (or inhibited) according to the individual's wider circumstances. This is achieved through structurally definable circuits within the brain (motivational–emotional systems); that is, different types of contextually contingent behavioural control systems, which are significantly affected by subjective inputs. Three qualitatively different motivational–emotional systems associated with self-preservation have been described. These are:

- The *pain* system, related to the maintenance of body integrity and functioning. This responds to the personal significance of actual or potential tissue damage.

- The *anxiety–fear* system, related to the comfort provided by predictable access to essential resources. This coordinates activity associated with the management of threats to personal or resource security.
- The *panic–grief* system, related to the protection provided by others and reflected in a need for social contact. This results in the potential generation of distress and actions directed towards maintaining or reestablishing contact when separation from an attachment figure and, to a lesser extent, other significant social contacts occurs.

With respect to motivational–emotional systems associated with exploiting incentives, the following have been described:

- The *desire* system. This takes the form of a common circuit for encoding the personal significance of seeking and consummatory activity directed towards different types of physical resource which have their own specific behavioural motivational systems. This includes activities such as feeding, drinking, environmental exploration and some forms of solitary object play, but not social play. The specific behavioural system engaged at any given time is dependent on the integration of a range of internal and external factors, with the *desire* system providing a common currency for evaluating potentially competing behavioural motivational systems (Figure 2.7).
- The *frustration* system, which integrates the personal significance of a failure to meet expectations relating to resource acquisition or control (including territorial integrity) and the consequences of restraint. The system serves to invigorate behaviour directed towards establishing the expected level of control in the situation. The associated motivational–emotional predisposition is reflected in a need for control over certain resources or situations.

In addition, there appear to be three specific systems involved in encoding important subjective information relating to different types of social interaction:

- A *lust* system, associated with subjective input directed towards the organisation of the reproductive needs of the individual, ranging from the attraction or selection of a mate through courtship and any associated bond to mating with a sexual partner. The associated motivational–emotional predisposition is reflected in a need for sexual activity.
- A *care* system, associated with facilitating a personal significance in acts of recognisable parental care or nurturance towards others. The associated motivational–emotional predisposition is reflected in the importance of maintaining the bonds to the individual.
- A *social play* system, which integrates the personal significance of interactions in this context. During social play, a large amount of important information relating to the individual's own social competence and potential in relation to others can be acquired without the risks inherent in agonistic encounters. Much of the information gained through rough-and-tumble play cannot be obtained through another route (Figure 2.8). The associated motivational–emotional predisposition is reflected in a social playfulness.

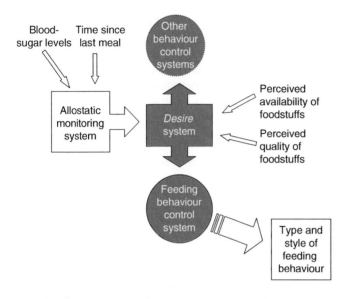

Fig. 2.7 Schematic representation of the integration of some subjective and absolute factors affecting feeding behaviour and the central role of the *desire* system, which must also mediate between competing activities.

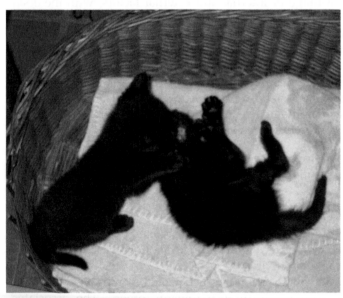

Fig. 2.8 Many social skills and much social information are gained through rough-and-tumble play.

As illustrated in Figure 2.7, these systems allow the integration of subjective information into the behavioural decision-making process, and this affects not just the likelihood of a given type of activity occurring over another but also the way it is expressed. One of the ways in which this individualisation of response can manifest is in the emotional intensity of the behaviour. Some subjective information affecting this may be derived from learned experiences relevant to the particular motivational–emotional system, but in other instances it may stem from more endogenous experiential factors. For example, in the case of feeding behaviour, personal preferences may be partly derived from experience of what tastes good, but also (especially in the young) from prenatal exposure to certain nutrients in utero. Thus two individuals may show very different emotional responses to the prospect of the same foodstuff, despite similar levels of hunger. However, differences in hunger due to absolute factors (such as blood-sugar levels) may also result in responses of differing emotional intensity, due to the perceived importance of feeding at a given time. In the case of the motivational–emotional systems relating to social interactions, the quality of the personal relationship between individuals will be a particularly important influence on the emotional content of the associated behaviours.

The important point to note here, from a clinical perspective, is that *certain events can be linked to motivational–emotional systems* and that the behaviours which follow as a result have the *potential to vary in their emotional intensity*. In some instances, problems arise because certain stimuli linked to a particular motivational–emotional predisposition are so important that the related system is much more readily engaged than is desirable in a given circumstance (i.e. there is a problem with the qualitative aspect of the response), whereas in other cases it is not the motivational– emotional system being engaged but the level of arousal that follows which is problematic (i.e. there is a problem with the intensity of the response). Therefore, in many cases, identifying the role being played by motivational–emotional systems in a given circumstance is at the heart of the diagnostic process.

The neurobiological substrate of most of these systems (albeit with a slightly altered nomenclature and a different perspective on their role in relation to behavioural control) has been described by Panksepp (1998) (see also Table 2.3), with a useful review of the neurobiology of *pain* described by Craig (2003). These systems reflect a range of 'needs' with a clear neurobiological basis, and it is interesting to note how well they map on to Maslow's hierarchy of needs (Chapter 1).

## 2.5.2   BEHAVIOURAL STRATEGIES AND SPECIFIC ACTION

So far we have examined how an animal prioritises its different needs and how this process can result in emotional behaviour. But this does not explain exactly what behaviour is going to be shown. The link between emotional decision-making and behavioural expression is not a direct one. In the first instance, an animal must decide upon its strategic priorities in relation to and within different motivational– emotional predispositions; only then can it execute a behavioural plan directed towards achieving a specific goal. Let us take a simple example to illustrate this point. Imagine a dog who is living in a safe environment at home, who is well looked after in many ways but who has a very strong attachment towards his owner. He detects that his owner is picking up his coat. This is perceived as a highly significant event to this dog, who finds it difficult to cope without his owner. As a result his *panic–grief* predisposition may be given priority and strategies directed towards preventing separation may be prioritised within this system (an alternative might be to seek contact with and comfort from the owner

Table 2.3 Key neuromodulators associated with activation and inhibition within different motivational–emotional systems. Adapted from Panksepp (2006).

| Motivational emotional system | Activating neuromodulators | Inhibitory neuromodulators |
|---|---|---|
| Desire | Dopamine, glutamate, opioids, neurotensin | |
| Frustration | Dopamine, glutamate, substance P, acetylcholine | |
| Anxiety–fear | Glutamate, diazepam-binding inhibitor, corticotrophin-releasing hormone, cholecystokinin, alpha melanocyte-stimulating hormone | Neuropeptide Y |
| Lust | Steroids, vasopressin, oxytocin, Luteinising releasing hormone, cholecystokinin | |
| Care | Oxytocin, prolactin dopamine, opioids | Opioids |
| Panic–grief | Corticotrophin-releasing hormone, glutamate | Opioids, oxytocin, prolactin |
| Social play | Opioids, glutamate, acetylcholine | Opioids |
| Pain | Glutamate, substance P, neurokinins A and B | GABA, opioids |

Norepinephrine increases arousal and serotonin has nonspecific inhibitory effects on central systems.

at this time). He may bark and then run around the owner, interfering with the owner's preparations to depart. These are the dog's behavioural decisions, and their emotional content, will depend on their perceived significance in the context of what is going on. Barking and running around the owner are not behaviours uniquely associated with *panic–grief*. For example, the former might be used in association with *desire* in order to receive a reward, and the latter might be used as a prelude to *social play*. Thus the behaviours are not exclusively bound to specific motivational–emotional systems; rather they can be recruited when relevant to the ongoing predisposition system. This means that behaviour alone cannot be used to infer regulating systems, but in combination with its emotional association it may be much more informative.

Let us take another example, relating to a suite of behaviours directed towards a particular goal, to illustrate this point further. Apparent attempts to escape may be associated with different motivational–emotional predispositions depending on the personal circumstances. For example, they may be associated with an attempt to reestablish contact with an attachment figure who has departed (*panic–grief*), with a frustrated attraction towards something outside of the current boundaries (*frustration*) or with an attempt to move away from something perceived as unpleasant in the current environment (*anxiety–fear*). Close behavioural analysis is beginning to reveal recurring but subtle differences in the behavioural style associated with different motivational–emotional predispositions. Specific examples will be given in some of the chapters relating to specific presenting complaints in Part II. For now we can make the following generalisations. Many behaviours performed in the context of *panic–grief* tend to involve a higher level of tension (these vocalisations are often higher pitched) or have a more extended performance than their expression in relation to many of the other predispositions. Acts performed out of *frustration* have a particular vigour, while there is an intrinsic variability in the responses associated with *desire* and invariability in those associated with *anxiety–fear*. Thus when an animal is trying to acquire an incentive it will often vary its behaviour each time; if it escaping from an aversive, this is less often the case. Taking note of such measures in certain situations may help us determine whether an animal is primarily motivated to escape from something it finds unpleasant or to move towards a place of safety. If it is the former, the behaviour will appear in much the same way each time, but if it is the latter we would expect more variability.

Thus a range of behavioural strategies may serve, but are not bound to, specific motivational–emotional predispositions. These strategies are themselves composed of a series of nonexclusive behavioural action units, which may need to be assembled in a flexible way in order to be executed efficiently in relation to the overall strategy (Figure 2.9).

This means we have to go beyond behaviour in order to make a diagnosis, and use all the available evidence relating to the form and context of the behaviour to help us make logical inferences about what is going on. The diagnosis should be built around recognising what motivational–emotional system(s) are being engaged and the level of their intensity, as well as the strategic objectives of the problematic behaviour within the need.

## 2.5.3   *ADDRESSING SEVERAL NEEDS THROUGH A SINGLE BEHAVIOURAL ACTION*

In the examples given so far, for the purposes of clarity we have presented scenarios in which the controlling motivational–emotional systems are active in absolute and exclusive terms, for example where an animal is motivated by *panic–grief* rather than *anxiety–fear*, but this may not be the situation in reality. Indeed, mixed emotional activity may well be the norm. Accordingly, the emotional elements of a display can be ambivalent. For example, in the case of an animal trying to defend one of its resources against a competitor, it may show aggressive behaviour with elements of *frustration* and *anxiety–fear*; that is, elements of offence and defence, since the decision to defend is not without risk. Aggressive threatening may however serve both needs. A careful analysis of the circumstance and sequelae

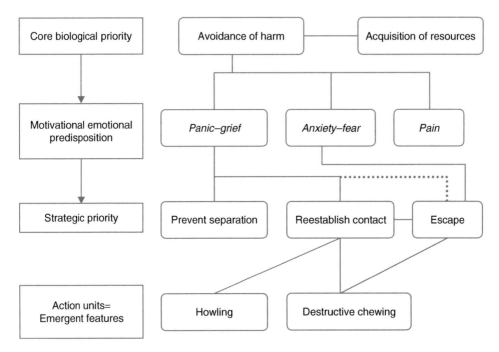

**Fig. 2.9** From biological priority to behavioural action. The left-hand column shows the hierarchical organisation of the decisions which ultimately lead to the expression of a specific behaviour. To the right are specific examples of potentially competing processes at each level. Note that the behavioural elements are not necessarily exclusive to a higher functional system. See text for further explanation.

of a display will help to identify exactly which systems are being engaged. This in turn will help us make more informed proposals about the specific treatment strategies available. For example, if a dog is making an aggressive display because it feels threatened then providing it with food will not reinforce the behaviour but may actually help to eliminate the response. This is because the motivational–emotional system underlying the display is not directed towards resource acquisition but towards obtaining relief. We can predict that only acts which bring relief, such as our backing away, will reinforce the behaviour. If food is accepted in this context, we would predict that the presenting behavioural strategy has not been satisfied, but rather the underlying motivational–emotional state has been changed. In this case, the state is not compatible with fearfulness, so we have effectively counterconditioned it. By contrast, if an animal is making an aggressive display to acquire a resource then yielding or providing it with a more valuable resource might exacerbate the problem, because the motivational–emotional goal is being achieved. This is why it is important to focus on the emotional background of a presenting complaint rather than simply the behaviours being displayed. Such an approach is difficult to explain from a purely behaviorist perspective. This does not dismiss the value of accurate behavioural descriptions and their circumstances (or *stimulus-response associations*, as they are often called), but rather emphasises their importance, since it is in the context of these that we can make sounder inferences about the underlying psychological state. This is perhaps one of the contradictions of the 'behaviorist ideal' – although it emphasises the importance of focusing on behavior, it typically fails to describe that behaviour with the necessary resolution to differentiate between the underlying subjective processes which it believes cannot be evidenced. As a result, progress has been slower and less productive than might otherwise have been the case had there been greater acknowledgement of these fundamental processes.

## 2.5.4   HELPING ANIMALS TO MAKE THE RIGHT BEHAVIOURAL DECISIONS

So far, it has been suggested that the structured motor outputs which make up behaviour (or *modal action patterns*, as they are sometimes called) are the means whereby different strategies relating to specific priorities or needs are achieved. However, as illustrated earlier, a given behaviour may be used to serve different goals, although it can vary in style according to its underlying emotional content. So the link between motivation and behaviour is not as direct as is often presented. Historically, many models of motivation have focused on the physical factors that might be related to specific behavioural goals; the current proposal, while acknowledging the importance of these physical factors, suggests that a more general psychological need (which may not be conscious) is the key intervening variable determining which goals are pursued. In relation to a given goal, there may be different strategies between which an individual has to choose, depending on the circumstances. While it may seem intuitive that the brain simply energises the most appropriate behaviours to achieve these goals, neuroscience offers a different perspective. The default situation is not one of dormant behaviours waiting to be activated, but rather one of active behaviours being continually suppressed, with their expression being the result of a release from this inhibition. This may also explain why a given behaviour can incorporate more than one emotional characteristic; that is, its inhibition is being relieved by several systems. From this perspective, voluntary behaviour is actually the decision not to do something, and thereby allowing the expression of a different path of action. While this might seem academic, it has very important implications in the management of behaviour. Much behaviour therapy has tended to focus on encouraging particular behaviours in certain circumstances in order to achieve a desirable outcome, because, in effect, it makes their inhibition harder. This is only one way of addressing the problem and more general training for inhibitory control may be of great importance in helping animals to make the right choices. This is not the same as the suppression of behaviour through punishment, but rather relates to the control of impulsivity. Recent work at University of Lincoln suggests that impulse control, at least in dogs, is a transferable skill that can be learned through relatively simple exercises. Thus a deeper understanding of neuroscience can help to open up new perspectives which might lead to the development of new and more effective treatments for behavioural problems. A less impulsive animal is more able to attend to a broader range of signals in the environment and so is more likely to make the choices we desire if we structure the environment appropriately. This requires us to ensure that the signals are there for the outcome we want, together with acceptable forms of reinforcement; that is, effective communication with the animal to be educated.

## 2.6    OTHER CONSIDERATIONS RELATING TO EMOTIONAL AROUSAL

### 2.6.1    AROUSAL LEVEL

Emotional processes are associated with changes in arousal, with the balance between the parasympathetic and sympathetic nervous systems being an integral part of this change. The intensity of arousal provides a quantitative aspect to the emotional process, setting a tone for the associated behavioural responses. Together, the valence (positive versus negative) and level of arousal constitute what has been referred to as *core affect*.

When it is anticipated that a significant energetic investment is necessary to achieve a strategic goal, high arousal can be expected as part of the process of preparation for action. If this reflects a typical way of responding for the individual, it may be referred to as an active coping style. By contrast, low-arousal states are more typical of a greater acceptance of events and more passive coping styles.

Therefore, the encoding of autonomic arousal within emotional processes reflects the predicted effort necessary to achieve the desired outcome. Low arousal might suggest an acceptance of the situation in either an emotionally positive way (satisfaction) or a negative way (resignation, as occurs in learned helplessness); alternatively, it may reflect the confidence an animal has in its ability to control the situation. For example, some potentially very dangerous animals can appear very calm before they strike, and this is an important feature to note when considering the overall risk of the situation. However, it should also be noted that just because a client reports they were unable to predict aggression or that an attack seemed to come from nowhere does not mean the animal was actually calm or showed no signs of heightened arousal beforehand. It may simply reflect poor observation skills by the client.

It is worth emphasising again that the arousal level and quality appear to be processed and stored separately and therefore they need to be evaluated individually, because they require different treatments. If the level of arousal (i.e. excitability, reactivity, activity) is the primary issue then systematic desensitisation may be particularly important within the behaviour modification intervention; however, if the primary issue is the quality of emotion (i.e. the type of negative or positive associations) then respondent counterconditioning may be particularly useful. While the two methods can be combined into a single programme, neither is very easy for many owners, and it may therefore be useful to make the distinction in order to determine whether it is possible to simplify the treatment protocol by emphasising the use of one over the other.

Another point to appreciate from an applied perspective is that a change in arousal may not be a consequence of emotional processing alone, but might also result from the processing of perceived events. For example, if animals are administered the beta-blocker propranolol, which inhibits the effects of the sympathetic nervous system, aversion learning may be disrupted. These drugs can also be used clinically to assist in the management of fears, since by reducing arousal they potentially reduce the magnitude of a perceived threat, but they will not change the qualitative aspect of the emotional response. They must be used as part of a more complete behaviour-modification plan.

## 2.6.2   THE EXPRESSION OF EMOTIONAL AROUSAL

The expression of emotion may play a similar role to arousal in providing feedback to the individual, which influences the emotional response (*biofeedback*). In humans it has been found that if you subconsciously manipulate their facial expression (by asking them to hold a pen horizontally using just their lips either at the front of their mouth or across their back teeth, to create more of a frown or a smile, respectively) then their judgement of ambiguous stimuli may be biased in line with the expression associated with a given emotion; that is, it will be perceived as more positive when smiling and as more negative when frowning. This phenomenon is also exploited clinically within the field of animal behaviour modification by encouraging animals to adopt relaxed postures during systematic desensitisation in order to create an emotionally positive bias and minimise emotionally negative arousal to ambiguous levels of the problematic stimulus.

The expression of emotion also has communicative value to both conspecifics and heterospecifics; for example, it has been found that dogs are sensitive to different emotional facial expressions in both dogs and humans; they also respond differentially to commands with different emotional qualities spoken for the first time by an unfamiliar trainer. The potential influence of experience in these phenomena remains uncertain, although the ability to read human faces does appear to depend on early immersion in an environment with people. This ability, while cognitively complex, provides clear biological fitness advantages, helping animals to avoid potentially harmful individuals and to exploit the opportunities provided by those more willing to interact.

## 2.6.3   PREPARATION FOR ACTION

The influence of emotions on the preparation of the body for action is diverse. As should already be clear, emotional responses bias the type of action taken. Additionally, emotional arousal may also prepare the body to learn about certain types of association; for example, conditioned avoidance when scared. This affects the animal's future preparation. The type of emotional arousal that occurs during learning may also affect the variability of the response learned, and this has adaptive significance. Where an animal has escaped an aversive, behavioural variability is often undesirable as it may result in a less efficient response the next time the aversive is encountered, which could have disastrous consequences. However, variability of response is adaptive in relation to learning about resource exploitation, as it allows the animal to determine the minimum energy expenditure necessary for the desired gain, after learning what works in the first instance.

The importance of emotional arousal to learning varies with the task involved. Emotional influences may be minimal in certain forms of procedural learning that do not align closely with a particularly important motivational–emotional predisposition – for example, the acquisition of a specific motor skill, such as how to manipulate objects in the environment – although motivation can be increased by increasing the emotional content of the event through enthusiastic encouragement and praise for success. Likewise, learning about what behaviour is considered acceptable to a conspecific (through a negative encounter) is likely to involve significantly greater emotional content, regardless of the behaviour of any third party.

### 2.6.4   *MOOD AND TEMPERAMENT*

So far, we have emphasised the importance of the emotional responses that occur in relation to specific events bound to particular motivational–emotional priorities, such as the identification of a potentially dangerous stimulus. However, the underlying motivational–emotional circuitry associated with a particular predisposition is always active to a greater or lesser degree. This is evident from the animal's mood and temperament. These phenomena have a more pervasive effect on behaviour and they may be distinguished from the emotional reactions discussed earlier on the basis of their temporal stability. From an evolutionary perspective, there are clear advantages to biasing attention, perception, cognition, arousal and behaviour according to prevailing conditions in the medium and longer term. An *emotional reaction* may be considered the immediate affective response to a new situation, a *mood* may be considered a particular emotional predisposition to behave in a certain way over a longer time span and *temperament* may be considered a trait which describes the affective style of an individual, and is the most stable emotional process. Although the distinction between these three emotional processes may be considered somewhat arbitrary, it can nonetheless be conceptually useful (Table 2.4).

Moods are less clearly defined qualitatively than specific emotional reactions, and it may be that there are basically only two moods: a positive, optimistic one associated with a prevailing opportunity to exploit resources/incentives and a negative, pessimistic one focused on a prevailing risk from aversives. However, some may argue that there are specific social moods associated with some of the related motivational–emotional predispositions, such as being in love, which is associated with seasonal *lust activity*. Moods generally last longer than specific emotional reactions and are less closely associated with specific events or intense arousal and expression, but they still play an important role in biasing cognition: shifting information-processing priorities. Moods may bias perception: we tend to

Table 2.4  Distinction between emotional reactions, mood and temperament. Adapted from Goldsmith (1994).

|  | Emotional reaction | Mood | Temperament |
| --- | --- | --- | --- |
| Temporal and other associations | Short-lived after removal of eliciting stimulus | Episodic and often related to a series of events with a particular quality | A general disposition or trait of the individual, activated by particular contexts |
| Cognitive components | Stimulus appraisal and selection of a particular behavioural response | Management of emotions and stimulus attribution | Interacts with a wide range of cognitive processes during development to produce personality |
| Antecedents | Species-typical or learned stimuli of personal significance | Cumulative effect of emotional reactions and endogenous biochemical states, such as diet or chronobiological effects | Genotypic and early experiential interaction |
| Universality vs individuality | Universal species- typical phenomenon | Universal states, individualised with respect to management of emotions | Contributes to the definition of individual differences |
| Development | Specific reactions at different early life stages | Unknown | Emergence of organisation and stability, especially during maturation |

pick out the features of the environment that are consistent with our mood. Moods also potentially alter the accessibility of information, so we find it easier to retrieve information consistent with our mood and harder to retrieve information that is incongruent; likewise, it is easier to elicit emotional reactions that are consistent with a given mood state than those that are not. Thus, within a negative mood state the negative attributes of a situation may be accentuated, there may be a bias to behave negatively or cautiously and access to positive memories and emotions may be reduced. In short, mood seems to provide some additional preparatory arousal based on recent experience. Mood will not usually shift as a result of a single experience and so if a problem behaviour includes an element of mood, more substantial intervention may be required, such as the restructuring of the environment to ensure it delivers many opportunities for positive experiences, or the use of psychopharmacological agents to elevate mood. This might be particularly important during the firework season for an animal which suffers from a sound sensitivity; that is, there is a need to treat both the noise reaction and the underlying mood in order to safeguard the welfare of the animal in the short term. Of course, in the longer term the sound sensitivity will need to be specifically treated in its own right with an appropriate behaviour-modification plan. Likewise, if we can change the mood, we may alter the probability of a particular emotional reaction occurring, and this may be useful therapeutically (see Chapter 1).

Temperament is a particular emotional predisposition within the individual. The term is often used interchangeably with 'personality', but there is some value in making a distinction between the two in the context of understanding emotions in animals. This is a personal view, since there is no widely accepted definition of 'personality' or 'temperament', even within the human psychological literature.

We wish to apply the term *personality* to describe the biologically based behavioural tendencies of an individual. It describes a relatively stable phenotype relating to motivational–emotional predispositions arising from the neurological changes associated with patterns of interaction between the genotype and the environment early in development and typically before maturation. This results in consistencies in behavioural style, but also serves to differentiate the individual from other members of the same species. Personality gives rise to general, consistent behavioural responses (habits) that are correlated to form traits, so if an individual habitually responds in a positive way to other individuals, we might say they score highly on a sociable personality trait. As noted earlier, we need to recognise that certain behaviours may be related to different traits depending on the context in which they are elicited, and so a given behavioural habit on its own may be relatively poorly predictive of the personality of an individual. For example, aggressive behaviour towards other dogs does not generally correlate with aggressiveness towards people, so neither can be used on its own to determine the aggressive personality of a dog. It is the traits which define the personality of the individual; in the latter example, this means that aggressiveness must be assessed in a range of contexts if we wish to try to say anything about the animal being aggressive. Traits and habits are not synonymous. For example, if an animal runs away from umbrellas when they are opened, it has a *habit* of avoiding opening umbrellas, but if it tends to avoid a range of other unusual circumstances then we may say it is neophobic, or fearful of new things, which would be a *trait*. A habit is a behaviour that is shown repeatedly in similar situations, whereas a trait is a predisposition to react in a certain way to certain situations. It is also important to distinguish personality from ability: a dog may appear to be very unreactive to a range of visual threats, but if it has poor vision then we need to appreciate that we have not assessed any aspect of its personality. It is only once it has perceived the threats that we have a potentially meaningful measure.

By contrast, we propose to use the term *temperament* to refer only to relatively stable emotionally related behavioural dispositions. We suggest these relate to a difference in relevant neurobiological substrates, for example a difference in the underlying balance in dopaminergic versus serotonergic activity. Variations in both dopamine receptor (especially D4) types and the serotonin transporter have, for example, been shown to be associated with stable individual differences in the tendency to exploit incentives (*desire*) and to avoid aversives (*anxiety–fear*), respectively. Thus, from this perspective, anxiousness, for example, may be considered an aspect of temperament, but cognitive flexibility cannot, although it can be considered an aspect of personality.

The development of temperament as a result of genotype–environmental interactions early in life has clearly been a biologically useful process during evolution, but it may become problematic in the domestic situation. In nature, the environment in which an animal grows up is likely to be similar to the one in which it lives as an adult, but this may not be the case with a companion animal born and reared in one environment and then sold to someone living in a very different one. The genotype of an individual reflects that of its parents. These parents have obviously been biologically successful, since reproductive success is a pinnacle of biological fitness, and so the offspring are likely to be well set up genetically for the environment in which they initially live. Further adaptive modifications in behavioural tendency may then occur based on this genotype as a result of early experience, which will make the animal even more efficient on the balance of probabilities; thus the development of temperament reflects an evolutionary adaptation to environments with differing levels of incentives and aversives. In domestic environments, however, a mismatch in temperament and environment can give rise to significant welfare problems, as an animal either struggles to adapt to the opportunities it is given or constantly seeks to take advantage of its situation. For example, an animal raised in a very quiet rural environment may not cope if it is then moved to live in a busy city centre. Problems arising from such a mismatch need to be recognised as they carry a generally poorer prognosis, unless medication is used to bring about a more fundamental biological change in the animal.

## 2.7   CONCLUSION

Panksepp's model of emotional systems provides a useful framework for conceptualising the behavioural processes subject to significant emotional influence in many terrestrial vertebrates. This emphasises that different levels and types of emotional arousal occur as a result of the varying subjective importance of behaviours associated with a number of important biological circumstances, namely:

- Resource (including information) investigation.
- Resource access and defence.
- Threat and harm avoidance.
- Social attachment.
- Sexual partnering.
- Opportunity for motor and cognitive refinement of future social behaviour.
- Parental behaviour.

We have slightly modified Panksepp's terminology in order to reduce the risk of confusion in a clinical setting and have proposed an additional biological circumstance, which can give rise to its own form of significant emotional arousal:

- Tissue damage.

Not all behaviour has a significant emotional element and highly predictable but nonharmful events will often result in a relatively unemotional or habitual response, whether or not it is associated with a potentially significant stimulus. Examples of potentially emotionally salient stimuli include:

- Resources that the animal wants.
- Resources that the animal wishes to keep/defend.
- Barriers to control of resources (including restriction).
- Stimuli perceived to be a potential threat to the individual.
- Stimuli which cause potential tissue damage.
- Attachment figures.
- Perceived potential sexual partners.
- Social-group members.
- Perceived dependents.

An important task for the clinical animal behaviourist is to identify which, if any, of these circumstances are relevant to the problem, and their impact.

At any given time, an organism may perceive a diversity of potentially emotionally salient stimuli, but these will normally need to be prioritised. In some circumstances, conflict may arise from an uncertainty as to which event to prioritise, whether a particular stimulus should be approached or avoided (e.g. in the case of novel or inconsistent stimuli) or what action to take in response to the circumstances (e.g. to take flight or defend a resource) – in these cases, conflict-related activities such as displacement behaviours or ambivalent behaviours and emotional expressions may become apparent.

An important role of the clinical animal behaviourist might be to remove any such emotional ambiguity and ensure that the animal is provided with emotionally consistent signals which result in appropriate behaviour in the problematic circumstances. In this context, 'appropriate' means an acceptable type (quality) and intensity (quantity). This requires an analysis of the motivational–emotional control of behaviour and its strategic function. It is also within this context that we should consider the range of possible treatment interventions; that is, the *specificity* and *precision* of their effects on the strategic and motivational–emotional priorities of the individual and how these relate to the management of the presenting problem.

In summary, an initial reflection on the role of affect in a problem case might take the form:

- Is there problematic emotional arousal with specific events?
  - If yes:
    - What are the circumstances causing this arousal? That is, stimulus quality and contingency (appearance, disappearance, predicted appearance or disappearance).
    - Is it the quality or the intensity of arousal that is problematic?

- How can this be changed?
  ○ If no:
    - Can emotionally salient stimuli be introduced to break the habitual response?
- Is there problematic emotional arousal associated with mood?
  ○ If yes:
    - What are the circumstances leading to bouts? That is, what events are occurring together or with sufficient frequency to bias affect (note, chronic pain is a common cause of negative affect)?
- Is there problematic emotional arousal associated with temperament?
  ○ If yes:
    - What sort of intervention is necessary to bring about more fundamental long-term physiological changes?
    - Advise the owner of the need for a permanent or semipermanent intervention to reshape temperament.

As we shall see in the next chapter, pheromonal semiochemicals may be particularly important in the regulation of affect, and so pheromonatherapy may have a significant role to play.

## REVIEW ACTIVITIES

- Behaviorism, in its purist form, predicts that behaviour is reinforced by any important resource, whereas a motivational–emotional perspective predicts that only resources relevant to the underlying arousal state will reinforce behaviour. Consider the implications of this when it comes to controlling the management of behaviour.
- Predictability and unpredictability can have both useful and problematic effects on animal behaviour. List examples of each.
- If pheromones affect motivational–emotional predispositions, what sort of messages might they convey?
- Examine video clips of animal behaviour from the Internet. For each clip, consider the motivational–emotional arousal that is evident. On what basis do you make this inference (consider both the circumstances and behaviour signs)?
- What role does arousal have in the appraisal of an event?
- Draw a diagram to show how emotional reactions, moods and temperament are related.

## REFERENCES

Craig AD (2003) A new view of pain as a homeostatic emotion. Trends in Neurosciences 26: 303–307.
Goldsmith HH (1994) Parsing the emotional domain from a developmental perspective. In: Ekman P, Davidson JJ (eds) The Nature of Emotion – Fundamental Questions. Oxford: Oxford University Press. pp. 68–73.

Panksepp J (1998) Affective Neuroscience. Oxford: Oxford University Press.
Panksepp J (2006) Emotional endophenotypes in evolutionary psychiatry. Progress in Neuropsychopharmacology and Biological Psychiatry 30: 774–784.

## FURTHER READING

Gray JA (1987) The Psychology of Fear and Stress. Cambridge: Cambridge University Press.
Kringelbach ML, Berridge KC (2010) Pleasures of the Brain. Oxford: Oxford University Press.
Mendl M, Burman OHP, Paul E (2010) An integrative and functional framework for the study of animal emotion and mood. Proceedings of the Royal Society B 277: 2895–2904.
Mills DS (2003) Medical paradigms for the study of problem behaviour: a critical review. Applied Animal Behaviour Science 81: 265–277.
Pilley JW, Reid AK (2010) Border collie understands object names as verbal referents. Behavioural Processes 86: 184–195.
Ramos D, Ades C (2011) Two-item sentence comprehension by a dog. PLoS ONE 7: e29689.
Rolls ET (1999) Brain and Emotion. Oxford: Oxford University Press.

# Chapter 3

# Communication and Information Transfer

## 3.1  INTRODUCTION

In this chapter, we consider communication in animals, with a view to providing a deeper appreciation of its importance in effective behaviour management. In addition, the chapter pays particular attention to the often underestimated significance of chemical cues in the environment, which also underpins the practice of pheromonatherapy.

The chapter is broadly divided into two parts:

- In the first part, some principles of communication are considered, including the nature of information transfer between animals, the constituents of a signal, the way animals send signals to each other and the rules governing information transfer.
- In the second part, the different types of signal that animals can send and how they are integrated is considered, with particular emphasis on the role of chemical signals. Pheromones form part of this latter group, and so their role is explained in this context.

## 3.2  COMMUNICATION

*Communication* may be defined as the transfer of information from a sender to a receiver, where both sender and receiver map a signal to a particular meaning. This mapping of the meaning of a signal does not require consciousness, but means that a signal is not simply anything that has an effect on the receiver, but rather that its specific transmission has a function for both the sender and the receiver. Signals differ from cues as they can be varied by the sender, whereas cues are typically permanent features. Thus, in a biological context, the yellow and black stripe of a wasp and many other unpalatable insects is a cue that it might be better not to eat them, but the change in colour associated with the ripening of a fruit to attract seed dispersers is a signal. There is therefore an intrinsic additional

*Stress and Pheromonatherapy in Small Animal Clinical Behaviour*, First Edition.
Daniel Mills, Maya Braem Dube and Helen Zulch.
© 2013 John Wiley & Sons, Ltd. Published 2013 by John Wiley & Sons, Ltd.

energetic cost to the communication of a signal, and some signals are more expensive to produce than others. This may be one of the factors which affect the channel being used for signal communication, as it is most efficient to use the least energetically demanding signal that effectively communicates the required message.

Since we have to go beyond simply assessing if something has an effect on something else in order to fully appreciate whether it is a meaningful signal, a change in the behaviour or physiology of the receiver may be a necessary condition for communication, but it is not sufficient on its own. The behaviour of one individual may affect that of another by pure coincidence, and this should not be considered an act of communication. For example, the behaviour of a prey animal may affect the behaviour of the predator, but we do not consider that the prey is communicating with the predator. However, as every owner will testify, communication between different species (interspecific communication) does occur, but this is a two-way process, and often we need to help owners read the signals being sent by their pets.

### 3.2.1    FUNCTIONS OF COMMUNICATION

Broadly speaking, we can consider three major functions of communication:

- *Identification of an individual and its status*: This might be its sex, group membership, emotional or reproductive status.
- *Group organisation and coordination*: This helps to ensure that different individuals efficiently fulfil their roles and so helps to reduce unnecessary tension between individuals.
- *Manipulation of others*: This is for the more specific benefit of the sender and usually occurs between members of the same species, but may involve members of other species, such as humans, especially in pet animals. It is perhaps uncomfortable for many owners to think about this, as they will tend to consider it in terms of conscious manipulation and scheming, but this is not necessarily the case, and the type of long-term scheming which is so often done by humans does not seem to be possible for pet species. Nonetheless, in evolutionary terms, it often pays for an animal to express behaviours which manipulate the behaviour of others to its own benefit. This does not mean that the animal is being deceitful or wicked or evil.

### 3.2.2    PRINCIPLES OF COMMUNICATION

As already mentioned, communication may occur within a species (*intraspecific*) or between species (*interspecific*), but the principle remains the same. One party or individual sends a signal containing information, which is transferred to another individual or another party (Figure 3.1). This information is processed and becomes the message that is received. In many cases the individual receiving the information will not receive the whole of the signal that is sent: often there will be gaps, which the receiver will have to fill in. Thus the signal sent and the message received

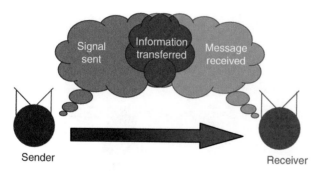

Fig. 3.1 Principle of communication. The sender sends a signal (blue), which may be only partially perceived by the receiver (purple: 'Information transferred') but is used to form the basis of the message received (red).

are not necessarily the same. The mapping to meaning which forms the basis of the information transferred is an active process that will be affected by the circumstances, by the clarity of the sender's information and by the receiver's expectations. Brains try to determine patterns and have to fill in gaps relating to the available information, and this is where misunderstandings can occur. The art of good communication requires that clear, unambiguous and complete signals are sent, in order to minimise the amount of processing required by the receiver and so the risk of misunderstanding. Quite often signals involve the use of several sensory channels, where one channel might dominate (although exactly which may vary with context and species involved) while the others interact and aid the interpretation of the actual message that is received. However, if there is a contradiction (either between or within a channel) then the receiver must either decide which element to prioritise and accept or decide that the message is ambiguous or uncertain and act accordingly.

An important principle to appreciate is that the response of the receiver will depend on the message received rather than the signal that was sent. An animal's behaviour tells us about the messages it is receiving, not necessarily about the signals that are being sent from any particular source. This explains why some animals do not obey or respond in the way their owners would wish, and why some owners think their pets are being wilful or spiteful. In reality, assuming the animal knows a given instruction (which is not always the case), there may be a contradiction from the perspective of the receiver's needs or desires in the signals being given by the owner, such as a request for proximity with a threat of punishment (Figure 3.2). As discussed in Chapter 2, the signals of punishment will naturally override the other priorities of most animals, as they seek safety first. So the animal will choose to avoid the owner, following an assessment of its interests and associated risks, rather than wilfully disobey the owner as a gesture of defiance or social dominance. It is important that our body language, our tone of voice and the verbal instruction we are delivering are congruent (i.e. all give the same message).

Similarly, a chemical signal might convey a message of safety, but if this does not agree with the visual signals being received at the same time then the animal may be confused and at best will choose to stay away and at worst might panic. This is quite important when we consider pheromonatherapy, because the pheromone does not simply release an innate response – it biases the emotional processing of the message. Thus it is only part of the overall message being received from the

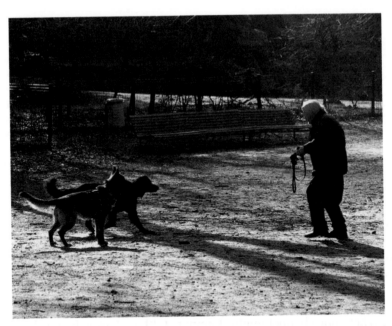

Fig. 3.2 Look carefully at the signals being sent in this interaction involving an owner trying to recall his dogs. The owner's body language has elements of threat (not to mention his tone of voice) as he tries to approach the dogs. As a result, the message the dogs receive is ambiguous, and you can see that the German shepherd has stopped and is trying to reassess the situation (the signals being sent). This might be interpreted by the owner as the dog refusing his demand, and lead to further antagonism. The other dog is cautiously approaching, with a slightly lowered body posture, but may well suddenly run off if the anger of the owner increases.

surrounding environment. This is discussed further in Chapter 4. The significance of other environmental inputs relating to the perception of the environment can be one of the reasons why the application of pheromonatherapy may appear ineffective in some cases. It is often most effective in novel situations where there are no learned contradictory signals competing with the chemical ones being transmitted.

### 3.2.3   THE BIOLOGY OF INFORMATION TRANSFER

### 3.2.3.1   CHANNEL USED

Signals differ according to the channel of communication that is used for the transfer of information, whether it be visual, chemical or so forth, and different species have different biases in the channel they use to convey certain types of information. Cats and dogs clearly use chemical signals to interpret the world around them more than humans do. Of the two, the cat is perhaps the more influenced by chemical signals in the environment, which is not to say that cats have a better sense of smell than dogs, but simply that they appear to bias their response more on the basis of information conveyed in this type of signal. The type of channel that is used in any given situation usually depends on the function of the message and the energetic cost of using a particular route versus its necessity. Quite often several channels may be used simultaneously, in order to maximise the efficiency of communication, especially when the risks associated with trying to convey a message using just one channel are significant. Alternatively, a signal may be shown with a more notable intensity or frequency within a single channel in order to make it stand out from the background 'noise'.

Important considerations with regard to the selection of a preferred communication channel include the following:

- *Distance to be travelled/area to be covered*: Chemical signals, for example, can be transmitted over very long distances, as can visual signals – as long as there is nothing blocking the view – and auditory signals. However, chemical signals are longer-lasting and typically have the potential to cover a larger area; for example, a dog can probably detect a bitch in oestrus several miles away.
- *Energy necessary to produce signal*: Different signals also require different amounts of energy to produce them. Body movements are energetically quite expensive, whereas chemical signals are often relatively cheap to produce, since they are simply secreted from the body.
- *Speed of information exchange*: With chemical signals, the exchange of information is often quite slow, whereas with visual signals, information literally travels at the speed of light, facilitating rapid exchange of information between individuals. Likewise auditory signals travel at the speed of sound, which is still quite rapid.

We discuss some of the pros and cons of different channels in this section.

## Visual signals

These normally travel reasonably well and allow a very rapid exchange of information, but they may easily be blocked by physical obstructions. The identity of the signaller is very obvious if the signal is given by means of a body gesture, but may not be clear at all in the absence of other signals; for example, a scratch mark needs to be accompanied by a chemical signal for its meaning to be appreciated. Nonetheless, the visual signal helps to guide animals to a place where they can gather further information. We can use the location of the signal as a basis for its categorisation, contrasting signals apparent from:

- *A particular signaller/individual*: What might be referred to as 'body language'.
- *A particular substrate (e.g. a specific object)*: Information conveyed with the help of an object, such as a scratch or urine marks.

In either case, the visual signal may be associated with the release of pheromonal secretions.

The energy required to produce visual signal is very variable. In some cases the information is an incidental byproduct of another process (e.g. the vulval 'winking' of a mare in oestrous has its origin in the act of urination required to release the important sex pheromones indicating her sexual receptivity), in others a visual display may be highly demanding (e.g. the sexual displays of a male trying to attract a female, since the energy of the display is used as a marker of the fitness (and thus desirability) of the male).

In order to fully understand the affective element of visual (or any other) signals, we also have to consider their context and circumstances. For example, a dog may show signs of fear in its owner's presence but not in other contexts and not around other people when the owner is not present, indicating a specific emotional reaction (fear of a specific individual) and not a temperamental problem (see Table 2.4).

## Auditory signals

Like visual signals, these have the potential to travel a long distance and allow a rapid exchange of information. They are not as easily blocked by physical obstacles in the environment, but they generally require a lot of energy to send. The signaller is often relatively easy to identify: for example, vocalisations are typically phonetically quite distinct, but other auditory signals such as foot stamping in rabbits are less individually identifiable. For these reasons, auditory signals are quite often used in similar circumstances to visual signals, but when the features of the environment would block the information conveyed by a visual channel. Animals like pigs do a lot of grunting in their communication because they have evolved to root around in woodlands, where visual signals might not be as effective for communication as auditory ones. Similarly, dogs howl when isolated because they wish to communicate with companions whom they may not be able to see because of distance or physical barriers such as the walls of a house.

Generally, we do not have a very good understanding of the different auditory signals that are used by cats and dogs, although we are beginning to get a better insight into them, as a number of recent studies have started to investigate vocalisations in more detail. Barks of certain characteristics can be described which are consistently associated with certain types of emotional content on the basis of the circumstances in which they arise and the characteristic behaviour patterns at such times. Interestingly, it seems that humans are also intuitively very good at recognising these, especially when they occur in the context of:

- *Threats of personal intrusion*: These barks are relatively low-pitched noises that are loud and repetitive, with little variation in pitch or loudness. They typically occur in response to disturbance or entry into the territory or personal space of an individual. They therefore represent the consequence of activation of both *anxiety–fear* and *frustration* circuits. The properties and contexts of these barks fit with the observation (discussed in Chapter 2) that behavioural persistence and rigidity are characteristic features associated with the elimination of an aversive event, and repeated negative reinforcement will ultimately lead to a habitual response.
- *Isolation*: These barks tend to be higher-pitched and have more tonal qualities than those occurring in response to threats of personal intrusion. They also vary

more from one bark to another. They often occur as singular barks, rather than in clusters. These are signs of potentially high emotional distress, associated with activation of the *panic–grief* system (see Chapter 2), and function to encourage the reestablishment of contact with other individuals – hence the pause after each bark, to allow reciprocal vocal communication.

- *Social play*: These sounds may superficially appear quite similar to the isolation barks (i.e. high-pitched) but they do not sound as tense and usually occur in clusters rather than singly. They may be interspersed with other vocal sounds, such as a form of breathy exhalation which has been referred to as the 'dog laugh'.
- *Denial of an incentive*: When denied access to something that the dog wants, it may issue powerful but medium- or mixed-frequency barks of more variable pitch. These are perhaps the least well studied of the barks described.

Barks may also become quite individualised, with more subtle but reliable differences occurring in emotionally related but contextually distinct situations, or in other situations that blend different emotions, such as when the animal is isolated and also frustrated.

In cats, we recognise a number of different types of call. There is obviously the purr, which some people perceive as a sign of intense pleasure, but which also occurs in very sick or terrified animals too. It is thought that it is more likely to be a care-soliciting signal (*care* system): a sign that the animal is seeking contact or company. Another type of call that a cat makes with its mouth closed is the trill or the chirrup, which is a greeting call (*desire*). There is also, of course, the meow with the mouth open: it has been found that the intensity of meow varies with the context, such that owners recognise more demanding meows when the animal wants something, such as to be fed (*frustration*). Many types of meow are used in social interactions with other cats and with owners, and it is probable that meows are used by cats in a similar way to how barks are used by dogs, and so may be associated with a range of motivational–emotional-system activation. There are many other auditory signals that we recognise as well, such as the hiss, which is a sign that the animal is trying to break off an interaction. It is perhaps surprising how little we know about auditory communication in cats and dogs given how much time we spend with these animals and how much time we spend chatting to them ourselves.

## Tactile signals

These require close contact between individuals for their transmission and are easily blocked by any physical obstruction. However, they allow for a rapid exchange and accurate identification of the signaller and are a relatively low-energy option. They are therefore useful in the transfer of relatively intimate information, such as in mutual grooming. In this case, a combination of channels may be being used: the tactile contact may have a directly calming effect, while the use of the tongue, for example in cats, may also allow both the deposition and the uptake of chemical signals on the coat. The deposition of saliva may help in the generation of a shared social odour, while the uptake may help identify both the individual and features of where it has been. As with licking, when cats rub against each other they are not only exchanging tactile signals but also depositing chemical signals. When cats rub their chins on inanimate objects it is a form of chemical and visual communication (since the deposit is visible), but not tactile, as while there is a tactile element on the part of the sender, there is no transmission of the tactile element to the receiver.

Tactile signals are widely used by owners towards their pets, such as when they stroke cats and dogs. They are also commonly utilised by these species amongst themselves, probably far more frequently in cats and dogs than we generally recognise. In some behaviour cases, it is useful to ask an owner to watch their cats' behaviour in order to identify the level of social integration that exists within the group. By asking the owner to record which cats rub against and lick which, you can often help identify members of the same social group and define whether one cat is an outsider. Owners often do not realise this until they go through the actual exercise of recording their interactions. They may then see that they actually have two groups of cats, or perhaps one group of cats and one who does not really fit in with the others, or perhaps even a collection of individuals, and no social group at all.

## Chemical signals/semiochemicals

These are discussed in more detail throughout this text, but at this point it is important to appreciate that they can travel over long distances, although they are typically relatively slow to exchange. The sender may or may not be easy to identify, depending on the inclusion of an individual identity element. Chemical signals are relatively cheap, energetically speaking, to send, and are traditionally divided into:

- *Tastes*: These are typically detected in the mouth, and especially by the tongue (oropharyngeal region), with information relayed to the medulla, thalamus and ultimately gustatory areas of the cerebral cortex.
- *Smells, odours or aromas*: These are mainly detected via the main olfactory epithelium, especially around the back of the nasal chambers (but also via less well-known specialised chemosensory structures within the nasal cavity, like the septal organ of Masera). They mainly relay information to the main olfactory bulb.
- *Pheromones*: These are typically thought of as being detected via the vomeronasal (Jacobson's) organ (VNO), which is situated in the palate between the nose and the mouth. However, there are other structures, such as the Grunenberg ganglia and main olfactory epithelium, which may also respond to some of these chemicals. The VNO connects with the nasal cavity, but depending on the species may also connect with the mouth via an incisive duct (e.g. in dogs and cats, but not horses). Information is relayed from here to the accessory olfactory bulb of the brain, which is part of the limbic system that regulates emotional processing.

Not only may the chemical channels operate in conjunction with other channels to improve the transfer of information, as already mentioned (see also Figure 3.3), but they may also operate in conjunction with each other.

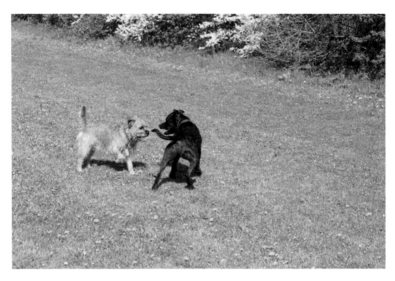

Fig. 3.3 These two dogs have just met. They are clearly using a lot of visual signals, but they are also exchanging chemical signals. The Border terrier has a raised paw, and while this may be read as a sign of uncertainty, it may also increase the exchange of semiochemicals from the pad (which may be the origin of the visual signal); meanwhile, the straight tail of the Staffordshire bull terrier exposes the perianal glands, which are also highly important in chemical signalling, including individual identification.

Thus taste and smell are integrated to provide the quality of flavour. This is why if we have a cold we often find that food seems bland. Similarly, odours may combine with pheromones to enhance the detection of emotionally significant molecules or provide greater emotional salience to certain chemical signals. Since the use of the VNO is an active process, requiring what is known as *flehmen behaviour* (Figures 3.4 and 3.5), unless the chemicals are presented at a high concentration (as may occur when artificial versions are used clinically) it is often important for there to be some other signal to encourage the use of the VNO, such as the scratch mark of the cat, the winking of the mare, or the inclusion of a certain odourant in the case of urine. Thus these chemical senses and the associated semiochemicals are not as distinct or independent as might often be implied.

## 3.2.3.2   *INTEGRATION OF SIGNALS TO CREATE A MESSAGE*

It is important to appreciate that while it is possible to break down signals into their component parts, in reality most communication is multichannel and all aspects of it are functionally integrated. This means that certain signals may naturally go together, but also that certain signals may not. If we return to the example of the scratch mark: it consists of a visual signal, which may be informationally important in its own right, but which may also attract an animal's attention to the area and

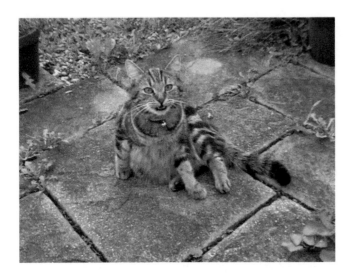

Fig. 3.4 Flehmen in the cat is often called a grimace or gape, as seen in this image (picture courtesy of Jenna Kiddie).

increase the chances of detection of a chemical signal released from the pads at the time the scratch was made (Figure 3.6). The two signals are synergistic in the process of information transfer (i.e. they go together): the visual signal is integral to the investigation of the chemical signal, which carries an important message.

Some signals do not go together and may actually be antagonistic. For example, cats do not typically face mark where they scratch. This can be used clinically, because we may be able to employ synthetic components of the face mark to deter cats from scratching a particular area.

However, in some situations inappropriate integration can cause problems. For example, if an animal is presented artificially with a chemical signal that says 'everything is okay' (e.g. the product 'Felifriend®') but there are visual signals signifying that 'this is something really aversive' (e.g. someone who has an established history of antagonism with the cat) then the message received is incongruent and potentially confusing. There may be a highly aggressive rejection of the confusing social stimulus. This is a potential risk that needs to be appreciated when trying to restructure the messages received from the environment in the modification of behaviour. That is not to say we should not try to restructure interspecific communication as part of behaviour modification, since, in appropriate circumstances, it is not only a very effective way of bringing about change, but also much easier for owners to implement than the alternative, which might involve the application of a complex behaviour-modification programme. In general, problems arise when the salience of contradictory signals is similar; if one signal is particularly salient (i.e. it is strong or produces a natural attentional bias) then the risk is lower, as less-significant conflicting signals will tend to be ignored.

When trying to analyse communication between animals involving conflicting signals, it is important to work out which signals are most important and which are potentially redundant. In the case of contradictory messages, an animal's behaviour tells us which signal it is responding to, because behaviour does not lie. However, many signals do not convey all-or-nothing messages (i.e. they are not

(a)

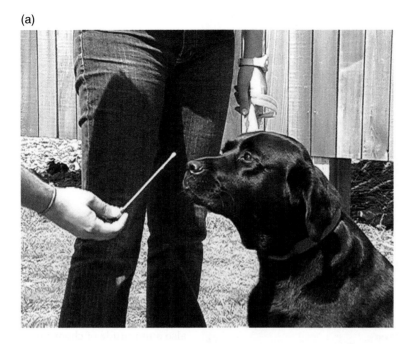

(b)

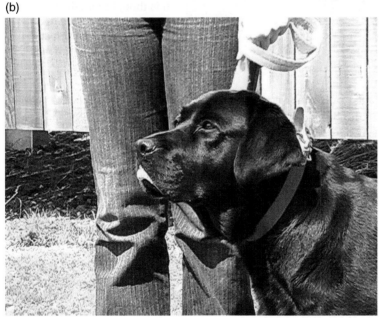

Fig. 3.5 In these pictures, a dog is being presented with the odour of another dog. In (a) the dog sniffs it and begins to engage the VNO. Ongoing flehmen behaviour can be difficult to spot in a dog, although a puffing of the cheeks might be seen. However, when it is over, fluid may be apparent, dripping from the dog's nose and foaming around its mouth (b). The dog will often lick its nose and lips at this time as well.

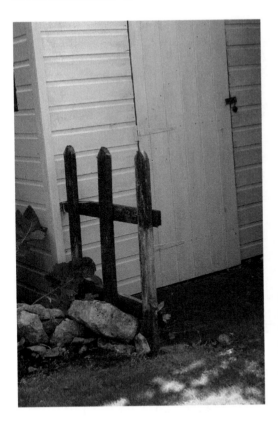

Fig. 3.6 When a cat scratches an area such as this fence post, it not only leaves a clear visual signal but also a multitude of chemical ones. It is thought that the visual signal serves to attract the attention of cats to the more important chemical message contained within.

*discrete signals*) but rather contain information of qualitative value (i.e. they are *graded signals*). These two terms are discussed further in Section 3.3.

When we use semiochemicals in a clinical setting, we might load the environment with higher levels than occur in nature, the idea being that by doing so any conflicting visual or chemical signals from the environment should be overcome, or else evaluated within the context of the prevailing chemical message. In effect, the aim is to chemically create an overwhelming sense of security, which causes the animal to relax and adjust to the environment and thereby to reevaluate the stimuli that it would otherwise have perceived as potentially threatening. As a result of repeated exposure in this context, the animal can learn to accept certain stimuli even in the absence of the pheromone signal.

## 3.3  SIGNAL CONTENT

### 3.3.1  *DISCRETE VERSUS GRADED SIGNALS*

*Discrete signals* are either present or not. These might include the chemical signals associated with oestrus: Certain chemicals present in a bitch's or queen's urine during this time indicate that she is ready to breed. Similarly, vertical scratch marks as visual signals are either there or they are not; there is no evidence to suggest that the style or amount of vertical scratching is important to their meaning. By contrast, *graded signals* vary in their intensity. This might be achieved through qualitatively different displays which indicate different intensities in the same message, for example in an agonistic interaction: much of what we consider to be aggressive behaviour is the animal trying to communicate its preference not to engage in physical conflict (avoidance of the situation). It may end up resorting to actual harm because the other, more subtle, signals have not been read effectively and the threat is either ignored or perhaps escalated. In dogs, such a series of signals has been described by Shepherd (2010) as 'the ladder of aggression', with individual elements sometimes referred to as 'calming signals' by others, such as Rugaas (1997). Neither term may be entirely accurate, as one such signal is not necessarily followed by another in the manner of the rungs of a ladder, and the signals' function may not be so much to calm as to avoid conflict (Figure 3.7), with the grades reflecting avoidance in different circumstances. Alternatively, a graded signal might simply be a change in the quantitative intensity of a single signal. For example, the amount of a certain amino acid, such as felinine, might be an indicator of the biological fitness of an individual. The time-dependent decline in intensity of an odour might also be a form of graded signal, indicating how recently a given individual has been in the area.

As a general rule, the more costly a signal is to send (i.e. the greater risk it poses to the animal or the more energy it requires), the more likely it is that it is honest, because either it cannot be faked (an individual who is not fit enough cannot create the most costly signal) or because the risks of bluffing are too high, unless there has been learning to the contrary. Hence, more expressive threats of harm are usually very honest signals, as bluffing in this context is a very risky strategy. A display signalling a willingness to engage in a fight if the receiver does not move away contains an acceptance of the chance of being injured if the problem is not resolved. However, in an agonistic interaction the exchange is not simply about the willingness to engage in a fight. There is an emotional signal, which is both more complex and more subtle. The following messages may need to be communicated in this sort of situation: the desire to claim the resource which is leading to the conflict/the willingness to give this resource up, any perceived need for self-defence (i.e. protection of the self rather than the resource) and any frustration at being denied the focal resource, among others. Failure to recognise the risk associated with the signals contained within any of these messages may lead to injury.

Animals tend not to bite for no apparent reason or without good reason. A good reason is unfortunately all too often that the signals indicating a willingness to yield have been ignored or frustrated. If the animal had been given the opportunity to escape it probably would have done so, unless either it had learned that fighting back was the only option or the cost of walking away was perceived as too great. What is important is that we learn to read the relevant signs and respond to them appropriately in order to be able to manage the situation and to avoid anyone being bitten or scratched.

In order to fully understand the message associated with a signal, it is often necessary to understand its context, and a failure to appreciate this can lead to serious problems, as discussed in the next section.

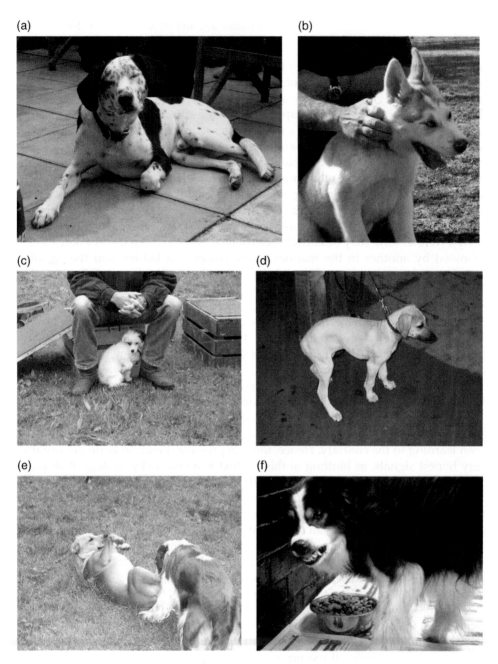

Fig. 3.7 The images here may be variously described as 'calming signals' or elements of the 'ladder of aggression', but they are best understood as graded signals associated with avoidance in different circumstances. (a) Blinking is a relatively straightforward way to break off an interaction with another and so is a sign of avoidance. (b) When an animal is in a state of conflict, displacement behaviours may arise. This might be the origin of yawning as a signal used in signs of conflict. The irrelevance of the behaviour may help to signal a lack of harmful intent to another and so be another sign of avoidance. (c) Paw lifting may help the transmission of a chemical signal from the pads that reinforces a lack of harmful intent. This may be useful when there is uncertainty or when there are more overt threatening signs present.

### 3.3.2   SIMPLE VERSUS COMPOSITE SIGNALS

*Simple signals* have a unique and specific meaning on their own, whereas *composite signals* are made up of two or more elements, so the meaning of one part may be dependent on its context. Of particular interest in this regard is the recognition of play. During play, animals may express and practise a range of skills and behaviours which are important in life, but without the associated risks. It is therefore important in the case of social play that partners recognise the context of the behaviour. Thus a play growl or rough-and-tumble fight is not a serious threat of harm. Dogs use a variety of signals to indicate that they intend to engage in play, ranging from a prancing approach–retreat style of behaviour to specific signals such as the play bow (Figure 3.8).

*Metacommunication signals* set the context for the message that follows; in the case of the example in Figure 3.8, the play bow says that everything which follows is an act of play (in cats, a lateral lie in front of another might serve a similar purpose). A growl following a dog's play bow is an example of a composite signal and the message can only be understood if the whole of the composite signal is recognised. Similarly, the chase that followed the encounter in Figure 3.8 (shown in Figure 3.9) was an act of play and not a genuine attempt to repel the Border terrier. Without recognising the play signal, this could be viewed as a very threatening and dangerous thing for an animal to do. These dogs are having a great time, but unfortunately if an owner misreads the situation and intervenes inappropriately, which sometimes happens, problems may result, as play or interactions with other dogs may become associated with aversive interactions with the owner.

Not all composite signals are separated in time: in some cases they may simply involve signals being delivered through a variety of channels, as occurs with the scratch mark mentioned previously.

### 3.3.3   SEMIOCHEMICALS AND PHEROMONATHERAPY

In order to understand the potential and limitations of pheromonatherapy, this section explores the use of chemical signals (*semiochemicals*) in more detail, ahead of a more specific discussion of pheromonatherapy in Chapter 4.

---

Fig. 3.7 (*cont'd*) (d) The tucking of the tail may help to reduce the transmission of chemical signals from the perianal region that might antagonise another, and so it is not surprising to see it in a fearful situation. (e) Rolling over sends a very clear signal of nonharmful intent in an antagonistic encounter, but if ignored will result in self-defence (e.g. if misunderstood as an invitation for a 'tummy tickle'). (f) A snarl is a sign of willingness to risk harm in order to resolve a dispute. By signalling this, the intention is to actually avoid physical harm, by communicating to the receiver how important this matter is to the sender. An important point to note is that all of these signals can only be understood in a given context, since the same behaviour may have a different function in another context.

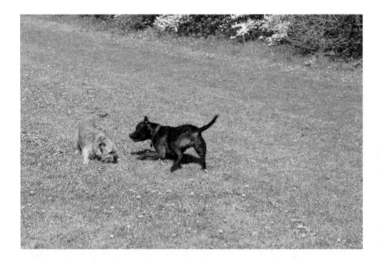

Fig. 3.8 Staffordshire bull terrier showing the typical play-bow metasignal, which indicates that what follows should be evaluated in the context of play.

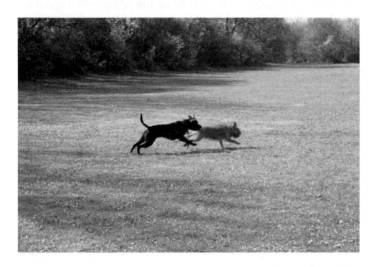

Fig. 3.9 This chase occurred in the context of a play, as it was preceded by the play metasignal illustrated in Figure 3.8.

## 3.3.3.1   *ADVANTAGES OF CHEMICAL SIGNALS (SEMIOCHEMICALS)*

*Semiochemicals* are, energetically speaking, relatively cheap to produce and so perhaps a preferred communication medium if there is a choice, particularly versus visual or auditory channels. They are also of specific value in certain contexts, including in materially dense environments, when an animal is isolated or when signals need to be sent to relatively immature animals who perhaps do not yet fully understand the complexities and subtleties that can be conveyed in the rapid exchanges possible with visual or auditory communication. For example, a dog may not see any other dogs but it might be useful to let them know that it is in the area, and so it will often scent mark by cocking its leg. Similarly, cats often engage in a lot of communication to minimise contact with unfamiliar cats and the risks associated with it, using chemical signals extensively to facilitate their spacing. As previously mentioned, newborn animals have to build up knowledge of what is safe and what is not, and semiochemicals may aid this process in a variety of ways. Odours which are associated with positive experiences, such as the mother's identity and suckling, may be used to identify desirable areas. This is a learned process. However, chemicals which create an intrinsic perceptual bias extend the possibilities further. This is the putative function of the appeasines: they provide a simple mechanism for identifying safety that does not require learning. By creating a reassuring environment, the young animal can both rapidly assimilate information about specific stimuli associated with its environment, which need not be feared, and explore further with confidence. As this information is accumulated, it provides a platform for further learning and more precise discrimination, which allows more refined decision-making and success in the complex environment in which the animal lives. When puppies and kittens are first born, they are blind and deaf. This should not be considered a handicap (such a situation would not arise or survive as a general biological feature in nature) but rather a useful condition for the efficient development of the brain. The initial restriction of sensory input to the chemical, thermal and tactile channels may help the animals to exploit the information and learning opportunities available from living in a nest. It may help their brains to focus and refine their development in specific areas in an orderly way in order to build greater perceptual competence. This exploitation of the circumstances allows the animals to become more skilled and cognitively flexible later in life. As the animals develop, there may be less need and dependence on such chemical signals as they become more able to integrate information from other senses, such as vision and hearing, which allow them to engage in more rapid information exchange. This is an important developmental process, which helps to maximise behavioural competence in the ecological niche occupied by cats and dogs.

Chemical signals are also particularly useful because some have the potential to be long-lasting and so they are often used to label a particular area or group. But because they also decay with time, they can convey more precise time-dependent information: they can indicate not only that somebody has been somewhere but also how recently. If an animal has a large territory, it would be inefficient to run around its borders all the time to show it was in the area, so chemical signals can be used to efficiently indicate an active presence. In this way, potential intruders may be deterred and conflicts avoided.

Time-coding is particularly important in the case of sexual markers. A female in heat, for example, wants to signify that she is in oestrus at this particular point in time. She may be out of season 3 days later, and attempts to seek her to reproduce then will be pointless. It is therefore not surprising that the chemicals used to signify heat very rapidly change with time. Once they have changed, the chances are that the female who deposited them is no longer willing to breed.

## 3.3.3.2   TYPES OF INFORMATION CONVEYED BY SEMIOCHEMICALS

### Individual characteristics

Chemical signals related to individual characteristics include:

- *Identification of the species*: The chemicals produced by a cat, for example, are different from those produced by a dog.
- *Group membership*: Some animals share a collective group smell or group odour. Individuals entering into a group that lack the group smell may be rejected because of this. That is why some dogs and cats may be rejected when they come back from the groomers or from the veterinary clinic – they smell different to when they left. The creation of a common scent may be particularly important to cats and useful in the resolution of social disputes. Normally a common scent is created through *allorubbing*, especially involving males, or mutual grooming, but this can be artificially imposed by using a common cloth to collect the scent from different individuals. This may be useful in reducing aggression when introducing a new cat to the home, or even in cases where the cats appear to attack on sight. A pheromonal component (feline facial fraction F4, available as the product 'Felifriend®' in several countries) may be an important adjunct to this process, biasing social acceptance.
- *Gender*: Different sexes may have different odours as well, especially after maturity. Odour changes may occur after neutering, which can give rise to relationship problems between previously familiar animals.
- *Age*: Approximate age or precise lifestage may be signified through chemical odours.
- *Health status*: The chemical signals an animal produces can vary with its health. Not only can sick animals produce slightly different signals, but the flora of their skin and related glands can be very important in producing appropriate odours. A long course of antibiotics may actually destroy the surface flora of bacteria of the treated animal, which can change its odour and precipitate social problems, such as aggression within a group of dogs. If a group of dogs that normally lives together quite peaceably suddenly starts fighting, it is worth checking whether one has been put on a course of antibiotics and whether any of them have an infection in their anal sacs or ears.
- *Social relationship and associated emotional predispositions*: It is well established that certain aspects of a social relationship, such as social status, can be conveyed through chemical signals. However, the extent to which related significant emotional predispositions may be conveyed by mammalian semiochemicals is less clearly understood. It seems that a composite signal consisting of chemicals which identify a specific individual together with those that induce a particular motivational–emotional bias may be important in the perception of a range of biologically important relationships, such as that existing between a mother and her offspring. Similarly, dogs who tend to take control of the group's resources are not only recognised in terms of their individual identity, but may

also produce a pheromonal signal which provides reassurance to the others. Recent work suggests that these chemicals are released from around the ear region. Again, animals with chronic ear problems who are put on long courses of antibiotics or have chronic changes in their ear may have problems with chemical communication at this level. This pheromone is identical to the appeasine of the bitch produced shortly after whelping. Therefore, disruption to the production of this pheromone may result in increased anxiety and social instability within a group of dogs in the home.

## Spatial organisation and arrangement

Chemical signals can be important not only in conveying information to allow individuals to space themselves within a particular area so that they do not come into conflict, but also in identifying the personal significance of particular areas (e.g. the core territory). However, chemicals are used to mark not just the *core territory* (the main area defended by an individual) but also the *home range*, which is the full area covered by an animal and the paths within this linking different functional areas. Some of these signals may act as a deterrent to potential intruders, while others possibly provide reassurance to the occupant and so potentially allow it to conserve attentional resources for other activities. The core area, in which most activity occurs and in which the mother breeds, will also have characteristic odours and pheromone deposits. Appeasine is produced by the mother and is widely used in pheromonatherapy.

## Growth, development and maturity

The chemical signals that animals produce change with age and with sexual maturity. The presence of adult-related chemical signals can also be important in promoting sexual behaviour and maturation, affecting not just physical development but also the development of a whole motivational–emotional predisposition. Individuals reared in either total isolation or simply isolation from the opposite sex may mature later or show aberrant sexual behaviour due to a lack of exposure to important semiochemicals.

### 3.3.3.3  SEMIOCHEMICAL DETECTION

Although the vast majority of chemoreception is via chemoreceptors in the relevant regions of the nose and mouth already discussed, these are not the only structures that might be involved in the detection of semiochemical signals. Other means of detection relate to:

• Direct neurostimulation of non-olfactory nerves, especially the fifth cranial nerve – the trigeminal nerve. Stimulation of this nerve is usually associated with irritants in the environment, which might include certain types of semiochemical used in defence. Stimulation of the trigeminal nerve is linked to the sneezing reflex, and also to changes in heart rate.

- Direct absorption into surface capillaries. Most of the olfactory epithelium is very highly vascularised, which, at least theoretically, makes it possible for some semiochemicals to cross through the mucous membranes directly into the blood, where they might be able to have direct effects more generally around the body. This aspect of chemical communication is largely unexplored, but may become an important research area in the near future.

## 3.3.3.4   *STRUCTURE OF THE VNO*

The VNO (also referred to as 'Jacobson's organ') is one of the specialised structures used for the detection of specific semiochemicals of motivational–emotional significance. Given its importance in pheromonatherapy, it is worth considering its structure in a bit more detail. The VNOs of the cat (Figure 3.10) and the dog are broadly similar at both a gross anatomical and a histological level. They appear as a crescent-shaped tube either side of the nasal septum.

The epithelial lining is largely made up of two regions, one consisting of respiratory-type mucous-secreting cells and the other of sensory cells; the area around the organ is well vascularised, and changes in the surrounding haemodynamics allow the opening of the lumen of the structure. Air does not normally flow over the surface of the structure, so animals engage in a range of oronasal pumping actions (flehmen – the exact form of which varies with species – Fig. 3.4) which encourage the circulation of air into the blindly ending tubes. This is typically accompanied by an increase in seromucous production, and the animal may appear to drool, froth at the mouth or drip from its nose as a result (Fig. 3.5). The nerves associated with the VNO synapse in the accessory olfactory bulb (part of the limbic system), unlike those extending from the main olfactory epithelium, and this, at least in part, explains how stimulation of the receptors in the VNO can have such a marked (involuntary) effect on emotional arousal and the behaviour that follows as a result. However, as mentioned above, the VNO does not operate in isolation from the other chemical sense organs. Some of the molecules used in pheromonatherapy are quite abundant in nature, but it appears that at least two requirements must be met for them to have a pheromonal effect: their presence in a given mixture combination and the detection of this by the normally quiescent VNO.

The functionality of the VNO does not relate to the olfactory ability of a species. Thus dogs have nearly 900 intact genes for olfactory receptors, but only 8 for the primary family of VNO receptors (V1R), which is amongst the lowest in the terrestrial vertebrates. By way of comparison, cats have around 30 V1R genes, cows 40 and mice 187, but humans have only 5 V1R genes and less than 400 olfactory receptor genes. The small number of V1R genes in the dog is not a function of domestication, as the wolf has only 9; it might however reflect a move away from a dependence on pheromones for the regulation of behavioural decision-making in many contexts, perhaps associated with more advanced social cognitive abilities.

(a)

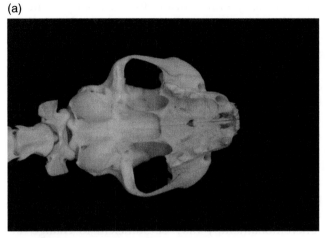

Respiratory epithelium

(b)

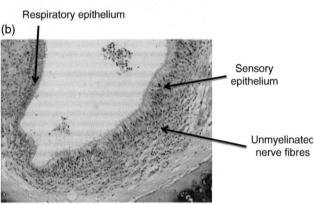

Sensory
epithelium

Unmyelinatec
nerve fibres

Fig. 3.10 The vomeronasal organ (VNO) is a bilateral crescent-shaped tubular structure situated in the rostral part of the hard palate either side of the septum. In the cat skull (a), the location of the duct joining the nasal and oral cavities is clearly illustrated by the fossae just behind the incisors. Ciliated respiratory epithelium lines the lateral and dorsal regions of the structure, while the medial and ventral parts are lined by a thicker receptor-dense sensory epithelium with unmyelinated nerves (b) (picture courtesy of Patrick Pageat).

### 3.3.3.5   *PHEROMONATHERAPY*

*Pheromonatherapy* involves the use of semiochemicals which have an emotional impact within a clinical context to manage the behaviour of animals. These are typically derived from the signals used in intraspecific communication. Pheromonatherapy is discussed more in Chapter 6, but it is worth discussing some points in the context of the current chapter. The concept of chemicals conveying emotionally important information is sometimes difficult for some scientists to appreciate when referring to conditions like anxiety or separation-related distress, but it is really no different from the idea that chemicals in the urine of a female in oestrus cause sexual arousal in males, since this too is obviously an emotional quality (associated with activation of *lust*). Similarly, when distressed, many species produce alarm signals, which are also emotionally significant in their quality. The production of these chemicals from the pads of a cat's or dog's paws in the veterinary clinic means that it is important to clean the area with a detergent that will remove all traces of these chemicals – otherwise, in the absence of other signals to the contrary, the next animal coming into the clinic is likely to detect these chemicals and become distressed straight away.

To understand the uses and limitations of pheromonatherapy in creating messages to help make the behaviour of animals more predictable, it is important to appreciate their biological context, and to recognise that chemical signals are only part of the signals surrounding an animal in its environment and that their significance will vary with other contextual features. Thus pheromonatherapy is a form of complementary therapy in the true sense of the word; that is, it complements other therapies that we might use to manage behaviour problems in cats and dogs. Pheromonatherapy has a sound scientific basis and may be considered a form of environmental management that encourages more acceptable behaviour. In some cases, the use of pheromonatherapy may be sufficient to change an animal's perception of its environment and thereby also its response to specific stimuli. In other cases, these chemicals may be used less specifically to relieve anxiety or create a sense of safety and thereby encourage appropriate attention to facilitate essential training.

## 3.4   CONCLUSION

In conclusion, communication in the species with which we deal is a multimodal process in which information with a particular meaning is sent by one individual and interpreted by another. This interpretive process typically depends on the integration of all information of perceived relevance to the animal at that time, in the context of its previous experience. To this end, emotionally relevant information may be used in the final subjective decision made by the animal with regards to its strategic priorities. Emotionally relevant information which causes a subjective bias may be conveyed through any sensory channel and its potential impact may relate to biologically predefined stimulus properties, which do not require prior learning. For example, in the absence of training to the contrary, the looming gesture is typically perceived as threatening, as is the hiss of many species; similarly, there are certain chemicals which can have a strong emotional impact because of their biologically predefined meaning, through their direct link and processing by the limbic brain. Some of these chemicals are related to the generation of negative affective states, while others may create a bias towards a more positive mood. The evolution of these can be understood in the context of behavioural and developmental optimality. In the next two chapters, we present a perspective on an approach used for the assessment and management of problem behaviour, which helps to lay the foundation for understanding pheromonatherapy (Chapter 6) and, when manipulating chemical signals, may or may not be effective in bringing about behaviour change. We then go on to consider specific presenting complaints and challenges in Part II of the text.

# REVIEW ACTIVITIES

- Observe communicative exchanges between two or more animals. What signals are being sent and which elements do individuals appear to be responding to the most?
- Consider the reasons why different types of information are communicated using a particular sensory channel.
- Watch the behaviour of animals in different contexts, paying special attention to regions associated with chemical-signal production. Can you identify a link between possible visual and olfactory communication in these contexts? What is the value of each in these contexts?
- Review videos from the Internet of animal vocalisations in different contexts. What common features can you identify and what differences occur within a species?
- Consider ways in which humans may send contradictory signals that have the potential to result in ambivalent messages to cats and dogs. Which element is the animal likely to attend to and why?

# REFERENCES

Rugaas T (1997) On talking terms with dogs: calming signals. Legacy by mail. Carlsborg, WA.
Shepherd K (2010) Behavioural medicine as an integral part of veterinary practice. In: Horwitz DF, Mills DS (eds) BSAVA Manual of Canine and Feline Behavioural Medicine (2 edn). Gloucester: BSAVA. pp. 10–23.

# FURTHER READING

Adams DR, Wiekamp MD (1984) The canine vomeronasal organ. Journal of Anatomy 138: 771–787.
Dusenbery DB (1992) Sensory Ecology: How Organisms Acquire and Respond to Information. New York, NY: WH Freeman & Co.
Pongracz P, Molnar C, Miklosi A, Csanyi V (2005) Human listeners are able to classify dog barks recorded in different situations. Journal of Comparative Psychology 119: 136–144.
Salazar I, Sanchez Quinteiro P, Cifuentes JM, Garcia Caballero T (1996) The vomeronsal organ of the cat. Journal of Anatomy 188: 445–454.
Simonet PR (2001) Laughter in animals. In: Bekoff M (ed.) Encyclopaedia of Animal Behaviour (Vol 2). Westport, CT: Greenwood Press. pp. 561–563.
Wyatt T (2003) Pheromones and Animal Behaviour. Cambridge: Cambridge University Press.
Yin S (2002) A new perspective on barking in dogs. Journal of Comparative Psychology 116: 189–193.

# Chapter 4

# Assessment of the Problem-behaviour Patient

## 4.1 INTRODUCTION

When evaluating a case of problematic behaviour for a client, it is important to have a logical framework for the necessary analysis, so that rational conclusions can be made on the basis of the available, but often incomplete, information. Central to this process is an appreciation of the following questions:

- What makes a behaviour problem? That is, what is the nature of a behaviour problem?
- What is the purpose of the consultation and why do behaviour consultations tend to be such lengthy affairs?
- How do you undertake a consultation in order to gather reliable information from which to draw inferences and hypotheses about the cause of the problem?
- What is the relationship between behavioural and medical issues, when considering problem behaviour? The two often overlap and the distinction may not be as clear as it is often portrayed.

These subjects form the basis of this chapter. In addition, it is essential that we can clearly, and preferably effortlessly, recognise the differences between our observations and the inferences we draw from these during this process, since the latter should always be open to reexamination in light of new information.

## 4.2 RECOGNISING THE NATURE OF A PROBLEM BEHAVIOUR

What is a *behaviour problem*? Askew (1996) states, 'the problem is not the animal's behaviour per se but rather the problem that the behaviour poses for its owner'. This means that the definition of problem behaviour is inherently subjective and not necessarily biologically distinctive. The behaviour may be perfectly normal but it is a problem for the owner to cope with. For example, imagine a puppy that

*Stress and Pheromonatherapy in Small Animal Clinical Behaviour*, First Edition.
Daniel Mills, Maya Braem Dube and Helen Zulch.
© 2013 John Wiley & Sons, Ltd. Published 2013 by John Wiley & Sons, Ltd.

house soils when it is left alone for long periods of time. The reason for this might simply be that it is not mature enough to hold on to its bladder and bowels for that length of time. It is perfectly normal, then, for it to urinate or defecate wherever it has the possibility, which in this example is in the house; however, if the owner does not appreciate this they may report it as a problem. On the other hand, some behaviours are genuinely dysfunctional. For example, a *phobia* is a fear response that is out of all proportion to the actual threat, and this response interferes with the normal functioning of the animal. It is not adaptive and so is a problem for the animal, as well as for its owner.

If we accept that a behaviour problem is defined by the problem it poses to an animal's owner, this means that the solution to the problem also lies with the owner. It does not mean that the owner is the cause of the problem, but they are certainly key to its resolution. The problem arises from the interaction between pet and owner and the conflict of interests that may result. From this perspective, there is rarely a single cause of a problem in a developmental sense (though there may be specific triggers in a regulatory sense), but rather the problem arises as a result of certain risk factors relating to the animal and its circumstances.

Owners with a problem pet often feel guilty and blame themselves, and therefore it is essential when dealing with behavioural problems not to blame the owners, but to provide them with reassurance and support in order to help motivate them to bring about the necessary changes to resolve the problem. Owners need both encouragement and the skill base required to make the necessary steps to resolve the issue – knowledge is not enough. As the owner is seeking help, it is also important to let them know that their problem is being taken seriously. That is why veterinarians should consider scheduling a special behaviour consultation rather than trying to dispense behavioural advice within a general short medical appointment, for anything other than routine matters. There is an old adage that says, 'Free advice is cheap advice', and there may be some truth to it: if you give casual advice, owners will probably just ignore it, but if anything goes wrong you will still be liable. This means it is important to make sure that consultations are always conducted in a professional and safe manner.

## 4.3   THE CONSULTATION

### 4.3.1   *AIMS OF THE CONSULTATION*

The consultation appointment has several aims:

* *Assessing the problem*: It is important when assessing the problem to recognise that the current behaviour has almost inevitably been modified from the original performance which gave rise to the initial concern of the owner. How the owner, other people and other animals have responded and continue to respond to the patient's behaviour will have effects on the animal and influence future expressions of the behaviour. Animals learn in every situation, whether we want them to or not, so learning will always play a role in these cases. The sad

reality is that most owners only seek help several weeks, months or even years after the onset of the problem. It is when they have reached breaking point that they are most likely to seek professional help. The assessment of a problem is an interpretation of events, and in order to provide a scientifically sound explanation it is essential to gather good data.

- *Explaining the problem and offering rational treatment advice to the client*: If a client understands the nature of the problem, they are more likely to be able to cope with it and will be more willing to engage in the methods necessary to resolve it. There will often be a variety of solutions to a given behaviour problem, and it is not the aim of this book to cover every possibility; rather, it aims to lay out the principles that should be followed, with a special emphasis on the need to create a way of being together which is acceptable to both owner and pet. The details of specific behaviour therapies can be found in other texts (see References and Further Reading at the end of this chapter). We emphasise here the importance of recommending precise treatments and implementing good management practice, which is often overlooked, despite being much easier for many owners than more generic training programmes. When dealing with behaviour problems, it is not as simple as just recommending appropriate treatments, because these treatments will almost inevitably depend on the owner's implementing them; the simpler and more precise we can be, the greater the likelihood of success.
- *Maximising owner compliance*: Another very important aim of the consultation process is to try to maximise owner compliance and owner buy-in to the resolution of the problem. Owners need to be motivated to change their ways or adopt unusual strategies in order to resolve the problem and prevent it from coming back. This may require both counselling and coaching skills, which are discussed in more detail later.

## 4.3.2   INTERVIEWING SKILLS

Interviewing in order to get clients to disclose useful information is a vast subject in its own right. In this section, we provide a brief overview and highlight a few important areas for consideration. Most individuals working with animal-behaviour problems are not human-behaviour specialists or clinical psychologists and so if the process appears to be particularly challenging, consideration should be given to either referring or working alongside another appropriate professional. This may be particularly important if some form of mental-health problem is believed to be affecting the ability of the client to have a satisfactory and healthy relationship with their pet.

When interviewing a client, there is generally a lot to be learned about their perceptions, but it is important not to appear critical as this is likely to result in resistance, which is counterproductive to our aims. These are to encourage clients to discuss things and reflect upon what they are saying in order that they can discover the issues and the potential solutions for themselves. In order to do this, it is important to ensure that not only are any interjections well timed, but that the questions asked are precise and focused. To this end, the clinician should try to keep them simple and singular. The key skills involved in interviewing can be summarised in the acronym OARS. This stands for:

- **O**pen-ended questioning.
- **A**ffirmation.
- **R**eflective listening.
- **S**ummarising.

Open-ended questions – that is, questions that cannot be answered simply 'yes' or 'no' – encourage greater dialogue than closed questions. In general there are two types of open-ended question:

- *Probing questions*: In which we want the client to enlarge upon their response, to provide greater context.
- *Focusing questions*: In which we want to encourage more detail, or to go into more specifics, about the situation being described.

The style of questioning can also have an impact on the willingness of the client to reveal information. Consider the following scenarios:

- You want to encourage the client to expand on something further. If you say, 'Tell me more…', you are giving an instruction, which can be intimidating to some clients. A more encouraging style would be, 'Please, can you say more about…'
- You want to encourage the client to examine more closely some aspect of what they have said. In this case there is a danger that you will come across as critical or unbelieving, but the risk can be ameliorated by phrasing your enquiry as something like, 'Can we look at why you believe this?', or perhaps by guiding the client to reflect upon the logic of what they have said.

Affirmation is aimed at helping a client to recognise the reality of the situation and to accept that they have a choice in how things are. In this process, it is important to communicate that the client is accepted for who they are and that the clinician is not going to judge or criticise. The client and their priorities must be respected even if they are not agreed with. Affirmation is an important aspect of the general empowerment of a client necessary for change. By highlighting that they have the power to make choices, clients are encouraged to face the reality of the outcome of these, and in so doing accept responsibility for their consequences. This can be an essential step in resolving conflicts of interest between a client and their pet and motivating change.

Reflective listening involves encouraging clients to express their concerns and highlighting any discrepancies in a nonjudgemental way, in order to encourage reflection and the motivation necessary for change. Both verbal and nonverbal signals expressed by the client are evaluated and reflected by the counsellor during bouts of reciprocal communication, which should include acknowledgement of the distress the client is feeling. Key reflective listening skills are:

- The expression of empathy through verbal reflection of the feelings of the client. For example, 'I can understand that it must be very distressing for you when…'
- The paraphrasing of factual content, in order to communicate and establish that you have understood key elements of the discussion. For example, 'So if I have understood you correctly, there have been three incidents in total…'

Summarising is an opportunity to demonstrate and test the counsellor's understanding of what has been said in a way that reflects the client's frame of reference and highlights the most important points revealed; for example, 'It seems to me that you feel your dog is trying to control everything that you do, and this is what you mean when you say he is a very dominant individual.' As with any interpretation of the client, it is important to express the evaluation tentatively, so that the client feels free to correct you if necessary, without creating conflict. Avoidance of language that could be seen as judgemental, unless it is a direct paraphrase of an owner's statement, can also be beneficial in assisting the owner to remain open rather than become defensive. For example, it is not constructive to say something like, 'You might think he is dominant because of the way he behaves, but I don't agree with you because…'

### 4.3.3   ASSESSING THE PROBLEM

As already indicated, one of the first aims of a behaviour consultation is to assess the problem, which usually involves quite a lengthy behavioural history. Some behaviourists like to ease the process by obtaining the history in the form of a questionnaire in advance of the consultation. This has several practical advantages, especially when starting out in the field. First, if an owner is asked to complete an extensive behavioural history form and return it in advance, the case can be reviewed before the consultation and extra assistance can be sought as necessary or a referral can be made without wasting either the consultant's time or the client's. Second, by completing the behavioural form and sending it in advance, a level of commitment and motivation for change has already been established.

Within the clinic, the first requirement is to *define the behaviour and its context and then postulate motivational–emotional reasons for why it occurs*. These are different processes. The first requires the gathering of accurate information; the second depends on sound scientific reasoning. Often owners will complain that the behaviour is unpredictable or happens for no apparent reason. The job of the clinician, then, is to try to determine the cues for the behaviour and *why* this is the case, in order to help the client eliminate or at least manage the problem. At the same time, the clinician and owner must be aware that the possible reasons for a behaviour remain hypotheses, which will be supported, challenged or rejected by the animal's behaviour in response to the treatment recommendations that are implemented.

Owners will often want to give their opinion of this, that or the other, but what we really need are good data: objective measures of what is going on. Clients should be allowed to express themselves and their feelings, but they may require guiding in order to produce the relevant information. It is then necessary to stand back from the problem and assess what is going on. Throughout the consultation, the clinician should engage in *active* listening in order to build a bond with the client and establish the quality of the information being obtained. Active listening means engaging with what the client is saying in such a way that they can recognise that the clinician is attending to what they are saying. This is communicated very effectively through body language and simple affirmations, such as 'I see' or 'That's interesting'.

# 4.3.3.1   *ASSESSING THE QUALITY OF INFORMATION OBTAINED*

There are a number of ways to assess the history in order to determine the reliability of the information being obtained. First we need objective information. Owners should be encouraged to be descriptive. They might say, for example, 'Well, he's aggressive whenever I go out', but what do they actually mean by 'aggressive'? For some owners, this might be a growl, for others it could mean the dog is simply standing in their way. These are very different issues. Another example might be the owner who says, 'Well, he messes everywhere'; 'everywhere' is not a very helpful descriptive term. In this case it can be useful to ask the client to draw a plan of the area and indicate exactly where they have found mess; a pattern to the mess might then be revealed, for example it may indicate that the animal is scent marking or that it has a problem with the litter box in the case of a cat. Never underestimate the value of a good drawing, picture or video. If it is safe to do so, it is useful to encourage owners to take video footage of their house, the behaviour, their interaction with the animal or their pets interacting with each other. In addition, in all cases where there is an interval between first contact and the consultation, a diary of daily events involving the pet's problem behaviour and the happenings within the home can deliver more objective data than reliance on memory. In some cases, and where possible, it might be necessary to undertake a house call to observe the animal in its own surroundings. The aim is to gather real data, in the same way that a chemist might want to examine the exact quantities of chemicals rather than talk in terms of broad amounts or 'a lot of this chemical and a lot of that chemical make this other chemical'; we are trying to define things quite precisely.

Just because data are objective does not mean they are reliable, and if we are to get as full an understanding of the problem as possible, the information needs to be both objective and reliable. There are a number of ways to assess the reliability of information in a clinical setting. The first is to ask the same question in a number of different ways. For example, imagine we ask, 'How often does your cat urinate outside the litter box?' The owner might say, 'Every day'. We can then ask later on, 'Over the last month, how often have you found patches of urine in the house?' To which they might reply, 'On fifteen occasions'. That would suggest that the cat is not doing it 'every day'. It is important when using this method not to make it obvious that the same information is being sought, since some owners may think that you are not listening to them properly.

Another approach depends on more than one person from the family being present. Each is asked to explain what they think is going on and verify what the others have said, in a nonconfrontational way. If this technique is to be used, it is important to try to identify early on who is more vocal in the family and ask them to speak last. Otherwise it is likely that other members of the household will simply agree with them. It is important to note when contradictions occur. Sometimes behaviours genuinely do occur differently with different people present, and often different people are attentive to different things, which might be an explanation for any inconsistencies. This should be explained and explored. If one owner does interrupt another, it needs to be pointed out that it is possible that the animal behaves differently with different people, and that everybody will get the chance to offer their opinion in due course.

It is useful to ask owners to describe at least three situations in which the problem has arisen. The first two are the earliest occasion they can remember and the most recent occasion. This allows an assessment of how the problem has changed over time and what role environmental (including owner) feedback might have. The third situation is usually the one that they can best remember. This will give the richest picture of what exactly is going on. If there are several people present in the consultation, we might ask them each to explain the episode they remember best, in order to get as much information as possible.

By far the most reliable way of getting true data is to directly observe the behaviour that is causing the problem. Obviously, this is not possible in all cases and is not safe in some cases. It should not be attempted unless a proper risk assessment of the situation has been made (see Section 4.3.5). In some instances, seeing the actual behaviour clarifies the situation. For example, when the behaviour of a dog that is presented for being very aggressive to other dogs is observed, the clinician may notice elements of play signalling and behaviour which have not been noticed or recognised by the owner. The dog might indeed get involved in fights, but actually, in this case, the problem relates to its management when it gets aroused in anticipation of play, the level of arousal shown and/or inappropriate attempts at punishment by the owner in the past. When the dog sees another dog coming, it may still want to play, but it may also be frustrated and anticipate that the presence of other dogs will bring punishment by the owner. As a result it tries to signal for the other dogs to stay away by growling. This mixture of signals is confusing for owners and other dogs, who may well respond aggressively, exacerbating the problem further. This is not an uncommon problem, and illustrates the value of direct observation or video footage. In such cases, it is important to make sure that the animal is well secured, to ensure the safety of all involved. It might be useful to secure the animal through a long line in order to make sure it cannot escape and cause any harm. At the same time, ask the owner to hold the dog on its normal lead (attached in addition to the line) and to act as they normally do. In this way, what the owner does can be observed, such as whether they jerk on the lead or tell the dog off.

Once a clear description of the behaviour giving concern has been obtained, we can start to evaluate how this gives rise to a problem for the owner, and then make a tentative diagnosis of the problem, which is our interpretation of or hypothesis about the reason why the animal behaves as it does. These matters are the focus of the next section.

## 4.3.3.2   IDENTIFYING CONFLICTS OF INTEREST BETWEEN PET AND OWNER

As already mentioned, a behaviour problem is not just the behaviour of the animal: it is also how the owner perceives the behaviour. It is therefore an emergent feature of the interactions occurring between owner, pet and the wider environment. The problem is that there is often a conflict of interests or a miscommunication of interests (i.e. misunderstanding) between the owner and their pet. It can happen, for example, that each wants something different, and when they work towards their own goals there is a tension in their relationship; that is, there is poor communication and poor recognition of each other's interests.

- Conflicts may arise because the owner does not understand the fundamental needs of their pet. An example of this might be the owner who has unrealistic expectations of how long a dog can be left alone without access to a toilet, or a desire for their cats to form a close social unit rather than live as a less closely knit group who simply tolerate each other. In these cases, developing realistic expectations is key to resolving the problem.
- In other cases, the conflict may arise because the pet has not been given guidance to help it perceive what the owner wants. An example might be the owner who complains that their dog jumps up to greet them, when they have never trained it to greet people as they would like. In this example, the end goal is a realistic expectation, but there is an unrealistic expectation of what needs to be done to achieve it. In these cases, developing realistic expectations around effective communication to facilitate the necessary training is key to resolving the problem.
- Quite often there is a misunderstanding by both the pet and the owner of the other's interests, with problematic behaviour occurring as a result – in this case, it might be argued that the problem behaviour emerges from the failure of each party to effectively communicate their own interests. Examples include many scenarios in which owners try to punish their pet. In these cases it is important for the clinician to help the owner recognise and reevaluate the mistaken beliefs they have about what they are achieving, and to do so in a noncritical and supportive way, in order to instigate a more effective pattern of behaviour and interaction.
- However, in some cases, both pet and owner may have some appreciation of what the other wants, but put their own interests first – that is, the conflict arises from active resistance to each other's interests. An example of this might be the dog who wants to play when the owner wants it to work, or the attention-seeking animal who the owner finds annoying at times. In these cases, it is important for the clinician to work as an arbiter of the interests of both pet and owner, and agree with the owner a realistic compromise which respects the welfare of all involved.

In each of these scenarios, it is necessary to create within the owner an understanding of and a *way of being* with their pet before considering specific behaviour-modification plans, since it is only on this basis that we can expect change to be sustained. Creating a way of being refers to the ability to encourage a routine style of interaction with a pet that is supportive of its needs, rather than specific training exercises. It may include addressing background stressors (see Section 1.4), as well as promoting specific enjoyable interactions for both owner and pet, such as playing informal games together. These are usually quite easy to instigate once the owner has a fuller appreciation of their pet's needs. It is important to identify all conflicts and assess whether each owner's expectations are realistic and their interests are sensitive enough to the needs of their pet. But, at the same time, we must evaluate whether the pet is oversensitive to certain stimuli and requires behaviour therapy. *The fundamental difference between training and behaviour therapy is that the latter is focused on altering the emotional responses of the individual while the former focuses on behaviour first and foremost. Therefore, training is appropriate where we simply wish to encourage an animal to respond in a specific way to a specific cue, but behaviour therapy is necessary when we wish to control and change the animal's reactivity.*

Most behaviour problems do not arise from single or specific trigger factors, but as a result of a number of factors coming together in a particular individual at a particular time. The more of these factors we can identify, the better the chance of being able to control the problem, due to the greater number of factors we can address in its management. It may well be that many of the factors arise because of a misunderstanding of the interests of the pet, and that by addressing these a way of behaving with the animal will be created which does not require the often more challenging and difficult option of behaviour therapy. Therefore, it is important to look at the needs of the animal and whether they are being met through its general management, living situation, social relationships, communication and so on, and to identify those factors where the interests of the owner and their pet conflict and give rise to distress.

## 4.3.4   *DIFFERENTIAL DIAGNOSIS*

On the basis of the information available, we can start to formulate different ideas as to what might be going on, especially in terms of its motivational–emotional basis (see Chapter 2). Any possible explanations for a problem are hypotheses and collectively form the differential diagnosis for the patient. Once we have a differential list in mind, we can formulate additional questions that explore these in more detail. As we do this, we will further develop ideas or hypotheses that we can test. When testing a hypothesis, it is important not only to ask questions which will support the ideas (this is what is done most commonly and naturally), but also questions that will help distinguish between other possible explanations of what is going on (this is more challenging). If the answer to a particular question contradicts what we would expect then we should consider other explanations of the behaviour and ask questions that will test our new hypotheses. It is also important to appreciate that more than one motivational–emotional system may be contributing to the problematic situation being encountered by the owner.

In many cases we can only get so far with a history, and further medical or behavioural tests may be needed to be able to differentiate between these hypotheses. When deciding which route to take with respect to additional diagnostics, we have to consider how much more information we will get, how expensive the tests are and what risks are involved in carrying them out. The available options should be discussed with the client and ultimately the decision rests with the owner as to what to do next. It is the professional's job to advise on the basis of their experience and expertise, and to offer the best advice accordingly. We cannot dictate a path to a client. In addition, when investigations are considered we must again be cautious about selecting tests that will simply confirm our own beliefs. The key point to bear in mind is that any information gathered must aim to differentiate competing hypotheses.

If we get to the situation where we have managed to exclude all competing explanations and are left with one possibility then we should think about accepting that hypothesis. This is rarely the case – it is not possible to rule out every differential with certainty – but we can make reasonable conclusions on the basis of probability. In reality, we are typically left with several possible explanations and may have to start treatment on the basis of minimising risk and doing no harm, perhaps using treatment itself to help differentiate between the remaining possible explanations for the behaviour.

The aim is to have a clear idea of the most important factors contributing to an explanation of the problem by the end of the consultation. Always bear in mind that common things are common and remember what we can actually eliminate during just a consultation and what will require further assessment (e.g. medical evaluations of possible pain foci). There is nothing wrong with recommending further tests before implementing behavioural treatment, if the risks have been carefully assessed and managed.

## 4.3.5   RISK ASSESSMENT

It is important to assess the risks associated with any problem. Risk assessment is necessary for many reasons:

- It helps establish priorities for protective measures so that resources can be deployed efficiently.
- It helps to identify where skill development is necessary (e.g. client training).
- It is a legal requirement that will protect against claims of negligence.

It is important for both clinician and client to appreciate that not all risks can be eliminated – owning a pet comes with a degree of inherent risk – and so the aim is to manage risk, identifying, analysing, addressing and monitoring risks in such a way that both the probability and the impact are minimised to what is reasonably practicable through a logical and systematic approach. Sensible risk management is about:

- Ensuring that individuals are properly protected from the risks posed by animals.
- Ensuring the benefits and risks are properly balanced to maximise the benefit to all from companion animals.
- Enabling responsible animal owners to enjoy the experience of animal ownership.
- Creating awareness of the real risks associated with companion animals and managing them responsibly, as well as promoting an understanding that failure to manage these risks responsibly might lead to more robust (e.g. legal) action.
- Enabling individuals to understand that as well as the right to protection, they also have a duty to exercise responsibility.

We therefore need to risk assess both the current situation and the agreed management plan for the problem, and ensure the assessment is communicated to the owner efficiently.

Risk is the product of the probability of an event and the severity of its consequences. That is:

$$Risk = Probability \times Impact$$

A simple method of risk assessment is to assess each of the elements as either high
or low. This gives us four possible types of risk:

- *High probability–high impact*: These are obviously the most serious risks and must
  be managed. An example is a dog that is aggressive towards children and whose
  owner is pregnant.
- *High probability–low impact*: Owners are often aware of these risks but can have
  a tendency to accept them, even when this is not appropriate. Relatively straightforward risk-management protocols should be put in place – aimed particularly
  at reducing the probability of an event – such as safe-management practices. An
  example is a dog that frequently barks at people but does not threaten harm.
- *Low probability–high impact*: There is often a tendency to dismiss these risks as so
  rare that they don't need to be worried about, but this is perhaps the area of
  greatest danger. Strategies aimed at reducing both impact and probability are
  needed, given the risk. An example is a neighbouring cat who comes into the
  garden and sees off the owner's cat, which only occasionally goes out.
- *Low probability–low impact*: These are the lowest-priority events and in some
  cases a client may simply need reassurance that this is your assessment. An
  example is a dog living in the city that runs after cows.

Risk needs to be individualised according to the circumstances. For example, if
young children or perhaps elderly or infirm individuals are living in the same
household as an aggressive animal, the risk situation is much higher than if these
individuals are not present. By way of further example, both big dogs and little
dogs will bite, but a bite from a large dog is potentially much more dangerous and
so carries a greater risk.

The risks of a clinical behaviour situation focus on three broad areas:

- *The risks to the patient*: In this instance, the harm that might occur to the patient
  associated with the problem and its management is the focus of attention. This
  is not simply the risk of physical injury, but includes potential threats to the
  animal's well-being, such as the risk of being given up to a rescue or euthanised,
  the risk of the owner harming the animal through punishment and the risk of
  inconsistent interaction producing anxiety or frustration.
- *The risks to immediate contacts*: In this instance, the focus is on those who typically
  come into contact with the animal, such as family, friends, neighbours, other
  animals and potentially other dog walkers. Again, this is not just focused on
  physical harm but includes their wider well-being.
- *The risks to others*: In this instance, the risks to wider society are considered.
  This will include consideration of the effect of the animal escaping or being
  rehomed. It is here that a judgement may need to be made that it is not appropriate for the animal to be given up for adoption and that euthanasia is the
  most responsible option.

There is a fourth area of risk which, although it does not fit within the traditional model of risk assessment (i.e. assessment of risk of harm), is nonetheless essential. This is the *risk of failure or relapse of the treatment programme*. If a treatment plan is recommended which the owner is either not competent or unwilling to implement, then it is not only ineffective but may actually produce an unacceptable risk. In that case, it may be best to recommend something simpler which, although not the preferred strategy of the clinician, is more realistic, if only in the short term, for the client. Thus the prognosis associated with the recommended treatments must also be evaluated as part of the risk-assessment process, and this assessment needs to be communicated to the client. In relation to this, it is also important to distinguish between measures which contain (restrict) the problem and those which eliminate (resolve) it. From a long-term management point of view, the goal should always be to resolve the problem (which might however not always be realistic or possible), but as an interim measure restriction may be necessary in order to minimise risk.

Having made an assessment of the problem, it is important to reflect upon our own abilities. If we feel out of our depth, it is essential that we seek further assistance as far as is reasonably practicable.

## 4.4    MEDICAL VERSUS BEHAVIOURAL PROBLEMS

### 4.4.1    *THE MEDICAL–BEHAVIOURAL DICHOTOMY*

In a classic and somewhat simplistic approach to behaviour problems, a problem like aggressive behaviour towards people might be divided into 'medically related' and 'nonmedically related' conditions. This implies that there is a sharp division between behavioural problems on the one hand and medical problems on the other. But in reality it is not this simple, and it is certainly very difficult to rule out every possible medical cause of behavioural signs. Nonetheless, there are indicators we can use that might help to guide us towards seeing how important medical factors are in a given case. If the problem is medically related, it is often assumed that the pattern of the behaviour is a little more erratic or perhaps slightly more disorganised than something that is more typically behavioural, which is usually much more predictable. However, even very predictable episodes of aggressive behaviour can be medically related, for example if they are associated with pain in certain contexts. If we have a pattern of aggressive episodes (after very detailed questioning aimed at uncovering predictability where owners are not aware it exists) that are very hard to predict through motivational–emotional explanations, this would tend to suggest that a purely environmentally based explanation is unlikely. This perhaps helps to emphasise the importance of looking to exclude factors rather than to consolidate a particular opinion. Predictability does not help us differentiate, whereas unpredictability does.

If we adopt a risk-factor rather than causal approach to the development of behaviour, as described in Section 4.2 and in Chapter 2, then the dichotomy between medical and behavioural problems seems less important, since health and behaviour considerations are always present. A commonly heard approach to behaviour problems is to say that a problem is behavioural if a medical basis cannot be found. However, it is not really reasonable to try to exclude *all* medical causes, and certain behavioural changes might occur before a physical problem is detectable. We do not do brain scans on every patient, and we do not exclude each and every rare condition before making a definitive diagnosis or starting treatment. A negative result also simply means no abnormality was found, not that none is present.

## 4.4.2   PROFESSIONAL OBLIGATIONS

In practice, many vets may not appreciate the behavioural aspects of some medical conditions. They might not recognise, for example, that an animal presenting for aggression may have an underlying lesion such as hip dysplasia that is making it irritable and so more likely to behave in this way, and hence do not look for it. There is much debate about the role of veterinarians and non-veterinarians in behavioural issues. Currently relatively few veterinarians undertake much behaviour work and so it is not surprising that a lot of non-veterinarians take on these cases. However, with the best will in the world, non-veterinarians are not qualified (under UK law, at least) to diagnose and manage medical problems, which means they can be put in very awkward situations when a potential medical issue is affecting behaviour, especially when they only see cases on referral. Responsible non-veterinary behaviourists should work both on veterinary referral – they usually require that a veterinarian has seen the animal and certified that it is 'healthy' (even though this does not guarantee that all possible medical causes have been excluded, as explained in Section 4.4.1) before taking on a case – as well as in close association with a veterinary behaviourist (a veterinarian who can evaluate behaviour within a medical context). This is because if a veterinarian does not know what they are supposed to be looking for, an animal might be certified as healthy when there is actually a relevant underlying medical problem.

So, although a non-veterinary behaviourist is not qualified to make a medical diagnosis, they should be able to evaluate whether medical problems might be impacting on behaviour, whether pain might be contributing to the problem or whether a problem has uncharacteristic features indicative of non-environmental features in its development. This again emphasises the importance of collaboration between non-veterinarians and veterinarians. For example, there are many medical reasons that might result in a dog showing aggressive behaviour towards humans, including:

- General irritability due to pain, discomfort, itchiness and so on.
- Increased frustration as a result of the increased effort required to compensate for a medical problem, such as a difficulty in breathing.
- Changes in sensory-organ functionality: the onset of blindness or deafness.
- Age-related changes, such as dementia.
- Metabolic changes, such as hypothyroidism or diabetes mellitus.
- Neurological problems, such as hydrocephalus or a brain tumour.

Not all of these are necessarily direct causes of a problem, but they will certainly contribute to the problem and their identification is important for the long-term success of treatment, particularly as it pertains to protecting the animal's well-being. Even when a lesion cannot be detected, there may be certain features which are suggestive of a medical problem, such as a change in temperament later in life, a change in mobility or voluntary routines and so on, which warrant caution in the behaviour-management recommendations that are made.

### 4.4.3  MEDICAL COMPLICATIONS OF BEHAVIOUR PROBLEMS

There have been a number of reviews of possible medical factors relating to behavioural problems over the years, and it seems that the more we look, the more we see. One of the first studies, by Voith (1981) in the USA, suggested that in her caseload nearly 5% of dog behaviour cases had an underlying medical problem. In the experience of one of the present authors (DM), who consulted in general practice before moving into academia in the mid 1990s, about 13% of cases had some medical factor involved in the problem. The subdivision of these cases shows that medical factors were far more common in cats, with nearly 20% of cat cases having some medical involvement. This relates largely to cases of spraying, with the involvement of urinary-system disease, although more recently the obesity epidemic in cats may have increased the involvement of pain in feline-aggression cases. In cats, obesity frequently results in arthritis, which, unlike in dogs, has systemic effects on health as well as causing pain. In dogs, too, pain is quite a common underlying factor, often leading to an increase in aggressive behaviour.

In the same author's own general practice caseload of dogs, the most common presenting complaints were long-standing, chronic cases. When there was no obvious lesion to cause the behavioural complaint, the most common underlying problems related to musculoskeletal and dental pain. It is therefore always worth examining a dog's gait and ability to turn and sit tidily, looking for chipped teeth and exposed pulp cavities, which might be painful, and asking about the dog's feeding behaviour or seeing how it chews on a chew toy or a chew stick. Dietary sensitivity, which may present as overactivity or perhaps aggression; anal sac infection and impaction, which can result in other dogs attacking the patient; and hypothyroidism are all also not uncommon.

Hypothyroidism is quite a controversial topic in relation to behaviour problems, since the normal blood values for different breeds of dog are not generally reported. This means that what might be a normal level for one breed may actually be a low level for another. In some cases, dogs with low or borderline thyroid levels improve their behaviour enormously with thyroid supplementation. However, this does not mean the cause of the problem is low thyroid, only that supplementation can improve things. This is a specialist area of behavioural medicine, and if such a case is suspected it is essential to engage the support of a suitably qualified individual.

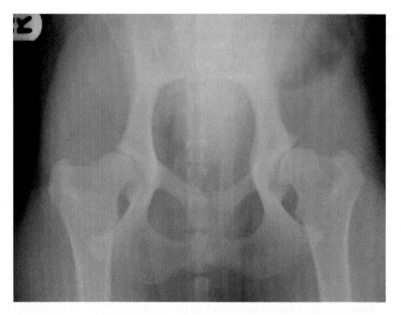

Fig. 4.1 Radiograph of a dog with hip dysplasia, which led to aggressive behaviour when the dog was asked to sit by its owner. The correlation between clinical signs of lameness and radiographic signs is not very reliable and therefore determining the significance of such changes can be difficult. However, if identified, the animal's well-being should be given the benefit of the doubt and risk management instigated accordingly.

Figure 4.1 shows an x-ray from a dog with hip dysplasia. The dog had shown resistance and sometimes aggressive behaviour when its owner tried to get it to sit, and this was mistakenly interpreted as a sign of dominance towards the owner. Obviously, the dog did not want to bend its hips because it was painful. When the owner pressed down on its back end, this made matters worse, which was the reason for the original complaint. This case also shows the interaction between learning and medical problems. Clearly, the dog has an underlying painful condition, but it has also learned that it can avoid contact with the owner by growling or snapping when the owner approaches it. This case is typical of the way medical factors are presented in behaviour problems, and while it may be possible to train the dog to sit for the owner, without analgesia the dog will still be in pain, so recognition of the medical condition is an important welfare consideration.

For long-standing cat cases in the aforementioned caseload where there was no obvious lesion, the most common causes of problems were:

- Chronic renal failure, for example in an old cat that has presented for house soiling.
- Cystitis, in relation to both eliminating outside the box and spraying problems.
- Some pain focus, such as arthritis.
- Hyperthyroidism, especially in older cats that suddenly became quite aggressive.

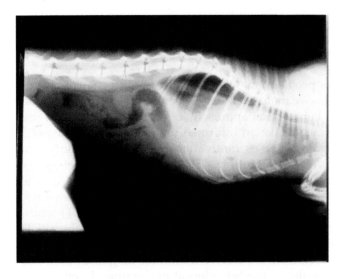

Fig. 4.2 X-ray of a cat with a hernia of the diaphragm, probably following a road traffic accident, which led to aggressive behaviour when the owner tried to pick it up.

Figure 4.2 shows an x-ray of a cat that was presented for sudden-onset aggression when the owner tried to pick it up. On closer examination, it was found that the cat's nails were frayed, suggesting that it might have been involved in a road traffic accident, and an x-ray of its chest showed that it had a ruptured diaphragm. It was not surprising then that when the owner went to pick it up round its belly, the cat reacted quite aggressively, as in effect they were forcing all its abdominal contents into its chest and nearly suffocating it!

### 4.4.4    MEDICINE AND THE ENVIRONMENT

The previously mentioned cases were all fairly obviously caused by ongoing medical problems. However, medicine and the environment can interact in other ways that are perhaps less obvious. Buffington (2002), in particular, has looked at the risks of a range of medical conditions in cats that are kept indoors versus those that are kept outdoors, as well as the effects of disturbance to their routine. The results of these studies suggest that a whole range of diseases are actually far more common in indoor cats, possibly as a result of stress. These illnesses include lower-urinary-tract disease, lesions of the teeth where the enamel is dissolved and the teeth start to break down, obesity and hyperthyroidism, which might be influenced by diet, exposure to fire retardants in the furniture and possibly chronic stress. We do not fully understand the relationship between stress and hyperthyroidism as yet, but, nevertheless, it remains an interesting point for consideration, which emphasises the importance of being aware of the impact the environment can have on the health of an animal. Cats experiencing changes to their routine have been found to be more likely to vomit and develop other minor ailments. Effective environmental management can help to minimise the risk of these problems and the need for costly medical care.

## 4.4.5   AN INTEGRATED RATIONAL APPROACH TO BEHAVIOUR PROBLEMS AND HEALTH

If we cannot divide behaviour problems into those that are purely behavioural and those that are medical, how do we manage them? Rather than exclude all medical factors and pursue a purely 'behavioural approach' to the problem, we must use professional common sense and make an informed judgement about the need for further medical investigation versus motivational–emotional exploration. Certainly, all cases should involve a careful physical examination by a veterinary surgeon and possibly further blood tests and/or urinalysis depending on the particular condition. However, the use of more specialist examinations, like x-rays, ultrasonography, neurological examination, computed tomography (CT) scans, magnetic resonance imaging (MRI) and positron emission tomography (PET) scans, obviously depends on whether or not they are indicated and how much more they can tell us. The information we receive from these diagnostic tools has to be balanced against the results of the behavioural exploration. In effect, we undertake a process similar to a risk assessment, in which we look at the probability and impact of identifying a medical factor relevant to the case. If the behaviour is very consistent and easy to explain on the basis of previous experience, there is little justification in doing a lot of medical tests in the absence of clear clinical signs. However, if the pattern is inconsistent from a historical point of view, or the reason for its consistency cannot be clearly identified, this may suggest a need for closer veterinary involvement and further medical tests.

There are a number of pieces of history and signs that might suggest the need for greater involvement of medical investigation:

- *Apparent potentially painful lesions*: If an animal has an obvious lesion which could be painful or a focus of pain that might at least partly explain the problem, the significance of this needs to be carefully evaluated.
- *Apparent neurological deficits*: If an animal has an overt neurological deficit (e.g. it walks in a strange way or perhaps crumples on its feet a little) then again this is a cause for concern.
- *Inherited and developmental neurological conditions*: Certain breeds are predisposed to certain inherited conditions, including a wide range of developmental neurological conditions. For example, dogs with a more domed head are at far greater risk of developing hydrocephalus, which in turn can lead to behaviour abnormalities, including aggressive behaviour.

Other factors in the history which might suggest medical involvement include:

- A sudden change in behaviour, particularly in a middle- or old-aged animal that previously demonstrated no behaviour problems.
- A history involving shifts in behaviour, which do not necessarily have to be related to the behavioural problem. An owner might state that the animal is 'moody' or perhaps that it has bouts in which it tends to demonstrate certain behaviours that at other times it does not show at all.

- Lack of generalisation of a behaviour. That is, the behaviour remains very specific and is not generalised in the way that we would predict from the animal's experiences.
- Very high or very low reactivity to the environment.
- Behaviours that do not seem typical for the ethology of the animal, such as licking a body part that is difficult to access.

Other factors that might act as flags for the potential need for further investigation include:

- *Age of onset*: Behaviour problems that start in rather old animals could be indicative of senile-related changes. So, for example, a case of separation anxiety that starts when the animal is eight years old, with no history of domestic trauma, of someone having taken a break from work or of someone having spent extensive time with the pet at home prior to onset is an unusual pattern and should perhaps raise concern regarding possible medical involvement.
- *Concurrent medication*: Any patient that is presented for a behaviour problem and is currently receiving any form of medication, whether it be for a behaviour problem or for any other problem, should be treated with special care. Recent work suggests that corticosteroids, which are widely used to control inflammation and pain, may bias the affective states of animals, making them more sensitive to aversive experiences.
- *Development of secondary behaviours*: Behaviour cases that present with a whole range of different behaviours, which may appear unrelated, also warrant closer medical evaluation. An animal that presents for aggression as well as sudden onset of some bizarre behaviours is certainly a cause for concern and may require extensive neurological tests to rule out a central-nervous-system lesion.

## 4.5   CONCLUSION

In conclusion, we should always treat clients with respect and sensitivity. Behaviour problems often make owners feel guilty and it is important to communicate clearly with clients to let them know that we care and that we will do what we can to help them with the problem. When investigating a problem, it is important to keep in mind the possible role of medical factors, and to think carefully about the full range of possible explanations for a given behaviour. Pain is an important motivational–emotional factor to consider in all cases. It is wise not to rush into drawing a conclusion without the evidence necessary to discount competing explanations, and it should be borne in mind that more than one form of motivational–emotional arousal may be active in a given situation. The aim of a behaviour history, an interview and additional tests is not simply to directly support an idea, but ideally to provide solid evidence by excluding other possible explanations. In order to do this, there may be a need for further expert help, and we should not be afraid to ask for this. Clients are often pleased to find out that a case needs further workup, because it affirms that it is genuinely challenging to understand and is not simply their fault.

## REVIEW ACTIVITIES

- Consider what criteria are used to label a presenting complaint as a behaviour problem and how confident we are that these criteria are met in any given case.
- When taking a history, it is critical to be able to differentiate between our observations and inferences. Consider examples of both of these and how they are related. How can we move from making observations to making inferences in a scientifically sound way?
- List the techniques available to you as a clinical animal behaviourist that can be applied to help gather more objective data regarding the presentation of a behaviour problem.
- Review the circumstances that would lead you to refer a case for further specialist evaluation and how you would identify these.
- List behaviour problems that might be caused by pain and how this might be identified.
- What aspects of the signalment and history would alert you to a higher risk of there being a medical component to a presenting behaviour problem?
- Undertake a risk assessment of some recent cases you have seen.
- How would you recognise a case that presents an unacceptable risk to you? What is your strategy for managing this and how will you implement this strategy?

## REFERENCES

Askew H (1996) Treatment of Behaviour Problems in Dogs and Cats: A Guide for the Small Animal Veterinarian. Oxford: Blackwell Science.

Buffington CAT (2002) External and internal influences on disease risk in cats. Journal of the American Veterinary Medical Association 220: 994–1002.

Voith V (1981) Profile of 100 animal behaviour cases. Modern Veterinary Practice 62: 483–484.

## FURTHER READING

Horwitz DF, Mills DS (2009) BSAVA Manual of Canine and Feline Behavioural Medicine. Gloucester: BSAVA.

Landsberg G, Hunthausen W, Ackerman L (2003) Handbook of Behavior Problems of the Dog and Cat. Edinburgh: WB Saunders, Elsevier.

Lindsay SR (2001–2005) Handbook of Applied Dog Behavior and Training (Vol 1–3). Ames, IA: Blackwell Science.

Mills DS (1995) Pathophysiological conditions in companion animal behavioural therapy practice. In: Proceedings of the 29th International Congress of the International Society for Applied Ethology. Potters Bar: UFAW. pp. 121–122.

Olm DD, Houpt KA (1988) Feline house-soiling problems. Applied Animal Behaviour Science 20: 335–345.

Stella JL, Lord LK, Buffington CAT (2011) Sickness behaviors in response to unusual external events in healthy cats and cats with feline interstitial cystitis. Journal of the American Veterinary Medical Association 238: 67–73.

# Chapter 5

# An Approach to the Management of Problem Behaviour

## 5.1 INTRODUCTION

In the previous chapter, we considered the assessment of the problem-behaviour patient. We focused on the skills involved in taking a behavioural history and the approach used to rationalise the available information in order to try to establish the most likely explanation for a given problem. In Chapter 2 we emphasised the importance of motivational–emotional considerations and in Chapter 4 we highlighted the potential significance of a range of medical aspects of the presenting complaint. It is also important for the clinician to clearly distinguish between those measures which serve to restrict a problem and those which offer longer-term resolution.

Restriction of the problem consists of measures aimed at the immediate minimisation of risk. The first priority is risk management. Once this is in place, greater consideration can be given to the implementation of longer-term strategies that address the motivation for the problem. At this time the primary concern is the welfare of the patient within the context of the risk-management recommendations.

Resolution consists of interventions which affect an animal's reactivity and style of response in the face of problem stimuli. These typically take some time to take effect, but should be the ultimate goal for clients if they genuinely care for the interests of their pet. Clients will normally engage with this process even if it is quite demanding of them, so long as they feel they have the necessary skills to do so and understand that it is important for their pet's well-being. In this context, the clinician may have to act as an advocate for the pet's interests, so that their importance is fully recognised, but they must also ensure that the client is properly equipped to cope with these demands.

### 5.1.1 FIRST PRINCIPLES

In this chapter, we consider a conceptual framework for potential management options. The adage 'Treat the patient, not just the disease' is as true for behaviour as it is for other aspects of care. This means that the management recommendations

*Stress and Pheromonatherapy in Small Animal Clinical Behaviour*, First Edition.
Daniel Mills, Maya Braem Dube and Helen Zulch.

need to be tailored to the individual patient within their domestic setting (the 'system' which includes the patient, as described in Chapter 1) as every client is different, with his or her own requirements and needs, which have to be considered in addition to those of the patient. Therefore it is important to provide management solutions that are suitable for both the individual patient and their family. There is no point overwhelming a client with tasks or suggesting things beyond their competence, and so we need to maintain a flexible approach to management, considering as many possibilities as we can, rather than specific 'recipes' for specific solutions. An important role of the behaviour counsellor is to try to help prioritise things for the client and advise them on both effective strategies for their given situation and their implications. In this chapter, we describe a framework for organising management options and reflecting on their impact on the welfare of the patient. These management options are focused on behaviour change, but it must be remembered, as discussed earlier, that ensuring owners have realistic expectations is essential, and in some cases management may focus solely on this, without the need to directly change the behaviour of the patient.

The first rule of management is, 'Do no harm'. Our intervention should not increase the risks discussed in Chapter 4 or make matters worse. When we consider the different management options that are available, it is important that the owner understands what is required and why. If they understand the reasons, they can also understand some of the common pitfalls. It helps enormously to be able to demonstrate the different techniques, rather than just instruct the owner about what needs to be done or give them a handout. It is also important to recognise that owners must be motivated to bring about change. We should not dictate to them or order them about, but rather encourage them to take the necessary steps and reveal to them the advantages that can be gained from this. The best theoretical management option is useless if the owner is not motivated to actually try it. In some cases with a complex behavioural plan, it might be necessary to use counselling skills to bargain with the owner, for example by saying, 'Well, I know that this is really hard to do, but if you can just agree to try it for a week and see how you get on, we can review things then'. If the owner thinks they only have to commit for a week then they may be more willing to actually instigate the behaviour-modification plan, and initiation of change is often one of the greatest barriers to progress. If, as we hope, the animal starts to change its behaviour during that week, the owner will be more likely to continue with the behaviour therapy because of the difference they see in their animal's behaviour.

## 5.2   BEHAVIOUR-MANAGEMENT OPTIONS: STRATEGIES AND TECHNIQUES

In our approach, we distinguish between management strategies and management techniques.

- *Management strategy*: A management strategy broadly defines in what way the problem behaviour is going to be brought under control. It is the mechanism underlying proposed changes in behaviour.

- *Management technique*: A management technique describes the method used to bring about that strategic change.

So the strategy might be to encourage another behaviour (i.e. increase the likelihood that another response will be elicited within the context that includes the problem stimulus), for example teaching a dog who barks at people to instead sit and look at the owner. The technique used to achieve this strategic goal might be considered psychological, if it involves training the animal through operant counterconditioning to produce another behaviour in response to the problem trigger stimulus, for example by rewarding the dog when it looks at its owner when at a distance from other people. A primary aim of this chapter is to illustrate how different types of strategy can be implemented via a range of different techniques, using a range of examples of varying practicality, for illustrative purposes only, in order to develop a consistent way of thinking about how to manage a given case. When deciding what is appropriate for a given case, we need to balance two important considerations:

- Which management options are likely to be effective *in this instance*?
- What are the associated risks to the short- and longer-term well-being of the patient and their associates?

## 5.2.1   *STRATEGIES FOR BEHAVIOURAL CHANGE IN THE PATIENT*

Counselling and coaching the owner is an integral part of the case-management process. It can include avoiding exposure to the trigger of the problem to a greater or lesser degree, which may be important in reducing the stress of the situation while the owner learns a new way of behaving towards their pet when the problem arises.

Whether we are simply explaining the nature of the problem behaviour to the client (or how they might best accommodate the animal's behaviour) or proposing change, we must not simply dictate our opinion, but work with the owner and their resources. However, in this section we will focus on the consideration of options rather than on how to deliver them, which is covered briefly in Part II, with further details available from the texts listed in the Further Reading section at the end of this chapter.

The strategies used to bring about change in a patient's behaviour can be grouped into four broad categories. While it is useful to consider them independently, we may typically combine several within a given treatment programme. The four strategies are:

1 *Prevent the problem behaviour from being expressed*: This does not necessarily direct the animal to a new specific goal, but (depending on the method used) might stop it from continuing to perform the unwanted behaviour, controlling the immediate risk and giving the owner a chance to introduce a longer-term behaviour-modification plan. An example of prevention might be the restraint of an animal to control the risk of injury.

2 *Do something about the immediate trigger of the problem behaviour*: This approach can be subdivided into two options:
  - Aim to remove or avoid the trigger, if possible, for example by rehoming a dog that is aggressing towards another dog in the family.
  - Aim to alter the animal's perception of the trigger, because, ultimately, the animal's response depends on its perception of the stimulus, rather than the presence of the stimulus per se (i.e. the message received rather than the signal sent). In this instance we might in effect teach the animal to ignore the stimulus or to evaluate it differently from an emotional perspective. This could involve altering the ability to detect the salient stimulus or altering the animal's interpretation of it. In this latter regard, pheromones may be particularly useful, for example by desensitising an animal to something that causes it anxiety, or altering the intensity of its arousal by a given stimulus.

3 *Allow the expression of the motivation underpinning the problem behaviour in a modified form*: We might redirect the animal's behaviour on to a different substrate or train a different response to the same motivation, for example. This means in effect that we still allow the same emotional processes to occur, but direct them into an acceptable expression, for example redirecting the attention of an indoor cat that has been 'attacking' the owner's toes to a toy tied to a string.

4 *Encourage specific alternative behaviours to replace the problem behaviour*: The aim here is to make other, alternative behaviours more attractive to the patient when it encounters the trigger stimulus. It then chooses the alternative response when it encounters the stimulus and so the problem behaviour is no longer expressed. An example might be teaching a dog that runs after bicycles to go into a down when a bicycle passes.

One of the challenges when dealing with problem behaviour is that owners are often focused on trying to stop the problem (Strategy 1) rather than building a more comprehensive and appropriate solution that better respects the animal's interests. Part of the counselling process involves encouraging owners to reflect upon what they want their animal to do, rather than on what they want it to stop doing, so that we can move beyond prevention and avoidance. This can be facilitated by explaining the likely impact on the interests of the patient of a focus on prevention and the value of a more comprehensive programme (see Chapter 4). Prevention measures may have a place, but usually only in association with strategies aimed at guiding the animal towards more acceptable expressions. Most owners can recognise the value of working towards more specific goals, especially when this is explained in a supportive context, for both them and their pet. However, the techniques need to be acceptable, and so we will consider these next.

## 5.2.2   *TECHNIQUES FOR BEHAVIOURAL CHANGE IN THE PATIENT*

The techniques are the methods used to bring about behavioural change. There are four broad ways that we can do this:

- *Environmental manipulation*: This involves changing the physical and/or social environment around the animal, for example by making sensory alterations to the environment, including pheromonatherapy, insertion of barriers and specific enrichments and so on. These changes create a different interaction with the environment.
- *Chemical manipulation*: This involves the introduction of one or more chemicals *into* the animal, through drugs, herbs, diet and so on. These are assimilated by the body, where they have systemic effects on behavioural regulation.
- *Physical manipulation*: This involves some form of physical manipulation of the animal, such as surgery, massage, physiotherapy, osteopathy, acupuncture and so on, which alters its responsiveness.
- *Psychological manipulation*: This involves a programme of structured stimulus exposure, aimed at bringing about a specific change in response, such as behaviour therapy, training and so on.

The choice of technique will not only depend on what is feasible in the circumstances but may also be affected by client preference, with independent input from the counsellor about the likely success of a particular approach in the current circumstances and its impact on the interests of the patient. This latter point is considered further in the next section.

## 5.3 IMPLEMENTATION OF A MANAGEMENT STRATEGY AND ITS WELFARE IMPLICATIONS

Every technique has its own specific risks, and these need to be considered before a final recommendation is made. But first it is useful to reflect upon the broader welfare implications associated with the strategic approach being adopted. We consider in this section how each of the techniques described in Section 5.2.2 can be applied within the context of a given strategy. In some cases, the examples are extreme and would not be used in practice, but they are useful illustrations that should encourage a systematic way of thinking about the strategic options available and their putative welfare implications before any specific recommendations are made.

### 5.3.1 PREVENT THE PROBLEM BEHAVIOUR FROM BEING EXPRESSED (STRATEGY 1)

Prevention involves the inhibition of the problem behaviour. It does not guide the development of a new specific goal and at best it is an inefficient strategy if used alone. At worst it can result in further frustration and serious welfare concerns. However, it may be necessary in some instances, perhaps in the initial restriction of the problem and management of risk. It may also be necessary in the longer-term resolution of the problem, for example to encourage appropriate decision-making in the presence of acceptable alternatives.

Specific examples, drawn from each of the broad techniques described in Section 5.2.2, are given below. This is not intended to be an exhaustive list and is merely illustrative. As stated previously, these are not necessarily examples which the authors endorse.

- *Environmental*: The use of a muzzle or a lead to prevent an animal from biting.
- *Chemical*: The use of a sedative to impair an animal's motor response, for example in the context of a veterinary examination.
- *Physical*: In dogs, surgical debarking has been described in the literature as a way of preventing the animal from performing the behaviour, but it is illegal in many countries.
- *Psychological*: The application of physical punishment in association with a behaviour to reduce its motivation, such as the use of booby traps to prevent animals from getting on to table tops and so on.

## 5.3.1.1   WELFARE CONSIDERATIONS REGARDING THE PREVENTION OF BEHAVIOUR

From these examples, it should be apparent that prevention of the behaviour alone is unlikely to be a preferred option in many cases, although it is likely to be the strategy that most owners have considered or used. It is also worth noting that its effects on the well-being of those associated with the problem are not necessarily negative and the significance of this needs to be carefully considered in every individual case. The impact on welfare in both the short and the long term should also be considered, as on some occasions a negative short-term impact may be outweighed by a positive long-term impact. This section lists the general pros and cons of an intervention strategy based around preventing the problem behaviour.

### Positive effects on welfare

- The effective prevention of a behaviour reduces the previous risk of harm to the self or others caused by the problem. So, for example, by muzzling a dog we prevent others from being bitten.
- In the longer term, preventing a response which is reinforcing to the patient may help the patient to make good choices and learn that an alternative response can be just as or more reinforcing.

### Negative effects on welfare

Preventing a behaviour does not address its underlying motivation and so may increase frustration or result in other negative emotional states, such as fear (e.g. from the use of physical punishment). When a muzzle is applied in the absence of any other strategic intervention, for example, the animal is still motivated to bite when threatened and so may become very frustrated.

- Prevention of a behaviour will also typically reduce the ability of the animal to adapt in some other contexts. For example, the wearing of a muzzle or the inhibition of aggressive displays through the use of punishment may inhibit the ability of a dog to defend itself if attacked.
- Whatever intervention we use, we must appreciate that every management option carries its own specific risks. This is a factor that has to be considered for every intervention, no matter what strategy is used or what particular method is implemented to achieve it. The use of a muzzle, for example, may prevent a dog's ability to pant and hence to thermoregulate in hot weather.

## 5.3.2   DO SOMETHING ABOUT THE IMMEDIATE TRIGGER OF THE PROBLEM BEHAVIOUR (STRATEGY 2)

As mentioned in Section 5.2.1, if we wish to address the immediate trigger of the problem, we have two options: to try to remove it or to try to alter the patient's perception of it. Each of these is considered in this section.

## 5.3.2.1   REMOVAL OR AVOIDANCE OF TRIGGER FACTORS

Each of the broad techniques described in Section 5.2.2 can be used to achieve this strategy:

- *Environmental*: Rehoming one animal in a case of intraspecific aggressive behaviour in the home. Walking the dog at times when other dogs are unlikely to be encountered in the case of aggressive behaviour towards unfamiliar dogs.
- *Chemical*: The use of drugs to treat a skin allergy that is causing self-injurious hair-pulling behaviour.
- *Physical*: The use of surgery to correct a lesion causing joint pain which is making an animal irritable and aggressively self-protective when approached.
- *Psychological*: The use of an extinction programme to eliminate the perceived reward that reinforces and maintains a specific behaviour.

### *Welfare considerations regarding removal or avoidance of trigger factors*

Although it might seem ideal to remove the trigger of problem behaviour, in practice it may not always be practical or desirable for the owner, for example in the case of rehoming. Although in some ways the trigger might be seen as the 'cause' of the problem, it is important to appreciate that the trigger stimulus is not the same as the risk factors which lead to the behaviour. Risk factors include features of the individual and its historical and current circumstances, including the ongoing attempts at management of the problem.

## Positive effects on welfare

Removal of the trigger also removes any welfare issues linked to it. This is particularly important when the problem results from poor features of the environment. By addressing these factors, we have the potential to eliminate the suffering associated with living in that environment.

- From a human–animal-interactions perspective, the avoidance of the behavioural response may bring considerable relief to the owner in the short term, even if it is not feasible in the longer term. This can allow them to develop the confidence and skills necessary to bring about the required behaviour change using one of the other strategies.
- Removal of the trigger means that the problem behaviour is no longer expressed and so any harm caused by it is eliminated. However, this does not mean that new behaviours will not develop in relation to similar stimuli, which may also be harmful.

## Negative effects on welfare

Although there are no general negative impacts with this approach, the risks of any specific intervention need to be considered. For example, in the case of an extinction programme, one of the characteristics of the removal of the reward of a behaviour is an intensification of the behaviour before it starts to fade away (a so-called *extinction burst*). This may not be acceptable for certain behaviours. The removal of the reward can also generate frustration and in animals that are so predisposed may result in an increased risk from aggressive behaviour.

## 5.3.2.2 *ALTERING THE PERCEPTION OF THE TRIGGER OF THE BEHAVIOUR*

Again, hypothetical examples exist for each of the four broad techniques listed in Section 5.2.2.

- *Environmental*: The use of pheromones to encourage an animal to perceive its circumstances as nonthreatening, safe or secure.
- *Chemical*: The use of anxiolytic drugs or 'calming' food supplements, which act centrally to reduce the tendency to perceive something as potentially a threat or promote a positive mood which reduces potential sensitivity to negative events.
- *Physical*: The neutering of a male cat so that certain odours in the environment are no longer perceived as relevant and the tendency to respond to them in a potentially problematic way (such as by spraying) is reduced. A more drastic example is the use of olfactory tractotomy, in which the nerves relaying chemical messages from the main olfactory epithelium are obliterated. This has been described as a treatment for persistent spraying in the cat.
- *Psychological*: Systematic desensitisation, in which an animal is gradually habituated to the stimuli causing inappropriate arousal. This means that it no longer perceives the triggering stimuli as salient to the emotional reaction which causes the problem.

# Welfare considerations when using techniques that produce a modification in perception

## Positive effects on welfare

- Since the animal no longer performs the problem behaviour, welfare issues relating to that behaviour, such as its emotional associations or its impact on others, also disappear.
- In situations where the problem behaviour is associated with the animal's perception of the environment as being aversive, the alteration in perception means the animal may no longer perceive the stressors as significant threats to its well-being. However, the fact that it might still be in a poor environment is potentially an ethical concern.

## Negative effects on welfare

- By using techniques that cause changes in processing and reactivity to general events, we might alter the way an animal perceives other related factors as well, which could be problematic. For example, with the use of anti-anxiety medication, an animal may not respond appropriately when a real danger is present and so put itself at risk. In the case of the removal of the sense of smell to control urine spraying, the animal may experience appetite suppression.
- We also have to be aware of the specific risks associated with a given technique.

## 5.3.3  ALLOW THE EXPRESSION OF THE MOTIVATION UNDERPINNING THE PROBLEM BEHAVIOUR IN A MODIFIED FORM (STRATEGY 3)

Each of the four broad techniques given in Section 5.2.2 can be used to bring about the expression of a modified form of the behaviour, such as its redirection onto a new substrate or its expression in a less damaging form:

- *Environmental*: The provision of a scratch post or litter box.
- *Chemical*: The injection of lithium chloride into carcases. This has been described as a way of redirecting scavenging, since it makes the animal that consumes the meat sick, thus encouraging it to seek other food sources when motivated to scavenge.
- *Psychological*: The training of an animal to use a specific toilet area.
- *Physical*: Declawing, which does not prevent a cat from engaging in the behavioural sequence associated with scratching but does prevent damage. Similarly, amputation of the tail of a self-mutilating tail-chaser stops it from chasing its tail. Note such measures are not permitted under normal circumstances in the UK and certain other countries but are illustrations of what can be done.

## 5.3.3.1 *WELFARE CONSIDERATIONS REGARDING THE ALTERATION OF THE WAY IN WHICH A MOTIVATION IS EXPRESSED*

When only the form of behaviour is modified, it is important to recognise that the underlying motivation and emotional associations remain the same, and so the welfare of the performer has not actually changed in this regard. However, there are other welfare considerations associated with this strategy.

### *Positive effects on welfare*

- If the problem behaviour is causing harm or distress to others, then, by directing it away from them, we are resolving their welfare problems. So if we have a cat that is attacking other cats because it wants to play, we increase the other cats' quality of life if we redirect the attacker's play towards inanimate toys.
- If an animal is suffering reprisals from an owner when it expresses a behaviour in its current form, altering the behavioural expression in the short term may improve its welfare while other long-term measures are put in place.

### *Negative effects on welfare*

- The main concern here relates to the risks intrinsic to a given technique.

## 5.3.4 *ENCOURAGE SPECIFIC ALTERNATIVE BEHAVIOURS TO REPLACE THE PROBLEM BEHAVIOUR (STRATEGY 4)*

Encouraging the patient to do something else is the mainstay of most training programmes. An animal has a choice as to what it wants to do at any given time, and so often when we train an animal we are seeking to encourage it to make its decision in a particular direction: the one we believe is appropriate. This can be done by increasing inhibitory control of the problematic behaviour and/or increasing the tendency for a specific alternative to be expressed. We can encourage a particular behaviour through any of the four broad techniques:

- *Environmental*: The provision of food bowls where a cat soils, so that this area becomes a feeding station rather than latrine. Encouragement of the application of a feline facial mark where a cat has been scratching, by applying extracts of the normal facial mark in this location.
- *Chemical*: The use of serotonergic agents or their precursors to reduce impulsivity, so that the animal makes a carefully evaluated choice rather than a more immediate decision.

- *Psychological*: The use of either operant or respondent counterconditioning to encourage a particular behaviour in response to the problem stimulus. This might include focusing on the owner and letting them take control of the perceived problem.
- *Physical*: If a male roams or seeks conflict with other males then neutering reduces the motivation for sexually related roaming and associated behaviours and so allows other motivational–emotional considerations to become a greater priority.

## 5.3.4.1  *WELFARE CONSIDERATIONS WHEN ENCOURAGING AN ALTERNATIVE BEHAVIOUR*

### Positive effects on welfare

- When we encourage a new behaviour to be expressed, the problem behaviour should disappear, and with it any associated welfare problems. For example, with a dog that is jumping up at people, the risk of it injuring them, or upsetting children, disappears when the dog is taught to sit quietly instead.
- A new behaviour may be associated with a more positive emotional state. Thus we may replace frustration or anxiety in a given context by encouraging a positive motivational–emotional bias associated with the expression of the new behaviour. This approach also eliminates threats to the welfare of the performer associated with the original problem stimuli.

### Negative effects on welfare

- As with every strategy, there are specific risks associated with any management option. For example, neutering is associated with the risk of anaesthetic complications, wound healing and aftercare.

## 5.4  MANAGEMENT OPTIONS SHEET

By thinking about management options in this way, it is easier to brainstorm for possible solutions to a problem by simply asking the question, 'What specific methods can be employed using each of the possible techniques to achieve each of the five strategies?' Figure 5.1 presents the basis of this question in the form of a grid. This can also be used as part of a counselling aid, since different options can be presented to the owner and discussed with respect to their impact on the pet's interests according to which cell they fill. In some circumstances, adding some options which we know the owner will find unacceptable and which we would not really recommend (perhaps because they are too complicated or time-consuming) can help to encourage the owner to adopt other options which they might otherwise

| | Environmental manipulations | Chemical manipulations | Psychological manipulations | Physical manipulations |
|---|---|---|---|---|
| Prevent expression of the behaviour | | | | |
| Remove triggers of the problem | | | | |
| Modify perception of triggers | | | | |
| Alter expression of motivation | | | | |
| Encourage alternative activities | | | | |

Fig. 5.1  Management options grid.

resist because they perceive them to be personally demanding. It is also worth emphasising that for a given problem, several potential management options might fall within the same cell and it may be beneficial to implement more than one of them at the same time or in sequence.

## 5.5  BRINGING ABOUT BEHAVIOURAL CHANGE IN THE CLIENT

In order to change the behaviour of the patient, we probably need also to bring about a change in the owner's behaviour and in their beliefs and attitudes towards the animal and its problem. We may need to modify the animal's environment (owner's home or routines) to a greater or lesser extent and motivate the owner to change their behaviour towards the animal, although sometimes we might simply try to counsel the owner to accept the behaviour and adjust their expectations. The *transtheoretical model of change* provides a useful framework for evaluating the type of support a client will need at different times in order to bring about a change in their behaviour. This model was developed by Pochaska and DiClemente following an analysis of a range of psychotherapies. While popular with medical clinicians, it is worth emphasising that it is not without its critics. Within the model, there are five core constructs:

- *The stages of change*: It is proposed that there are six stages in the cycle of events that lead to long-term behavioural change (Figure 5.2). An important element of effective counselling is to identify at which stage the client is (different clients within the same household may be at different stages) and then use appropriate strategies to bring about the necessary shift. If a client is in a state of *precontemplation*, they may not even be aware of the need for change. An example is the

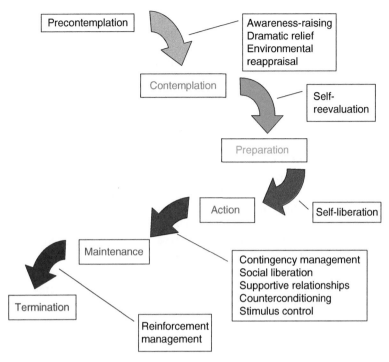

**Fig. 5.2** Stages and processes of change within the transtheoretical model. Arrows indicate the shift from one stage to another, while call-outs indicate the processes which may be necessary to enable this change.

client who has unrealistic expectations of their pets or expects the clinician to sort the problem out for them. During *contemplation*, a client is considering change, but is perhaps uncertain of exactly what change to make or how much is required. During the *preparation stage*, the client is beginning to commit to change by making some investment in planning for what they perceive to be necessary. During the *action stage* they are beginning to take the necessary steps to bring about a lasting change in their behaviour. During *maintenance* they are focused on establishing these new patterns on a more permanent basis. If this is successful, they exit the change process and the cycle is terminated.

- *The processes of change*: These consist of a variety of cognitive and behavioural processes, whose importance varies depending on where an individual is within the change cycle. Generally speaking, cognitive, affective and evaluative processes need to be supported early in the cycle, while conditioning, contingency management, appropriate relationships/commitments and control over the environment are more important in the later stages. To shift a client from precontemplation to contemplation requires the counselling skills associated with awareness-raising, such as encouraging a reevaluation of the client's environment or some form of emotionally significant event. For example, a client might suddenly seek help for their dog, who has never been good around children as a result of a near accident.

Before this, they did not really perceive the need for action. To move from contemplation to preparation requires the client to reevaluate their circumstances and acknowledge the changes that are necessary. It is important to establish that this has occurred before the end of the initial consultation, as otherwise change is unlikely to be made and the prognosis is very poor. The benefits of change and the new freedom it will bring the client are important motivating factors for the shift from preparation to action and will need to be emphasised by the clinician if the client's intentions for change are to become a reality. The development of action into a sustained pattern of behaviour is the area that is perhaps given most emphasis in traditional problem-behaviour-management texts. It involves processes such as enabling stimulus control, contingency management, counter-conditioning and the development of helpful relationships. Finally, in order to establish the new pattern of behaviours as an integral part of the norm for the client and terminate the cycle, attention needs to be given to the management of reinforcement during the maintenance phase. This is where support during follow-up and the celebration of success can be key.

- *Decisional balance*: This is the weighing of pros and cons, and often careful counselling is the key to tipping the balance in favour of change, especially when clients recognise the outcomes of a cost–benefit analysis of a change versus no-change scenario.
- *Self-efficacy*: This relates to the importance of empowering clients and building self-confidence in their actions. Making clients feel empowered and able to make change is among the most important requirements for a commitment to a change programme. Clients must feel they can implement the proposed management plan agreed with the clinician. For this reason, the counsellor must encourage clients to discuss any concerns they have, so that they can be addressed before the end of the consultation.
- *Temptation*: This describes the urge to engage in a particular habit in difficult situations. It is important to recognise when temptation to engage in old ineffective habits (such as trying to punish the animal) is likely to occur and discuss with the client how these situation will be more effectively managed. There may be a need for additional support at these high-risk times, and letting the client know that the clinician is available to help can be very useful.

## 5.6   CONCLUSION

In conclusion, it is important to tailor management plans and recommendations to the individual case, which can be done relatively easily with a systematic approach. By using the management-options sheet (Figure 5.1), we have a mechanism to think about a broad range of solutions to any given problem, and by considering the transtheoretical model of change (Section 5.5), we have a way to prioritise our counselling efforts. We must set realistic goals as a consequence.

With a range of options available, we next need to consider not only how effective they may be in theory but also how practical they are going to be in reality, as well as their impact on the welfare of the patient. It can be useful during the counselling process to discuss a range of options with a client and let them choose the ones they think are most suitable for themselves. In this way, we can help to empower them and so help them make the changes necessary in their own behaviour to resolve the problem. Finally, when treating a behaviour problem, a variety of different strategies may need to be combined in order to bring about change with maximum efficiency, but it is important not to ask clients to do too much at once as they may be overwhelmed, and to ensure that the recommendations are relevant, by being as precise as possible with our assessment. Clients asked to do too much often end up either doing very little or not doing things very well, neither of which is desirable or likely to be successful in achieving the goal of modifying the pet's behaviour. It is also unrealistic to expect the average client to become a skilled trainer as a result of a single session or demonstration, so it is often best to focus first on simple changes.

## REVIEW ACTIVITIES

- Create a prompt sheet of key factors to be borne in mind when designing a management programme for a patient.
- Consider a range of procedures commonly used to bring about a change in behaviour and where these fit within the management-options grid.
- Complete a grid for the management of a behaviour problem of your choice. Attempt to complete as many cells as possible, and evaluate each proposed strategy for its impact on the interests of the patient and of the client. It may help to systematically ask yourself what method could be used to implement a given strategy using a specific technique for each cell (e.g. 'How might I prevent the problem using an environmental intervention?' etc.).
- Consider the sorts of expression clients might use within each stage of the change cycle. How would you respond to these in order to either move the clients on or support them as necessary?
- Consider ways in which the process of change can be supported at different transition points in the cycle of change. For example, what might constitute a supportive relationship (and what would definitely not)?

## REFERENCE

Prochaska JO, Diclemente CC (1982) Transtheoretical therapy: toward a more integrative model of change. Psychotherapy: Theory, Research & Practice 19: 276–288.

## FURTHER READING

Blackwell E, Casey RA, Bradshaw JWS (2006) Controlled trial of behaviour therapy for separation-related disorders in dogs. Veterinary Record 158: 551–554.

Egan G. (2006) The Skilled Helper: A Problem-Management and Opportunity Development Approach to Helping (4 edn). Belmont, CA: Thomson Learning.

Horwitz DF, Mills DS (2009) BSAVA Manual of Canine and Feline Behavioural Medicine. Gloucester: BSAVA.

Hough M (2002) A Practical Approach to Counselling. London: Prentice Hall.

Landsberg G, Hunthausen W, Ackerman L (2003) Handbook of Behavior Problems of the Dog and Cat. Edinburgh: WB Saunders, Elsevier.

Lindsay SR (2001–2005) Handbook of Applied Dog Behavior and Training (Vol 1–3). Ames IA: Blackwell Science.

Todd J, Bohart AC (1999) Foundations of Clinical and Counselling Psychology. New York, NY: Longman.

# Chapter 6

# Principles of Pheromonatherapy

## 6.1 INTRODUCTION

In this chapter, we consider in more detail the nature of 'pheromones' used in clinical behaviour management, and their general indications. The circumstances in which 'pheromones' are not indicated are also discussed, since the effective use of pheromonatherapy depends on recognising when they are unlikely to be of assistance. This text aims to provide a fuller understanding of the potential and limitations of pheromonatherapy, about which there is still much to be learned; as discussed in the Introduction, there is confusion in the field, sometimes relating to the application of outdated and limited scientific approaches to the subject matter, which can lead to erroneous conclusions about the value of this mode of behaviour management, especially with regards to improving the welfare of animals with a range of problem behaviours. We should also empha- sise again at this point that we do not wish to be distracted by arguments over the meaning of words and the way they are used by different individuals. We will use the word 'pheromone' in places where some might prefer 'semiochemical'; by using 'pheromone' thus, we do not want to imply assumptions about the way these chemicals bring about their effects in other species or contexts beyond those discussed here.

## 6.2 DEFINITIONS OF PHEROMONES AND PHEROMONATHERAPY

### 6.2.1 PHEROMONES

The definition of *pheromones* has changed with time and indeed the terminology has developed as we have gained a deeper appreciation of the complexities and subtleties of chemical communication in different species. A classic definition was provided by Karlson & Lüscher (1959), who described them as 'substances secreted to the outside by an individual and received by a second individual of the same

*Stress and Pheromonatherapy in Small Animal Clinical Behaviour*, First Edition.
Daniel Mills, Maya Braem Dube and Helen Zulch.
© 2013 John Wiley & Sons, Ltd. Published 2013 by John Wiley & Sons, Ltd.

species, in which they release a specific reaction, for example a definite behaviour or developmental process'. If this reaction were a specific behaviour, the pheromone might have been called a *releaser pheromone*, but if it were a developmental process, then they tended to be called a *primer pheromone*. Pheromones were originally identified in insects, which are subject to simpler behaviour control, and because of their apparently predictable effect on physiology and behaviour, analogies were made with the hormone chemicals which are released internally. Indeed, in some texts the term 'ectohormone' has been used. However, even in insects we now recognise that behavioural control and development are much more complex than was envisaged over 50 years ago. A key feature of the scientific process is the acceptance of new evidence and the revision of ideas as a consequence.

In mammals, the first reported pheromones related to sexual behaviour, perhaps as a result of a superficially similar relationship between chemical signals and behaviour. Given the importance of the optimal timing of breeding behaviour, it is not surprising that chemical signals which indicate the optimal time for mating have evolved. These chemicals, which are often single molecules, are produced by the female according to her stage of ovulation, and cause sexual arousal in males and intensify sexual activity. The phenotypic similarities with the pheromones identified in invertebrates are obvious. A chemical stimulus appeared to trigger sexual behaviour in a typical stimulus–response style. However, we now know that this model of behavioural regulation is naive, and as discussed in Chapter 2, most behaviour is not subject to such simple control processes. It may be that because sexual behaviour is only expressed in very clearly defined contexts and is typically very intense (due to its biological importance in the ultimate determination of the fitness of an individual at a genetic level), the complexity of its regulation has often not been appreciated. An important scientific development in the study of pheromones and the chemical regulation of behaviour has been the recognition of the importance of a range and mixture of semiochemicals in this process; that is, that some of these signals are chemical mixtures rather than single compounds. As a result, the term 'social odour' is preferred by some when referring to pheromone-like substances in higher animals. We will continue to use the term 'pheromone', for reasons explained previously (see Introduction), and the discussion that follows relates to these chemicals in animals with a limbic brain. As different types of chemical signal are used to convey different types of message, it would be a mistake to consider that they all act through a similar mechanism. For some signals, such as those released in response to alarm, there is clearly an advantage if they intrinsically induce an emotional (affective) bias, which can shift the attention or ongoing priorities of the animal, for example towards strategies associated with harm avoidance, such as increased vigilance, caution or even overt flight. The bias allows the animal to operate more efficiently in uncertain situations (e.g. when it lacks direct information about the presence of a threat, such as a predator); it does not replace attention to clear, unambiguous stimuli, but rather helps in the calculation of the balance of probabilities.

Some have suggested that the term 'pheromone' be abandoned, as they believe it is an artificial and somewhat arbitrary distinction in semiochemistry. They argue that since we do not generally distinguish between signals conveyed using other channels that evoke a strong behavioural response and those that are more informational, we should not do so for chemical signals. They suggest it is inconsistent to refer to a chemical that induces sexual arousal as a pheromone when an image that has the same effect is not classed as a special class of visual signal (a 'visuomone', perhaps). While there is some merit in this argument, in that it highlights that there is some inconsistency in terminology between different disciplines, we suggest that its conclusion is not useful. It argues for a simplification of chemical communication, which will inhibit a deeper understanding of this subject. It might also be suggested that it oversimplifies the study of visual perception, in which a distinction is made for certain visual signals that seem to have specific dedicated processing systems, such as the configural processing associated with face perception. Indeed, perhaps certain visual signals that might have an intrinsic emotional quality, such as changing velocity during approach or looming over an animal, should be distinguished. Thus, in our opinion, the conclusion we draw from the inconsistency should not be the need for greater simplification, but rather a need for greater diversity in our description of signals.

An important point to appreciate is that the affective bias associated with a pheromone signal is the default position in the absence of signals to the contrary or other learned associations. It may be that if one of these signals is reliably paired with a clear signal that evokes a different emotional response, the bias will be lost. At present we have no data one way or the other, but it seems a reasonably likely possibility in mammals, given the flexibility of their behavioural systems.

A second important aspect, related to the preceding point, is that just because a chemical signal induces an emotional response it is not necessarily a 'pheromone'. Other semiochemicals used in a social context may produce no intrinsic emotional bias but still be very important to individuals, such as the chemicals associated with individual identification. The chemical identification of a specific individual may evoke contrasting emotional responses in different animals, according to whether that individual is associated with positive or negative experiences; that is, whether they are a 'friend' or a 'foe'. The emotional impact may be strong, depending on the intensity of the associated experiences, but these associations are learned and not intrinsic to the properties of the molecules used for individual identification and how they are detected; hence mixtures such as this are not considered pheromones.

The situation of chemical perception is further complicated by the finding that in many social situations a blend of pheromones and nonpheromonal chemical signals may be provided (not to mention signals using other channels). Again, depending on the signal that the animal is communicating, this is an efficient strategy. So, for example, if an individual decides to initiate an affiliative interaction with an unknown other, the combination of chemical signals indicating identity together with signals that induce a positive bias will increase the likelihood of this being reciprocated. By contrast, if an individual seeks to distance itself from others, the combination of identity with an intrinsically aversive stimulus may help to avoid unnecessary conflict. Unlike taste and olfaction, which are more 'open' senses of chemical detection – that is, there is extensive incidental monitoring of chemicals the whole time, through the anatomical location of the relevant sense organs – pheromonal detection is more targeted and time-constrained. The vomero-nasal organ (VNO) is not open to chemical detection in the normal course of events, and therefore pheromone signals often need to be accompanied by some other signal, which may be a more typical chemical signal, such as a distinctive odour, or a signal engaging one of the other sensory modalities, such as vision. This accessory signal allows the affective element of the message to be recognised. This also means that it is possible for chemicals which may be more widely present in the environment at other times to act as pheromones, since their potential emotional impact can be limited to contextually relevant circumstances. The signal released only becomes a meaningful message once it is detected by the receiver (see Chapter 3).

A fundamental point to appreciate in the scientific debate concerning phero-mones is that phenotypic similarity is no guarantee of mechanistic similarity; that is, similar phenomena may arise from mechanistically different processes depending on the complexity of the system involved. Thus the regulation of behaviour by chemical signals in an ant may be quite different to that which occurs in a mammal, which processes much more information from its environment (see Chapter 2). Given the complexity of the process of chemical communication in mammals, it seems that the original definition of Karlson & Lüscher is not really appropriate. Therefore it may be that a term other than 'pheromone' would be useful to describe the chemicals that are detected via the VNO, such as 'limbic semiochemical', but at present there is no consensus on this. An alternative approach, which we favour, is to allow adaptation of the definition of the term 'pheromone', since there is a broad understanding of the general properties of these signals, and recognise a diversity of definitions in different contexts. This requires that a clear statement be made of how the term is being used in a particular situation. To this end, we propose the following definition for the purposes of this text:

> In animals with a limbic brain, the term 'pheromone' refers to chemical signals which are normally used in intraspecific communication, which are typically detected through the VNO and which appear to have an intrinsic effect on the emotional processing of the receiver.

Thus not only can we refer to 'alarm pheromones', which encourage a motivational–emotional predisposition towards *anxiety–fear*, and 'sexual pheromones', which that encourage *lust*, but also other types of pheromone that influence other motivational–emotional predispositions.

## 6.2.2 PHEROMONATHERAPY

The term *pheromonatherapy* describes the use of chemical signals normally involved in intraspecific communication within a clinical context to manage the behaviour of animals.

There are three features of this definition to note:

- *Range of chemicals used*: The definition does not limit pheromonatherapy to the clinical use of pheromones as defined in Section 6.2.1. It embraces a wider range of semiochemicals (but not all chemical signals), since some of the chemicals used may not have an intrinsic emotional impact, but rather regulate behaviour in other ways. For example, some of the chemicals deposited during scratching may simply encourage this behaviour at the given site. This signal can be used to redirect scratching away from furniture and on to more appropriate substrates, without necessarily containing an affective element. Such chemicals are included in pheromonatherapy, since like pheromones, they are not dependent on learning for their effect.

- *Species involved*: The chemicals we use in therapy are derived from the chemicals that are normally used in *intraspecific* communication; that is, the communication between individuals of the same species. However, we might use them in another context to that originally intended in nature; for example, we might use a cat pheromone to help a cat to accept a dog in the house.
- *Clinical context*: When we talk about something being used in the *clinical context*, we mean it is being used in order to treat the sort of problem that we would see in a clinic; we do not mean that we are dealing with a medical problem.

## 6.3 PHEROMONES: CREATING BIAS RATHER THAN TRIGGERING BEHAVIOUR

The female Asian elephant shares the same sexual attractant pheromone as over 140 species of moth – (Z)-7-dodecen-l-yl acetate – but mammals and insects are not likely to confuse each other when it comes to selecting a mate. This is not a frivolous point, because it illustrates a principle fundamental to understanding pheromonatherapy. Pheromonatherapy is used to bring about changes in the environment, not by dictating behaviour but by creating biases. In clinical pheromonatherapy, the species which are being treated are highly developed cognitively and so these biases are not typically at the level of specific behaviour, but rather at a higher organisational level such as motivational–emotional predisposition or functional strategy. Neurological studies aimed at elucidating the central effects of clinically used pheromones are currently very rare. At the time of writing, only one study has been published. This used positron emission tomography (PET) scanning to visualise in real time the areas of the brain affected by the pig-appeasing pheromone compared to a nonbiologically relevant odour (amyl acetate) and a negative control. This found that exposure to the appeasine rather than the control odour was associated with increased activity in the parietal lobe (24%), the hypothalamus (5.7%) and to a lesser extent the temporal lobe (1%) (Figure 6.1). Although we do not know exactly which processes in the brain were affected by this increased activity, it is interesting to note that the parietal lobe is a region that is (amongst other functions) involved in assessment of novelty, familiarity and the intensity of emotional responses.

Accordingly, pheromonatherapy needs to be used in consideration of the totality of information being provided by the environment, in order to try to help manage the situation. It is therefore useful to understand which pheromonal

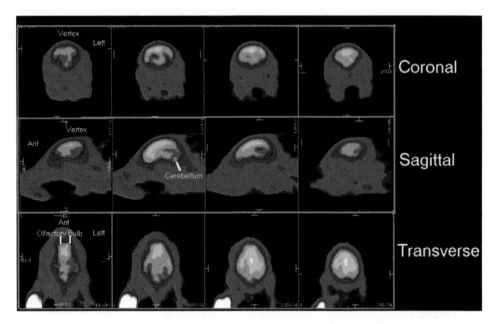

Fig. 6.1 PET-scan image of a pig exposed to pig-appeasing pheromone. Regions of greater neural activity are shown in lighter colors (Ant = anterior, i.e snout; Vertex = dorsal). The lighter areas indicate activation of the parietal lobe (images courtesy of John McGlone, taken from Anderson *et al.*, 2001).

signals are used to send which messages. Unfortunately, understanding the exact meaning of the signal being sent by the species with which we are concerned is an area lacking much specific empirical research, and so some of what follows is a personal perspective on a subject which will undoubtedly remain a focus for future research.

## 6.4   CHARACTERISTICS OF SIGNALS USED IN PHEROMONATHERAPY

Typically the semiochemicals used in pheromonatherapy have the following characteristics:

- They are generally secreted by specialised sebaceous, sweat or mucous glands associated with the skin or related ectodermal structures.
- They are organic molecules of variable volatility. Many of these signals appear to be based on fatty acids, though the steroid precursor, squalene, has recently been attracting attention too. Volatility is linked to the biological function of the signal.
- Naturally, very small amounts are produced, but when used clinically, much higher levels are required. This is to maximise the chances of the signal being detected, especially in the absence of an accessory signal to encourage the engagement of the VNO.

- They are generally *unconditional signals* insomuch as they bring about a change without there being a requirement for learning. However, as stated earlier, that does not mean that their impact is unaffected by learning or experience.

If an animal responds in a particular way to detection of a pheromonal signal, it may actually establish a new behavioural pattern that is maintained even in the absence of the semiochemical. This is a very important feature of pheromonatherapy, because by bringing about changes in behaviour in a natural multisensory way, the animal learns in effect to self-correct the problem behaviour and maintain the response in the longer term.

## 6.5   SOURCES OF PHEROMONES IN THE CAT AND DOG

Although there has been considerable work on sexual pheromones, these are not the focus of this text. In a clinical behaviour context, the semiochemicals involved in communicating other information are of more interest. These chemicals are released from a variety of different areas across the body (Figures 6.2 and 6.3).

A region of major clinical interest is the skin around the mammary glands. Shortly after a female gives birth, as the young become mobile, she seems to produce a group of chemicals which have a reassuring effect on the young. The signals, referred to as appeasines, seem to be based around a core of oleic, palmitic and linoleic acids, together with a species-specific signature. We think they help to orientate the young as they begin to move around their environment, as well as help them extend their perception of safe stimuli in the environment. By detecting this signal, the young can rapidly perceive and then learn using the other senses the features of a safe area, because wherever the mother has laid down and deposited the chemical in the vicinity of the nest, it is likely to be safe.

Another area of interest is the facial area, from which signals are produced in the perioral and cheek regions of the cat and the ear of the dog. In the case of the cat, there appear to be at least five common fractions, consisting of varying proportions of some well-known fatty acids (including azelaic, butyric, isobutyric, oleic, palmitic, pimelic and proprionic acid). The functions of the first and fifth fractions (F1 and F5) remain unknown; F2 appears to be associated with sexual marking and performance by males; F3 is involved in spatial orientation, antagonises urine marking and scratching and may be some form of familiarisation or safety signal; and F4 is involved in allomarking and may play a role in social acceptance.

Interestingly, the pheromone produced in the region of a dog's ear seems to be very similar to the appeasine produced by the bitch and may be some form of safety signal that provides reassurance. Dogs that are part of the same social group may be observed to sniff the ear, especially of those who tend to take the initiative in controlling the resources of the group, and may then flehmen. This 'safety' signal may help to coordinate group activity and allow individuals to conserve resources and relax in the presence of its sender.

By contrast, some of the chemicals that are produced from the foot pads of cats and dogs are associated with alarm pheromones and territorial marking.

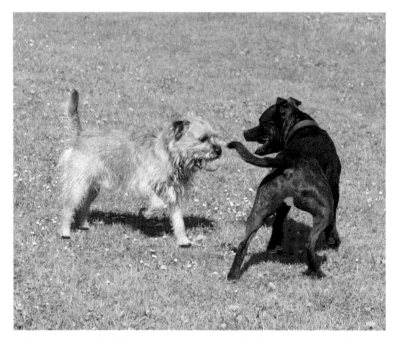

Fig. 6.2 Significant pheromone-producing regions in the dog: ears (blue), foot pads (purple), genitalia (green), anal sacs (red) and intermammary sulcus (not shown).

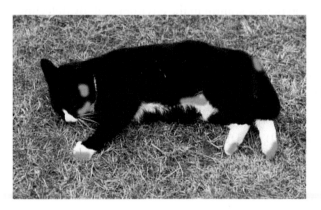

Fig. 6.3 Pheromone-producing regions in the cat, shown in blue: cheek and perioral regions, foot pads, tail base and intermammary sulcus. The significance of the flank as a pheromone site remains uncertain.

In a veterinary practice, a scared animal on an examination table may produce these signals and thereby leave a powerful message behind, which can be picked up by the next animal and perhaps encourage it to be anxious and try to escape in the face of uncertainty. It is therefore important to clean the table thoroughly between animals, with an agent that not only minimises the risk of infection but also denatures these compounds. As already mentioned, the foot pads in the cat also produce a chemical signal that encourages scratching behaviour.

Pheromones are produced by other skin glands in the perianal region. These include:

- *The supracaudal gland*: Production from this gland varies with sexual status and it is not uncommon in the tomcat for it to become infected – a condition called stud tail – which may affect its pheromonal activity.
- *The circumanal glands*: In the dog, this includes the anal sacs, which are a receptacle for the secretion of the surrounding glands. It seems the composition may change with circumstance, and bacterial activity on the secretions appears important in this regard. Both the circumanal glands of the cat and the anal sacs of the dog produce pheromones that are associated with alarm, in addition to a range of other chemicals such as those associated with individual identity. Raising and movement of the tail may help in diffusing and transmitting these signals between individuals. Infection of the anal sacs in dogs can alter the chemical signals they send, resulting in the attraction of other dogs or possibly provoking aggressive behaviour from them. This is probably due to a change in the resident bacterial flora or the products being released by these. While antibiotic treatment will eliminate the infection, it may also have an impact on the normal flora and change the signals being produced. If a dog is presented for getting involved in apparently unprovoked fights, it may well be that anal-sac infection or the use of antibiotics is playing a part in the problem, and this should be checked and addressed as part of the management programme.

Finally, a variety of pheromones are produced in the urogenital region, including the prepuce of the male and the lips of the vulva and clitoral fossa of the female. These chemicals convey information about sexual status in particular.

Not all the chemicals produced from these different glands are used clinically; in fact, the pheromone products that are currently commercially available for clinical use are derived from just two areas:

- The facial region in the cat (F3 and F4).
- The region around the mammary glands of the dog (dog-appeasing pheromone, DAP).

A new product is in development which is derived from the signals released by the pads of the cat, which can be used to encourage animals to scratch on an appropriate surface.

The theory behind the use of pheromonatherapy is that if we can use these chemicals in environments that might be perceived as uncertain and possibly overtly aversive, we can help communicate that they are less threatening than they might seem. However, the exact way in which the environment is perceived as aversive may be important to the efficient use of this treatment modality. This is why understanding the motivational–emotional predispositions of animals (discussed in Chapter 2) is so important. For example, trying to use a signal that is typically associated with a social interaction to treat a perceived threat to physical resources may not be effective. Pheromonal signals affect perception within a given context; this is also why we cannot simply refer to these products as having general psychoactive properties, such as being anxiolytic. Our diagnosis needs to be more specific and recognise not only different types of aversive emotional response (*pain, anxiety–fear, panic–grief* and *frustration*) but also their context (e.g. in relation to physical or social stimuli).

## 6.6   COMMERCIAL PHEROMONATHERAPY

### 6.6.1   *CHEMICAL IDENTIFICATION AND PRODUCTION PROCESS*

While rubbing a cloth on one animal has been used in the management of behaviour problems for many years, the French veterinarian Patrick Pageat has really led the development of pheromonatherapy as a clinical discipline by isolating the individual chemicals involved in clinical pheromone therapy from the complex that exists in the natural secretion.

The path from identification of natural secretion to clinically evaluated product is complex and spans many different disciplines, from analytical chemistry and chemical communication to clinical veterinary trials (Figure 6.4). There are many reports of the clinical efficacy of pheromones in a variety of conditions, and these are referred to in Part II in relation to specific conditions. This text will focus on those conditions for which clinical trials have been conducted and show good evidence of efficacy. While we understand the principles involved in pheromone therapy, it is fair to say we still have a lot to learn about the underlying mechanisms.

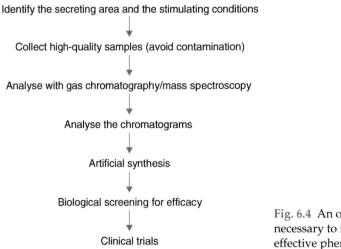

Identify the secreting area and the stimulating conditions

Collect high-quality samples (avoid contamination)

Analyse with gas chromatography/mass spectroscopy

Analyse the chromatograms

Artificial synthesis

Biological screening for efficacy

Clinical trials

Fig. 6.4  An overview of the stages necessary to identify and produce effective pheromone products.

### 6.6.2   *NATURAL VERSUS SYNTHETIC PREPARATIONS*

As already mentioned, once the natural chemicals have been identified it is necessary to artificially synthesise an effective formulation. There are several differences between the natural and the synthetic preparations:

- The commercial product is inevitably a simpler mixture than the naturally occurring one, and while clinical trials are used to establish efficacy, we cannot be sure that the message conveyed is the same as that when the mixture is contained in a larger complex of compounds.

- Often the commercial product is applied in a different way to the natural substance; it may, for example, be diffused into the air via a diffuser rather than applied on a specific object, since the distribution of the signal to a wider environment is desired. It is also easier for clients to administer the product in this way. DAP is also available as an impregnated collar. Thus the specific environmental contexts associated with the pheromonal signal are different.
- Because the products are generally used without an adjunctive signal (i.e. one that encourages the use of the VNO in the environment concerned), the concentration of the signal used in the clinical context needs to be many times higher than that which occurs naturally. In the case of one product ('Feliway$^®$' F3 spray), a herbal extract has been included to encourage the detection of the signal when sprayed on to a surface and the subsequent use of the VNO, but this is not the case for other formulations which include F3.

## 6.7   PHEROMONATHERAPY VERSUS PHARMACOTHERAPY AND AROMATHERAPY

Given that pheromone products are typically applied to the environment in which the animal lives, and from there are detected using the olfactory–vomeronasal apparatus, rather than being administered directly into the patient, these chemicals are quite different to medicines. This has both therapeutic and legal implications. As discussed in Chapter 3, the VNO is quite different to the main olfactory epithelium in terms of its innervations and projections, so pheromonatherapy is also different to aromatherapy, which typically uses nonbiologically active odours. We consider both of these comparisons in more detail below.

### 6.7.1   AROMATHERAPY VERSUS PHEROMONATHERAPY

Aromatherapy is the use of certain odours (i.e. chemicals detected by the main olfactory epithelium), especially essential oils, in a therapeutic context, often to achieve some degree of stress relief. The indications may therefore appear quite similar to those for pheromonatherapy. However, there are important differences:

- The word 'aroma' implies an intrinsic link with 'smells' detected by the main olfactory epithelium, which are not the focus of pheromonatherapy. Any odour used in pheromonatherapy is purely adjunctive, to aid the detection of the pheromone; that is, the primary sensory target is not the main olfactory epithelium.
- Aromatherapy uses much less refined preparations than pheromonatherapy, which involves the application of more precise mixtures identified within a secretion. This means that aromatherapy may include a wider mix of agents,

possibly including some products that are active on the VNO, but this is often incidental and unspecified. A notable exception to this is the terpenols in lavender oil, which have a known therapeutic effect on sleep.
- Aromatherapy often uses plant-based mixtures, whereas pheromonatherapy is based upon animal signals. Thus any effect through the limbic system is more incidental than engineered, whereas in pheromonatherapy this is central to its normal and clinical biological activity.
- Aromatherapy is also commonly used in association with various forms of touch therapy, such as massage, which may itself have relaxing effects. The effects of the odour may then be a conditioned association in some cases, whereas pheromonatherapy does not depend on such associations.

## 6.7.2  PHARMACOTHERAPY VERSUS PHEROMONATHERAPY

As already discussed, the interaction between external receptors and the pheromone chemicals means that changes in normal functional processes are produced, which in turn lead to a change in perception, and so any change in the behaviour of the animal is as a result of its normal functional physiological processes; that is, it is a self-correction by the animal. Thus, the disciplines centred around chemodynamics and chemokinetics are largely irrelevant to pheromonatherapy, beyond the issue of chemodetection by the surface receptors; however, understanding these processes is obviously critical to studying the therapeutic and side effects of drugs. Many of the drugs used for the management of behaviour problems act by changing transmitter activity in all associated receptor sites throughout the brain and the rest of the body or establishing a consistent level of a hormone. As a result, their use is often not only associated with changes in the functionality of a wide range of behavioural and physiological systems which may not be relevant to the problem behaviour but also with more fundamental structural changes to the body, such as direct changes in receptor sensitivity and a change in the endogenous production of the compound that the drug may be mimicking. This can explain the development of some of the unwanted side effects, dependencies and problems associated with withdrawal. The body may adapt to the provision of an exogenous supplement by producing less of the endogenous equivalent, so that when the drug is withdrawn, the endogenous production may not meet the need. Similarly, receptors may change their sensitivity, so that when the exogenous drug is removed, they are insufficiently sensitive to endogenous stimulation, as they have adapted to higher levels of stimulation from the therapeutic drug.

While animals may relapse after a course of pheromone therapy, the reasons for this are quite different to those described for pharmacological agents, and we do not have the same problems of withdrawal. Relapse following the use of pheromonatherapy often indicates that the treatment period was not long enough, that a more fundamental problem with the environment needs to be addressed or that a new problem has arisen with a similar manifestation.

Psychopharmacology provides a powerful method for bringing about central reorganisation of neurotransmitter activity related to problem behaviour, since in effect it reconfigures the animal's physiology to ensure a reliable behavioural response. There is often also a dose-dependent potency – that is, the level of effect is related to the level of the drug – whereas such an observation has not been made in the case of pheromonatherapy. Indeed, the level of efficacy appears to relate to the intensity of the stressor rather than the level of the pheromone; that is, pheromones will work up until a certain point, but if they do not then increasing the dose beyond the recommended therapeutic level is unlikely to make a difference. However, a downside to both the potency and mechanism of psychopharmacology is the risk of unwanted side effects. This is much higher with drugs than with pheromonal products. There are also many contraindications for the use of drugs, since they need to be metabolised and excreted efficiently (a feature of their pharmacokinetics) if they are not to become toxic. Again, such problems are not seen with pheromonal products, assuming they are indicated for the problem. This risk may be one reason for choosing a pheromone product in preference to a drug. It is not surprising therefore that drugs are only available through veterinary practices, whereas pheromonal products are more widely accessible. However, this should not be a reason for deciding between the two. If medication is indicated, it should be used, regardless of the clinician's professional training. A vet should be consulted if the clinician is not appropriately qualified to recommend the use of medication.

Individual studies have suggested some favourable comparisons between pheromone products and psychopharmacology, but many of these have been underpowered and so unlikely to pick up some potentially important therapeutic differences. Statistical meta-analysis provides a way of overcoming this problem. There have been sufficient studies of urine spraying in cats to allow a meta-analysis of treatments comparing drugs with pheromone products, but the conclusions are not as straightforward as we might like. It has been found that both modalities are effective, with the drug fluoxetine most effective, followed by clomipramine. However, closer analysis of the data reveals that the drug trials generally involved treatment over a longer timescale, so it is uncertain whether the difference is due to duration of treatment or the nature of the products used. Further studies are required before a firm conclusion can be drawn about this.

Pheromones are not alternatives to drugs, but rather an integral part of case management, which may include pharmacological intervention as well. The aim should always be to provide the most appropriate management programme for the case in question, not to advocate a personal preference. However, there are other factors beyond the clinician's immediate influence to consider relating to client preferences and compliance.

Some owners may look for a medical solution, and while there may be grounds for using medication in a case, for the reasons discussed earlier, it should be clear that pharmacology is not a solution on its own. It is important for clients to realise that a 'pill is not the solution', and neither is a collar or a spray; even if long-term medication or pheromonatherapy is required, it needs to be combined with an understanding of the nature of the problem, plus additional environmental and psychological intervention techniques as necessary to minimise dependence on these adjuncts and any associated risks. When medication has been prescribed, an integrated approach might include the use of pheromonatherapy or nutritional support to help minimise the necessity or possibly the dose of medication required.

At the other extreme is the client who is vehemently opposed to the use of drugs in the management of behaviour problems. While the final decision about the choice of specific therapies is the decision and responsibility of the client (in consultation with the clinician over a range of recommended treatment techniques), they should not simply dictate their preferences without discussion of the reasons why their stance may not be in the best interests of their pet, if the clinician is of the opinion that medication is necessary. Pheromonatherapy may be useful in this context, in a number of ways. First, some owners like the idea of using a 'natural' solution instead of drugs, which they perceive as artificial. Second, the recommendation of pheromonatherapy can be used as a counselling aid to allow the later implementation of medication as required. Thus it might be agreed that some adjunct beyond training and behaviour modification is required (e.g. to improve the well-being of the patient while the problem is corrected) and pheromonatherapy can then be used as a first line; in doing this, the clinician can guide the client to agree that if satisfactory progress is not made within an agreed timeframe (4 weeks is a typical recommendation), they will accept the need for further chemical intervention. Nutritional supplements can be used in a similar way. There is no strong evidence of a cross-reaction between any medication and pheromone product, but, anecdotally, it seems that DAP may potentiate the effect (but not affect the elimination and so toxicity) of benzodiazepines in some animals.

Another client-related difference between the two techniques concerns compliance. Delivering oral medication is inevitably more difficult than the environmental application of pheromones. Indeed, in some cases it may not be safe for the client to attempt dosing with tablets. However, in other cases the process of medication may itself become part of the behaviour modification plan, as it requires close interaction between the pet and its owner. Assuming this is safe to do, it may become a structured activity that helps to frame their relationship. Generally, however, client compliance is quite limited when it comes to medication. One study has suggested that if medication needs to be given once a day, 80% compliance can be expected; twice a day and the figure drops to just under 70%; three times a day and the figure drops below 40%. By contrast, pheromonatherapy requires, at most, daily or as-needed application of a spray to affected areas, and at best simply plugging in a diffuser and leaving it on for a month. However, there can be problems even with this. For example, in the absence of personal advice, many owners still do not read the instructions and so may not realise that there are two parts to the diffuser which need to be put together, that the device should be left on the whole time (not switched on and off) and that the reservoir level should be monitored and replaced as appropriate.

### 6.7.3 GENERAL CONSIDERATIONS FOR THE PRACTICAL USE OF PHEROMONATHERAPY

When using pheromones in practice, the following should be kept in mind:

* *Pheromones do not replace drugs*: Based on the differences between pheromones and drugs (see Section 6.7.2), one cannot be substituted for the other. In animals that are severely affected, it may be necessary to use both products together.
* *No treatment is without risk*: Toxicological studies have been conducted during the development of pheromone products to confirm their safety, but the occasional idiosyncratic response does occur. In the authors' experience, this is usually related to confusion over the combination of signals being presented to the animal, especially if there is a strong learned aversion to a particular stimulus and a pheromone is used to counteract this. The carrier used in the product formulation is generally safe, even for people with severe respiratory compromise.
* *Inappropriate use*: In the experience of the authors, the most widely encountered reason for an apparent lack of response to pheromonatherapy relates to the inappropriate recommendation of its use. In a very small number of animals there may be an 'increase in behavioural activation' associated with the use of pheromonatherapy, with an increased risk of 'frustration-related activities' as a consequence. In general, the currently available products do not appear to be very effective in conditions where frustration features as a significant motivational–emotional factor underpinning the problem behaviour, although this can be difficult to determine in some contexts. For example, if a dog is destructive when left alone, is it being destructive primarily because it is responding to the disappearance of an attachment figure (*panic–grief*) or because it is seeking something outside that it cannot get to (*frustration*) or for some other reason? This particular problem is discussed further in Chapter 8, with the general importance of identifying significant underlying motivational–emotional systems associated with the expression of a problem behaviour being discussed throughout Part II of the text.
* *Importance of appropriate location*: There are occasional reports of people placing pheromone products in inappropriate places. For example, they plug a device in behind the sofa only to find their animal wants to get close to it and so scratchess at the sofa and causes increased damage. This should not be mistaken for ineffective treatment.
* *Individual variation*: As with any treatment, not all individuals react in the same way. Generally, it is a good idea to tell the owner to observe their animal closely during the first few days after introducing the pheromones to the environment. Inflammation of the VNO has now been reported and this might limit the efficacy of products in some individuals, as might anatomical differences from selective breeding, but this requires further investigation.
* *Assessment of handler risk*: Since pheromones are administered externally, there is minimal risk associated with handling the animal while trying to administer the treatment. Also, there is no risk of owner abuse of the treatment, as can

unfortunately occur with some psychoactive medications. However, owners must be encouraged to adopt ways of behaving that are consistent with the chemical signals they are using in pheromonatherapy.

- *Interaction*: Pheromone products are reasonably species-specific, although there may be some crossover in closely related species. Also, the presence of one pheromone does not generally inhibit the detection of another, so if an owner has a cat and a dog who both require treatment, there is no risk of cross-reaction, or of any effect on themselves.
- *Behavioural control*: These products do not release or inhibit behaviour directly, but rather create certain biases in the individual which may encourage the expression of certain behaviour patterns depending on the circumstances. The goal is that these replace the undesirable problematic behaviour. Within pheromonatherapy, some chemicals might have more direct effects on behaviour, such as those that encourage scratching on a particular substrate, but these still work by way of communicating a message rather than through direct neurological control of behaviour.

## 6.8  PHEROMONE FRACTIONS USED IN DIFFERENT CONTEXTS

In this section we briefly review the different pheromone fractions that can be used in different contexts. In Part II, we will consider particular problems and problem scenarios in which pheromones can form a useful part of treatment.

### 6.8.1  FELINE FACIAL FRACTION F3 (FELIWAY®)

The F3 facial fraction is widely used as an aid in the management of urine spraying, in handling for minor procedures (e.g. putting in a catheter line), in the control of scratching and in the management of chronic interstitial cystitis. It is also used to reduce the impact of transport and hospitalisation stress and overnight roaming. For all of these indications, there have been clinical trials, with the exception of scratching, for which there is a lot of anecdotal evidence. This suggests that F3 used as a diffuser may reduce some forms of scratching and as a spray applied to specific areas will redirect the behaviour to another location. In general, certain forms of delivery are preferable for specific indications, as detailed in Table 6.1.

### 6.8.2  FELINE FACIAL FRACTION F4 (FELIFRIEND®)

There have been far fewer studies on the use of F4 than on F3. But F4 has been trialled in the following situations:

- Reduction of aggression towards unfamiliar people.
- Reduction of aggression between cats.
- Helping cats settle in shelters.

Table 6.1  Appropriate methods of delivery for specific indications for F3.

| Indication | Method of delivery |
| --- | --- |
| Urine spraying | Diffuser |
| Vertical scratching | Spray |
| In-clinic handling | Diffuser |
| Hospital cage | Spray (use 10–20 minutes before cat enters the cage) |
| Domestic disruption | Diffuser |
| Transport | Spray (use 10–20 minutes before cat enters the carrier) |
| Stress-related illness | Diffuser |

Table 6.2  Appropriate methods of delivery for specific indications for DAP.

| Indication | Method of delivery |
| --- | --- |
| Settling into a new home | Diffuser |
| Kennel-related problems | Collar |
| Puppy classes | Diffuser |
| Reducing stress in the veterinary clinic | Diffuser |
| Fear of fireworks or other noises | Diffuser in the home, spray on to a bandana when out |
| Aversion to novel stimuli in the home | Diffuser |
| Behaviours associated with distress during the owner's absence | Diffuser |
| Behaviour problems in the car | Collar, or spray on to a bandana |
| Anxiety while outside | Collar |

It seems that the F4 fraction is involved in social familiarisation; that is, helping a cat to accept new or existing members into its social group or at least tolerate their physical proximity with reduced distress.

### 6.8.3  DAP (ADAPTIL®)

DAP is available commercially as a spray, a diffuser and an impregnated collar, and has been reported to be useful in trials associated with the following behaviour problems: separation-related problems, sound sensitivity, adaptation to a new home, travel-related problems in the car, performance in puppy classes and the long-term outcome of such classes on the behaviour of the dog, adaptation to the veterinary hospital, barking and adaptation to the kennel environment. There are also a number of case studies relating to its use in a wider range of anxiety-related problems, including attention-seeking behaviour, some cases of owner and object protectiveness including certain forms of territoriality and some forms of compulsive behaviour; these all seem to be mediated by anxiety and insecurity. As with F3, different formulations are considered more appropriate for different circumstances, as detailed in Table 6.2.

## 6.9   CONCLUSION

In conclusion, pheromonatherapy is usually both safe and effective if used properly, but as with any intervention it is important to establish that the proposed indication is appropriate. The pheromone products currently available tend to help to reassure an animal about some aspect of its environment. In the case of cat pheromones, a useful distinction can be made between social stressors and physical stressors; that is, whether the cat's behaviour is motivated by physical or social considerations. If the problem behaviour is related to some threat to the physical environment (e.g. threat to resources), F3 is preferred, whereas if the behaviour is related to more direct social threats from other cats, people or other social stimuli, using the F4 fraction may be preferable. Having established which pheromone formulation is indicated, consideration needs to be given to the appropriate delivery system to be used; that is, to which will be most effective in the situation and easiest for the client to apply. The appeasines seem to provide a form of safety signal, possibly associated with the security normally provided by the presence of another animal.

It is also important to realise that *pheromones are not a 'cure all'* and often additional behaviour therapy will be required to resolve the problem. Therefore, it is important to monitor progress and adapt the treatment strategy accordingly. If good progress is being made, we would recommend continuing with pheromone treatment for at least a month after there is no noticeable change in the intensity of the behaviour being targeted. If progress is not made as expected, the case needs to be carefully reassessed and additional or alternative measures should be implemented as necessary. This may include the use of medication, since phermonatherapy and pharmacotherapy can be used effectively together.

## REVIEW ACTIVITIES

• Develop a client handout on pheromonatherapy to reassure them about its value in managing problem behaviour but also alert them to its limitations.
• Produce a diagram showing the main pheromone-producing regions of the cat and dog and the behaviours used in the transmission of the relevant signals to another animal.
• Create a list of presenting complaints for which pheromonatherapy might be considered.
• Discuss the indications leading to a preference for either pheromones or medical drugs in a given situation where the two might potentially be indicated. When might both be used?
• What is a safety signal and how does it differ from an anxiolytic?

# REFERENCES

Anderson DL, Bellon M, Chatterton B, McGlone (2001) PET studies of pig brain activity with biologically relevant and non-relevant odors. HiRes (Small Animal Imaging Meeting). Rockville, MD, 9–11 September 2001.

Karlson P, Lüscher M (1959) 'Pheromones': a new term for a class of biologically active substances. Nature 183: 55–56.

Mills DS, Redgate SE, Landsberg GM (2011) A meta analysis of studies of treatment for feline urine spraying. PloS ONE 6: e18448 1–10. Available from http://www.plosone.org/article/info%3Adoi%2F10.1371%2Fjournal.pone.0018448.

# FURTHER READING

Ceva Animal Health (2011) Adaptil Feliway Comprehensive References. Data compendium, available from Ceva UK.

Doty R (2010) The Great Pheromone Myth. Baltimore, MD: Johns Hopkins Press.

IRSEA (2010) 15th Anniversary International Symposium. DVD set available from http://www.biosemstore.com/fr/7-dvd-irsea.

Pageat P, Gaultier E (2003) Current research in canine and feline pheromones. Veterinary Clinics of North America 33: 187–211.

Wyatt T (2003) Pheromones and Animal Behaviour. Cambridge: Cambridge University Press.

# PART II

# Clinical Scenarios Involving the Management of Stress-related Behaviour Problems

This part of the book focuses on some conditions that can be stressful for cats and dogs and highlights the importance of recognising the diversity of 'stress' from an emotional perspective. We consider a number of presenting complaints and issues relating to the care of cats and dogs, and discuss how these can be managed more effectively if an assessment of the motivational–emotional basis of the behaviour is recognised. Special emphasis is given to the role of pheromonatherapy in this context.

*Stress and Pheromonatherapy in Small Animal Clinical Behaviour*, First Edition.
Daniel Mills, Maya Braem Dube and Helen Zulch.
© 2013 John Wiley & Sons, Ltd. Published 2013 by John Wiley & Sons, Ltd.

# Chapter 7

# Feline House-soiling Problems

## 7.1   INTRODUCTION

In this chapter we focus on house soiling by cats in response to stressors in the home. However, it is important to realise that a wide range of behaviours can present in response to different types of stressor in the home – some of these will be indicative of distress while others will be signs of adaptation. There is growing evidence to suggest that urine spraying by a cat is predominantly a behaviour expressed in response to a stressor, but it may not be a reliable sign that the cat is currently distressed. By contrast, frequent attacking of another cat over resources is clearly both a response to a stressor and a sign of distress. Either may be problematic for the owner, but obviously the welfare implications of the two types of behaviour are not the same. Pheromonatherapy might be useful in both cases.

## 7.2   WELFARE CONSIDERATIONS

### 7.2.1   *SOURCES OF STRESS IN THE HOME ENVIRONMENT*

In humans, one of the most commonly reported stressors is having to deal with people who do not seem to understand you, and this is probably just as important to pets. Understanding the needs and the methods of communication of our companions is at the heart of many harmonious relationships, and failure in either of these often leads to tension. There are specific events focused around a cat's territory which warrant particular attention:

- *Attempts to create a new social group for the cat*: For example, when a new cat is introduced and they are expected to socially bond and to share common resources, rather than simply tolerate one another (see Chapter 11).

*Stress and Pheromonatherapy in Small Animal Clinical Behaviour*, First Edition.
Daniel Mills, Maya Braem Dube and Helen Zulch.
© 2013 John Wiley & Sons, Ltd. Published 2013 by John Wiley & Sons, Ltd.

- *Changes in the surrounding environment which impact on the cat's resources*: For example, a new cat in the neighbourhood, or a high density of cats in the home or the neighbourhood.
- *Return of a (human or animal) family member that has been away*: For example, when a member of the family has to be away from home for a while, such as to visit the vet. This is likely due to a change in their odour or other chemical signals when they return, which the pets that stayed at home do not recognise (see Chapter12).
- *Unfamiliar odours, such as those introduced during DIY activities*: Sometimes, simply bringing new shopping bags home may result in spraying on them. Some cats tend to spray on electrical items, possibly because as they warm up they emit novel odours.
- *Inappropriate domestic facilities*: This includes minimalist homes but also things like toilet facilities placed in inappropriate areas or in insufficient numbers given the number of social groups.

The impact of some of these events on cats is the focus of this chapter.

The potential effect of a common stressor for humans on their pets was highlighted in a short case series from Australia relating to moving home. This reviewed the changes noted by 193 owners. Around 19% of cats were reported to show signs of anxiety prior to the move and 36% showed signs of anxiety following the move. The most commonly reported signs were:

- Increased vocalisation after the move (30%).
- Elimination problems (21%), especially in the first week after the move.
- Over-grooming (13%).
- Fighting with neighbourhood animals (32%).

The figures for dogs were worse (47% showing signs of anxiety afterwards), and only 33% of owners thought their pet was happier after the move. Although most animals settled within 3months, this is clearly a commonly overlooked stressor, which could be managed more effectively and simply with pheromonatherapy.

Another problem that is commonly reported by owners is a cat running away after a move, although no data seem to be available for this. However, one study from France reported that by using F3 the chances of this could be reduced.

## 7.2.2   *HOUSE SOILING AND WELFARE*

The term 'house soiling' is used here as a description of the presenting sign, since it literally means soiling in the house, without any inference as to why this might occur (this is not the case with all texts on the subject, so the reader needs to be careful). This is a serious problem, and according to one study was the main behavioural reason for the relinquishment of cats to shelters. The other main reasons were problems between pets, aggression towards the owners and destructive behaviours. House soiling can also be a sign of a more immediate welfare concern for the cat, since it may indicate certain painful medical conditions requiring

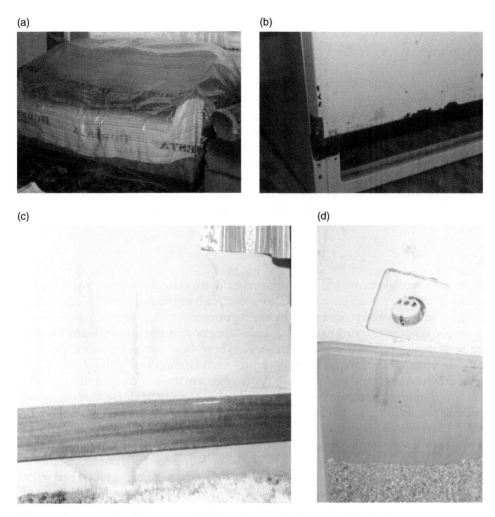

**Fig. 7.1** House soiling by a cat can lead to changes in the owner's lifestyle, such as having to cover up furniture (a). Urine spraying can damage the home, causing corrosion to items (b) or wall coverings (c). It can also be potentially dangerous, such as when a cat eliminates over an electricity socket (d).

veterinary attention or be associated with threats and other aversive features in the environment. The occurrence of the behaviour can lead to attempts at punishment by the owner, which is a further cause for concern.

The problem can also seriously compromise the owner's well-being, as illustrated in Figure 7.1, ranging from changes in their lifestyle to property damage or even electrical faults. This can damage the bond between the cat and their owner, which is stressful in its own right, quite apart from the cost of fixing any damage that is caused.

However, if treated appropriately, the outlook for cases of house soiling is typically very good.

## 7.3   THE BIOLOGY OF HOUSE SOILING AND EVALUATION OF THE PROBLEM

The first requirement when presented with a case of house soiling is to differentiate marking from elimination behaviour. The owner's knowledge or awareness of the problem should not be taken at face value. Any cat that is not using the litter tray may be described as spraying by an owner, or any urine outside the box thought to be due to a toileting problem. It is important to differentiate whether the cat is marking or showing latrine-related behaviour. To do this, it is useful to make reference to the natural characteristics of each behaviour and how they might relate to the current problem. Bear in mind that a cat may show both. However, if there is only one condition present, treatment can be more precise and easier for the owner.

### 7.3.1   MARKING BEHAVIOUR

Marking can involve urine and/or faeces and tends to occur in response to a perceived potential threat to resources or the environment. Such resources can include breeding potential, and so we can count sexual spraying in males in this category. When a male sprays, he is not only trying to attract females but also to protect this resource; that is, the opportunity to breed with a female. However, there are many other types of resource that might be threatened, and the presence of a new cat or some other change in the environment could be seen as a potential threat to these and trigger urine marking. It is important to remember that animals of concern may simply appear in the garden; they do not need to come into the house itself. Alternatively, the presence of new odours within the home can be perceived as a potential threat to the stability of the core area, which may elicit urine spraying. This is why shopping bags can be marked as soon as the owner gets home. The behaviour tends to be one that occurs at times of high arousal, and is associated with a characteristic behavioural sequence and posture (Figure 7.2). Typically the cat will smell an area first, possibly flehmen (an open-mouthed gaping which looks almost as if the cat is panting), before turning, raising and quivering its tail, and squirting a variable amount of urine. The volume of urine deposited is not a reliable indicator of marking or latrine behaviour. It is also important to note that an estimated 10% of neutered males and 5% of neutered females are reported to spray at some time. Marked areas are typically areas of prominence or significance to the cat and are separate to latrine areas.

### 7.3.2   LATRINE BEHAVIOUR

Latrine behaviour can obviously involve urine and/or faeces and typically occurs in relatively quiet or secluded areas towards the periphery of a cat's territory. Separate latrines are typically preferred for urine and faeces, and this may lead to the problem being presented with one type of elimination still occurring in the litter tray and the other not. Cats typically prefer to eliminate on soft, rakeable substrates, but individuals do vary in their preferences, and some problems arise

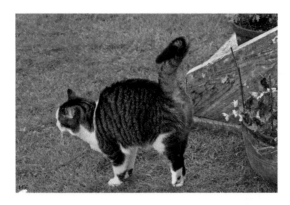

Fig. 7.2 Characteristic posture of urine spraying (picture courtesy of A Dossche).

not because of an overt aversion to the litter tray but because of a strong attraction to another substrate and location. However, if there is a problem with the latrine area provided by the owner, this can lead to the cat experiencing distress. There is growing evidence of medical problems among cats from households with litter-box problems, and this may reflect an influence of pain on the condition. If elimination in the box is painful, the cat may make an association between either the box or its location and pain, and then start to look for alternative sites. It is important to remember that the behaviour problem can persist as a learned behaviour long after the actual medical problem has disappeared.

Thus both failure to use a litter tray and marking behaviour can be seen as responses to stressors in the home environment, although these are qualitatively different types of stressor and so require different treatment regimes.

## 7.4    IDENTIFYING IMPORTANT CONTINGENCIES

### 7.4.1    LOCATION

An efficient way of finding out where the problem is occurring is to ask the owner to draw a map of their home and indicate where the eliminations are found, distinguishing between urine and faeces (Figure 7.3), and also to note the frequency and whether there has been any change in the locations over the course of the problem. This is very simple for clients to do and does not require great artistic ability but can provide a wealth of information. The distribution of the marks may help guide you towards the nature of the underlying problem, as might changes over the timeline of problem development.

### 7.4.2    IDENTIFYING THE CAT CAUSING THE PROBLEM

The owner may have their suspicions, but it is important to establish why they feel it is one particular individual and not another. They may assume that it is the new cat because the behaviour only started after the new cat arrived. However, it may

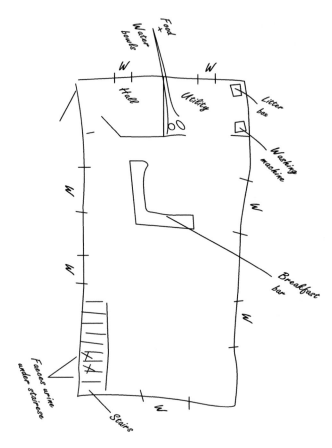

Fig. 7.3 Maps can be very informative in showing the location of the problem relative to the landscape of the environment. In this case of house soiling, it is useful to note that urine and faeces are being deposited in a more secluded area away from the litterbox, which is next to a washing machine and close to the feeding area, neither of which is conducive to a good latrine.

be that one of the original resident cats is distressed as a result of the new cat's arrival and is responding by marking. It is always useful to ask owners how the cats get on. If the owner has several cats, asking them to watch the cats and record which tend to rub against and lick each other, or sleep together, and which tend to have the odd 'spat' or simply avoid one another consistently can yield useful information about their social organisation. By recording this, the owner may become aware that they have two or three subpopulations within their home and that certain cats never interact closely. This can indicate that there is tension within the social group.

It is also worth asking the owner about the behaviour of the cats within the litter box, although even if they do not have a covered tray they may never have watched the behaviour with any interest. Cats with an aversion to the litter box tend to scratch less within the litter; they may go into the litter tray and come out without actually eliminating. If owners have observed these types of behaviour, this can indicate some problem with the litter box itself. Similarly, if they have never observed the animal going into the litter box, this may indicate a problem at that level as well.

In multi-cat households, it is also important to appreciate that it may be more than one particular individual that is creating the problem. There are many ways in which the animal(s) concerned can be identified.

## 7.4.2.1   URINE AND/OR FAECES

* *Isolation*: One method is to isolate the suspected culprit and to look at whether or not the problem stops. However, it may be that if one cat is taken away, other cats stop marking because the source of the problem has been removed. Hence, it is better to use other methods.

## 7.4.2.2   URINE

* *Observation*: If a cat consistently goes to a particular area, it is relatively easy to set up a video camera in order to try to catch it in the act. The owner may have actually seen the cat engage in the behaviour, but it would still be a good idea to set up a camera in case another cat uses the same area at a different time (especially in apparently refractory cases).
* *Fluorescein*: Fluorescein dye is used to identify ulcers in the eye, but if a few drops are applied to a cat orally, the dye is passed out in the urine. While this is generally a safe procedure, there are some problems linked to it, not least that the dye might stain light-coloured fabrics. Nonetheless, it may be a useful procedure. The dye is best detected using a Wood's light. Normal urine may also glow under this light, but usually less intensely. If Fluorescein is to be used, it is obviously important to treat one cat at a time and to allow several days in between treatments, so that all of the dye is eliminated from one potential culprit before moving on to the next. All cats should be tested, to check whether there is more than one involved in the problem.

## 7.4.2.3   FAECES

* *Coloured markers*: Coloured markers may also be used to help detect which cat is defecating. It is possible to add small shavings of nontoxic crayons to wet cat food. But, again, it is important to make sure that only one cat gets to eat one particular colour of crayon at a particular time.
* *Food colouring*: Alternatively, certain types of food colouring (including beetroot) may be administered orally. However, there is again the risk of staining furnishings, which needs to be explained to and accepted by the client if this route is to be used.

## 7.4.3   HOUSE-SOILING PROBLEMS AND DISEASE

House-soiling problems in cats have a close relationship with disease; perhaps more than any other problem occurring in relatively young animals. It is always important to ask whether the onset of the problem coincided with a known medical event.

A recent study in Brazil found that about a third of cats with house-soiling problems had some evidence of urinary system disease, with no difference between latrine-type problems and spraying. In control subjects from the same household, the figure fell to about 5% in sprayers, but it remained relatively high at around 20% in those from a household with a litter-box problem. One study in the USA suggested that nearly 40% of cats who were sprayers had some evidence of abnormality in their urine, suggesting that this was more common than in the general population, but another study using control subjects found no difference. In some cases, it may be that common stressors predispose cats to a house-soiling problem and urinary-tract disease, but in others it may be that the disease process itself causes the house-soiling problem, especially in the case of the development of a new latrine. In general, it needs to be recognised that urinary-system problems are common in these cases and careful veterinary attention is warranted, especially since bladder crystals can result in blockage of the urethra and ultimately prove fatal to the cat if not relieved. A refractory case may require an extensive medical evaluation, and this should be explained at the outset.

## 7.5   DIFFERENTIAL DIAGNOSES FOR HOUSE SOILING

In this section, house soiling is considered in relation to the various emotional systems discussed in Part I (Chapter 2), with the exception that pain has been combined with a range of medical issues, since these all require veterinary support. This approach helps to provide a logical approach to the most appropriate interventions for a given case.

### 7.5.1   *MEDICAL PROBLEMS RESULTING IN FAILURE TO USE THE LITTER BOX*

As already mentioned, all cats that house soil should have a clinical examination by a veterinarian to identify relevant conditions, and potentially evaluate the role of medical factors. A range of medical problems should be considered, which can be classified on the basis of the reason why they affect eliminative behaviour (rather than by diagnosis). It is essential that the specific medical conditions are treated by a veterinarian, although some behaviour modification may be needed too, in order to reestablish litter-box use. Of particular note are painful conditions, such as lower urinary-tract disease (especially if it involves crystalluria), inflammatory bowel disease and arthritis, which may predispose an animal to latrine behaviour outside of the normal box, result in a learned aversion or preference for another latrine area even after the condition has resolved (see Sections 7.5.2 and 7.5.3) or, in the case of feline interstitial cystitis or colitis, arise in association with stress-related factors. Therefore, close medical cooperation is important throughout the management of these cases. If a medical problem resulting in painful elimination is suspected, urinalysis and imaging of the bladder are usually recommended as a minimum before implementing a behavioural programme. Typically an ongoing painful problem will result in the use of multiple sites until a more comfortable elimination is achieved and a new association learned.

Useful pointers for identifying potential medical involvement include the following:

- A painful focus over the hindquarters, for example when stroking, or the cat showing a crouched body posture.
- An increased frequency and/or reduced duration of elimination behaviour (indicative of incomplete voiding) or history of straining to eliminate.
- A history of vocalising when eliminating, diarrhoea, colitis or constipation.
- Changes in mobility or movement, such as no longer jumping on to furniture.
- General features of sickness behaviour, such as a change in thirst or appetite.
- Indicators of cognitive decline.

In these cases, medical intervention is required alongside behavioural measures, which might include breaking the association between the current latrine and pain, for example by introducing a new litter box and litter type once any pain has been resolved.

## 7.5.2   *ANXIETY–FEAR AFFECTING LATRINE BEHAVIOUR*

There are several ways in which the presence or anticipation of something aversive associated with eliminating can lead to a latrine being developed in an undesired area of the home. This type of motivational–emotional arousal (*anxiety–fear*) may, for example, be evoked in response to the following:

- *A learned association*: For example, if the cat has experienced pain at some point in its life when eliminating into the litter box, it might have learned to associate the pain with the litter box and hence avoid it in the future. It is worth emphasising that there is a difference between pain as an initial cause (see Section 7.5.1) and an anticipation of pain. Both may lead to a learned avoidance related to the *anxiety–fear* system, or else to a preference for a nonpainful alternative (see Section 7.5.3).
- *Litter box type*:
  - Design. For example, covered versus uncovered.
  - Height of sides. It may be that the height of the sides is too great for the cat, particularly in the case of older cats, who may develop arthritis and have difficulty stepping in and out. That is, the box is associated with a fear of pain (see also Section 7.5.1).

- *Litter substrate*: For example, an aversion on the basis of:
  - Odour. The use of deodorants in the litter or other additives and cleaners. The odour will be intensified if the box has a lid on it.
  - Texture.
  - Absorbency.
  - Volume/depth.
  - Liners.

- *Litter-box cleanliness*: An aversion may arise from the urine or faeces of the individual itself or of other cats, or from an inadequate cleaning regime.
- *Immediate location*:
  - The position may be aversive because it is not consistent with a natural latrine, for example if it is close to a thoroughfare. It may be that there is a washing machine or a dryer nearby: the noise of these, particularly a washer that suddenly goes onto a spin-dry cycle while the cat is using the litter tray, can be very unpleasant. Some owners even put the litter tray on top of the washer or spin dryer, without realising what the impact might be for the animal, who may need to use the toilet while the machine is on. Many owners keep the litter tray close to the toilet or shower, and may scoop out the litter and flush it down the toilet. This practice is not recommended because the litter might block the system, but equally if an owner flushes the toilet or uses the shower while the cat is using the litter tray, this might cause problems for the cat.
  - Access and exit routes may make the latrine area aversive. This includes the potential blocking or defence of these routes by another animal.
- *Inappropriate interaction around the latrine environment*:
  - The owner petting the cat while it is using the litter box.
  - The presence of another animal or event while using the latrine. In some cases where a cat has access to the outside and so no indoor facility is provided, this might cause the cat to develop an aversion to going out to eliminate.

### 7.5.3    DESIRE AND PROBLEMATIC LATRINE BEHAVIOUR

Rather than an aversion to the latrine, it is possible for a cat to develop a positive preference for or an attraction to another area. In this situation, the underlying emotion behind the behaviour is *desire*, although it is worth emphasising that in some cases there may be a combination of *desire* and aversion. A hallmark of *desire* is that there is a consistent feature being sought for the latrine. Examples of latrine problems relating to this form of arousal include:

- Inadequate housetraining, which means an individual will seek its own preferred latrine.
- The number of facilities being insufficient for the number of cats in the household. As a general rule of thumb, one should provide one litter box more than the number of social groups within the household, each in distinctly different areas of the home. In the absence of this, a cat may simply prefer to make its own latrine elsewhere, although there might also be an element of aversion to using a facility in the core area of another animal.
- Specific environmental preferences for a specific location or type of substrate may lead an animal to prefer an alternative site to the litter box provided by the owner, such as an area with sand or a quieter, more secluded area of the home. If the current litter box is close to the sleeping area, it is likely that the cat will have a preference for an alternative site.

- Litter depth preferences. Cats tend to prefer a deep litter of a few inches, but many owners only provide a small depth in order to try to save on litter. Thus, if a deeper litter-type area is available elsewhere in the home, this may be preferred to the conventional litter box.
- Attention-seeking toileting behaviour is also underpinned by the animal working towards a desired goal, and can result in eliminative behaviour.

## 7.5.4   ANXIETY–FEAR AFFECTING MARKING BEHAVIOUR

When there is a perceived potential threat to resources, cats can change their marking behaviour and urine spraying. Horizontal urine marking or middening may occur as a result. These behaviours appear to help to identify familiar resources and to facilitate derousal in the presence of otherwise arousing stimuli and thus reassure the animal. Marking is not a direct defence aimed at deterring potential intruders and is definitely not a spiteful act. Once initiated, marking with urine or faeces might become self-maintaining, as marked objects remain important beacons for the behaviour (in which case the cat should no longer be considered to be motivated by the original motivational–emotional predisposition, as they are now self-reinforcing (*desire*) or more habitual in their performance). Thus the continuation of the behaviour might be due to the continued presence of the initial trigger stimuli or chemical factors associated with the scent marking, which encourage the animal to repeat the behaviour. Typical initial triggers of *anxiety–fear* include:

- Specific novel physical stimuli and odours introduced to the home.
- New social stimuli in the home, such as a new housemate – human, cat or other individual.
- General disruption to the home, such as a change in routine or moving home.
- New social stimuli near the home, such as a new cat in the neighbourhood.

Some cats will appear to mark when left alone. These cats are typically highly attached to their owners, but it seems that the elimination behaviour is not a *panic–grief* response. Instead it appears to be associated with providing reassurance, and so we suggest it is more appropriate to consider it under the category of *anxiety–fear* until further data become available, since beyond intervention aimed at increasing independence, the measures relating to this problem are aimed at reducing *anxiety–fear* in this context. Urine deposition in the context of owner separation is twice as common in females as in males, and occurs on the owner's bed almost exclusively (suggesting a marking function). Defecation in this context is also more common in neutered females, both urination and defecation occurring more typically in older (>7 years old) females. However, although less frequently reported for house soiling, male cats are in general more likely to show signs of separation distress (other signs include destructiveness, vocalisation and hair removal, some of which may be more *panic–grief* related; that is, aimed at reinstating contact with the owner).

### 7.5.5 *FRUSTRATION AND MARKING BEHAVIOUR*

When highly aroused, for example as a result of frustration, cats are often seen to pseudospray; that is, to go through the behavioural sequence of spraying without actually producing any urine. We think that in some cases this might translate into actual spraying, resulting in the two co-occuring. Circumstances that might lead to this form of elimination include the following:

- Denial of access to a desired physical resource.
- Denial of access to a desired social resource, such as the owner.

### 7.5.6 *LUST AND MARKING BEHAVIOUR*

Urine spraying can be a component of sexual arousal and so associated with the motivational–emotional system referred to as *lust*. In the case of the female, it may advertise her reproductive availability, while males may use this behaviour in courtship, though they might (at least theoretically) also engage in it because they perceive a female in oestrus as a valuable resource under threat from other males – in this sense, there may be two elements to sexual spraying by intact males: attraction of females and deterrence of competitors. Therefore, the high prevalence and frequency of urine spraying in entire males might relate to underlying activity in emotional systems characterised by *lust* and *anxiety–fear*. However, at present we do not employ treatments which allow us to differentiate between these, since most male housecats are neutered and stud cats are restricted in their access within the home. In summary, *lust* can relate to marking in relation to:

- Mate attraction.
- The response to a potential mate.

## 7.6 TREATMENT

In order to treat a given patient appropriately, it is obviously important to identify the cause of the problem. If the proper cause can be identified, the outlook is generally very good, with potentially more than 90% of spraying cats responding to pheromonatherapy intervention with F3 and a similar percentage improving with other interventions in the case of general house-soiling problems.

In all cases, whether the problem is due to latrine behaviour or marking, it is essential that affected areas be cleaned appropriately. We tend to recommend a regime based around making up a solution of biological washing powder, rinsing it off with water and wiping over the affected area with surgical spirit afterwards. A tablespoon of biological washing powder or its equivalent in 0.5 l of warm water is usually a strong enough solution. The area needs to be rinsed off well with water, especially if a pheromone product like F3 is going to be used on marked areas. This is important as any residual enzymatic action might break down the pheromonal signal; this and ineffective cleaning can explain some cases of failure of response of urine spraying to the use of the F3 spray. The enzymes in the biological washing powder help break down organic molecules within the urine, which may encourage reuse of the area. Wiping over with surgical spirit afterwards helps to lift these organic residues out. An inconspicuous area that is to be cleaned should always be tested first, and it should be noted that this regime can damage polished surfaces and some fabrics.

In cases where cats are eliminating on carpets, the soiling may soak through to the underlay, and wooden floors can absorb the urine. These cases can be difficult to treat and may require thorough scrubbing, resealing of the undersurface and possibly replacement of the underlay. It is important that owners do not use bleaches or ammonia-based detergents as these can be aversive to the cat in their own right and may actually make the matter worse or create a spraying problem in a cat that has a toileting problem. A recent study suggested that the fabric freshener 'Febreeze®' seemed to be better than most commercial products at removing cat-urine odour, and one of the advantages of using a commercial product like 'Febreeze®' is that it should not damage fabrics.

When considering treatment, we suggest following the 'three Rs' principle, namely:

- Risk assessment.
- Restriction of the problem.
- Resolution of the problem.

The aim is to resolve the problem, although some restriction measures are usually warranted initially in order to assist the owner in implementing the strategies for resolution without the cat continuing to practise the behaviour.

## 7.6.1  RISK ASSESSMENT

Obviously, in order to undertake a proper risk assessment, we must have identified the triggers and formed a clear 'motivational–emotional' diagnosis. Perhaps the most significant risks of failure to respond to treatment in this type of case relate to whether or not the right culprit has been identified and whether a correct diagnosis has been made. For example, a common treatment in the case of urine spraying has been the neutering of any entire male cats in the home, which is not going to do any good in the case of a litter-box problem.

## 7.6.2  RESTRICTION OF THE PROBLEM

Suggestions for restricting the problem include:

- Confinement when the cat cannot be supervised, which may be the normal way of keeping entire toms away from places where there should not be any spraying.
- Covering sprayed areas with heavy-duty plastic, in order to prevent further damage should occasional spraying still occur.

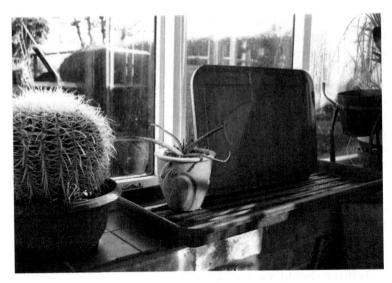

**Fig. 7.4** An L-shaped cat latrine built from a potting tray and a plastic lid, to catch the urine sprayed on a window within a conservatory. A judicious use of plants has also been employed to limit the problem behaviour to one area, so it can be more easily managed.

- Stopping all punishment, so as not to increase background anxiety, which might increase the risk of the problem.
- Creating cat latrines in soiled areas. If the problem relates to spraying then one tray can be placed on its end inside another to make an L-shaped container, or something similar (Figure 7.4). The cat can then spray against one box and the urine will run into the other.

### 7.6.3   RESOLUTION OF THE PROBLEM

In order to resolve the problem, we must usually address the underlying trigger and any related stressors. The management of certain stressors is where pheromonatherapy can be particularly important. It is clearly useful in relation to marking behaviour, and this was the first published indication. However, pheromonatherapy may also be useful in some cases of failure to use the litter box, because here too the animal may perceive the environment as insecure, as a consequence of having had unpleasant experiences. Nonetheless, we should determine whether or not any stressor relates to the litter box or a threat in the environment. Stressors around the litter box will tend to be presented as house soiling outside the litter box. Threats in the environment will tend to be presented as spraying. In Chapter 5 we described four different techniques for treating a behaviour problem:

- Environmental manipulation.
- Chemical manipulation.
- Physical manipulation (including surgery).
- Psychological manipulation.

All of these have a potential role to play in the control of house-soiling problems in cats. Examples of specific measures are given in Table 7.1, together with the suggested motivational–emotional activity with which they are most likely to help.

## 7.6.4   PHEROMONATHERAPY AND THE TREATMENT OF MARKING BEHAVIOUR

The use of pheromonatherapy has now become a routine practice in the management of urine spraying in cats. Several controlled studies show that in more than 70% of cases – and in some instances over 90% – of spraying due to some form of environmental aversive, are reduced when F3 is used in combination with the cleaning regime described at the beginning of Section 7.6. There is no scientific evidence as yet to suggest that pheromone products are more effective in the management of spraying associated with one emotion rather than another, although anecdotally it would seem that if there is a high degree of frustration, these products might be less effective. There are also data to support the use of pheromonatherapy in sexual marking. There does not appear to be a significant difference between the use of one delivery system over another, although the use of the plug-in is obviously simpler, as long as it is combined with effective cleaning of the problem areas. In this situation, very little other behavioural therapy is usually necessary, but it is important to identify the stressors triggering the response in order to achieve a long-term resolution without the continued use of pheromonatherapy. If relevant stressors are not controlled appropriately, the problem is likely to recur once the pheromone therapy stops. A summary of useful additional measures is given in Table 7.1, but we emphasise a few of the most commonly needed adjuncts here:

- *Treat conflict situations*: In a number of studies using F3, there has been at least a suggestion that in households where spraying is accompanied by overt aggression between cats, the pheromone product may be less effective and there will be a need for additional management measures. If there are specific conflict situations, these need to be treated. For example, if urine spraying is triggered by the arrival of another cat, all the cats involved need to be provided with an environment that at least allows them to tolerate one another. This means providing them with sufficient resources to have adequate control over their own piece of the environment. In some cases where there is consistent antagonism (as opposed to the odd spat due to an immediate conflict of interests), it may be necessary to desensitise the animals to each other as discussed in Chapter 11. In these cases, a pheromone product delivering F4 may be useful, in addition to odour-exchange exercises.
- *Elicit other behaviours in the sprayed location*: In some cases, the behaviour has become habitual. It may thus be useful to encourage other behaviours at the locations being marked, once stressors and triggers have been appropriately managed. For example, it may be possible to put a scratch post where the cat used to urine mark, or to feed the animal small amounts of food at this location. However, if the animal is spraying in a large number of locations, it does not make sense to have 40 food bowls scattered around the house.

Table 7.1 Techniques to prevent house-soiling problems in cats.

| Management procedure | Latrine-related | | | Marking-related | | |
|---|---|---|---|---|---|---|
| | Medical problems | Anxiety–fear | Desire | Anxiety–fear | Frustration | Lust |
| **Chemical** | | | | | | |
| MAOI: selegiline | cognitive dysfunction | | | x | ?x | |
| NSRI & SSRIs: amitriptyline, clomipramine, fluoxetine and others | | | | x | ?x | |
| Buspirone | | | | x | | |
| Cyproheptadine | | | | x | | |
| Diazepam | | | | x | | |
| Anxiolytic diets and nutraceuticals | | | | x | | |
| **Environmental** | | | | | | |
| Increase resources available to each household cat and strategically locate the resources for easy access by the various cats and social groups within the household | | x | x | | x | |
| Give the cat control over indoor–outdoor access, e.g. with an electronic-coded cat door. Prevent access to the home by outside cats (especially through cat flap) | | | | x | | |
| Install F3 diffusers | | | | x | | x |
| Use scent swapping to create group odour | | | | x | | |
| Encourage the cat to mark the area by using its cheek glands instead of urine by using cat combs | | | | x | ?x | x |

| | 1 | 2 | 3 | 4 | 5 | 6 | 7 |
|---|---|---|---|---|---|---|---|
| Promote litter-box hygiene, cleaning regime and odour control | x | | x | x | | | |
| Provide naturally attractive latrine features, including location and number of sites | x | | x | x | | | |
| Reduce access to potentially threatening stimuli, e.g. prevent inside cats from seeing out and clean doorways, paths and walls where nonresident cats are spray-marking | | | | | x | x | ?x |
| Expand territorial boundaries, e.g. install scratching posts, vantage points and latrines in the garden so that the territorial boundary is shifted from inside to outside | | | | | x | x | x |
| Control and manage resource distribution and linking paths, giving each social group its own distinct area | | | | | x | x | |
| Familiarise novel stimuli, e.g. apply a squirt of F3 to items when they are brought into the house | | | x | | x | x | |
| Provide spray stations (L-shaped litter boxes) | | | x | | x | x | |
| **Physical** | | | | | | | |
| Neuter | x | | | | | x | x |
| **Psychological** | | | | | | | |
| Habituate/desensitise/countercondition to potential stressors | | | | | x | x | |
| Appropriately structured interactions with owner | | | | x | | | |
| Provide house training | | x | | x | | x | |
| Employ deterrents, e.g. aversives or incompatible stimuli such as a food bowl at the site of soiling | | x | | x | | | |

- *Make locations aversive*: As long as the underlying stress is being treated, it may be appropriate to actually make the areas being marked slightly aversive. If done properly, this can help the animal in its decision-making without creating undue stress. Simply putting a bit of tin foil or double-sided sticky-tape in the area may stop the cat from approaching the wall where it urine marks, because it does not like the feel of the material. Caution is needed with odour deterrents or those which might induce higher arousal, such as noisy alarms. Deterrents alone are not a solution, since if the underlying stress is not treated, the cat is likely to simply spray somewhere else.
- *Eliminate internal views of outdoor cats*: Many cases of urine spraying are triggered by the arrival of a cat outside the home, who visits the locality. In some cases, the resident cats do not have access to the outside at all and simply see the other cat arrive in the garden, or else they might have access to the outside but only at certain times of the day. Seeing the other cat come into their territory can result in high arousal and possibly frustration, with urine spraying occurring as a result. In this case, eliminating the view of the outdoor cat can be helpful. If only as a temporary measure, many owners can be persuaded to use translucent static sheeting to cover the lower parts of windows so that their cat cannot see out of them. If something like a frosted-glass design is used, it can look quite attractive while still blocking the view of one cat by another. However, it should be remembered that cats use three-dimensional space in the home to look out of the windows, so the need for controlled access to some potential viewing platforms must be carefully evaluated.
- *Discourage outdoor cats from visiting the area*: An alternative is to discourage outdoor cats from coming into the area. This can be very difficult to do, although things like motion-activated garden sprinklers may be helpful if a discussion with the other owner regarding keeping their cat contained does not work.
- *Close cat flaps or limit access to the outdoors by resident cats*: Many cats enter other people's homes, unless their cat flaps have a regulating mechanism (e.g. collar or ID chip key). Owners are not always aware of this until they set up a video camera and see the neighbour's cat coming in. Nonresident cats entering homes can be the trigger of the problem. In this case, closing the cat flap or using a cat flap for which the resident cat has an automatic key may be effective. Spraying directed at specific entry and exit points is indicative of this type of problem.
- *Separate indoor cats*: If the problem relates to the stress arising from having multiple indoor cats then separating them for a while and providing them with their own essential resources (including a safe haven each) and their own connecting paths between these, and then gradually reintroducing them, may be required. In some cases, owners may simply have too many cats for the household and may have to be counselled to give consideration to rehoming one or more cats.
- *Medical intervention*: Drugs may also be used in the management of these problems. The specific serotonergic agents are particularly useful in this instance.

Treatment with fluoxetine for 16 weeks appears to maximise the chance of complete cessation, but the use of pheromones for a comparable period has not been reported in similarly controlled studies to date. Details on the use of medication can be found in texts listed in the Further Reading section at the end of this chapter. Pharmacology can be combined with pheromonatherapy but must always be implemented under veterinary supervision.

Most of the studies using F3 published so far have monitored the response of the animal over the first few weeks. Only one published study has examined the long-term outcomes. This was based on the use of the F3 spray. The study illustrates a number of interesting points regarding the treatment of behaviour problems: in particular, the fact that the therapist is managing the problem for the owner, rather than the behaviour of the cat. This is reflected by the finding that 10 months after the original study, only 14% of the cats were reported not to be spraying, while 77% were spraying less than before. Twenty-one of the owners – roughly half – had not used F3 for 7 months, even though some of their cats were still spraying a little. Thirteen of the owners were still using the F3, but none on a daily basis (as it had been prescribed). Given that the original study had shown a very high response rate to F3 treatment, it seems reasonable to suppose that the owners knew that by using the product they could get the behavioural problem under control. However, 10 months on they seemed to be willing to tolerate a higher level of spraying than occurred during the trial. One possible conclusion is that they did not feel the need to eliminate the problem completely. If they had wanted a lower level of spraying than they were living with at present, it would be expected that they would have been more likely to continue using the F3 as initially recommended.

The fact that no owners were using the F3 spray on a daily basis, as had been recommended and had been done before, might indicate a couple of further important points:

- Owners are not very compliant.
- These owners did not see the problem as so important that they needed to use the strict regime of daily treatment.

This is why it is so important to address owner expectations and hopes rather than our own goals, but also to consider the cat's interests and motivate owners accordingly.

## 7.6.5 PHEROMONATHERAPY AND LATRINE ISSUES

While it may not be immediately apparent, and there are no published clinical studies on the use of pheromone products in this context, pheromones do have a potential role to play in the management of this problem. It seems reasonable to suggest that F3 may be indicated where there is anxiety associated with the aversiveness of the latrine provided, in order to help improve reacceptance of the litter box. However, unlike urine spraying, with latrine issues the use of pheromones alone or with minimal behaviour therapy is unlikely to resolve the problem. Other measures, beyond the cleaning regime for soiled areas already discussed, are given in Table 7.1. Practical aspects concerning a few of these are emphasised here:

- *Clean boxes effectively*: A mainstay of treating latrine issues is owner consistency and good practice in cleaning the tray. It is essential that owners clean the boxes effectively; that is, very frequently and with appropriate cleaners that do not have a strong odour.
- *Offer a variety of litter types*: Owners should also offer a variety of litter types, especially if they have a multi-cat household, as different cats may prefer different litters. One litter-box site for each social group (recognised as individuals that sleep together and frequently lick or rub each other), plus one extra, should be made available in distinct suitable locations around the house; that is, not next to washing machines or alongside main routes.
- *Protect areas*: Soiled areas of the home may need protecting. Thick plastic or aluminium foil or double-sided sticky tape can be used to prevent access to these areas, while food or catnip can be placed in them to encourage different activities and change associations. In some cases an odour repellent may be used, but this should be considered only a temporary measure as it might itself induce spraying if it is not carefully managed.
- *Confine the cat for short periods*: In some cases it might be necessary to confine the cat for short periods, for example when it cannot be supervised or in order to facilitate retraining to a litter box.

Some texts suggest praising the cat when it is in the litter box, but in our opinion for many cats this can actually be quite stressful and unhelpful.

## 7.7   CONCLUSION

In conclusion, house-soiling problems are not necessarily exclusive to one form of behaviour and often involve pain or a medical issue as well. Cats frequently present with problems relating to more than one trigger; for example, they might have an attachment-related problem as well as incomplete housetraining. It is therefore important to have a thorough history that goes back, if possible, to the first episodes, as well as details of the current issue.

Disruption to the home or surrounding environment is quite a common precipitating cause of house soiling in cats. When considering how to manage domestic disruption, it is important to try to reduce the intensity of or, if at all possible, eliminate relevant stressors. This may not always be possible, especially if it relates to the presence of a member of the household. In this case, trying to reduce the intensity of the stressor by encouraging appropriate management methods and potentially using pheromonatherapy can be very helpful. The role of pheromonatherapy in disruptive stress in cats has to be carefully evaluated. If the problem relates to poor litter management, pheromonatherapy is unlikely to have much of an impact. Although it might reduce some of the stress, it is unlikely to get the cat back to using its litter tray.

# REVIEW ACTIVITIES

- Draw a map of a home with more than one cat in it. What measures help you to identify the number of feline social groups in the home, and how are these distributed within the home? Identify all key resources and associated pathways. Where is there overlap and what might be the implications of this?
- It is thought that F3 provides reassurance about physical resources in the home area. Consider the implications of this: when is the use of F3, and when is it not, indicated for the management of feline house soiling, and how might you determine this?
- An owner reports an unsatisfying response to a basic treatment programme using F3 for their house-soiling cat. What is your plan of action as a result?
- Discuss the implications for treatment of the different possible emotional states that can be associated with urine spraying and/or problematic latrine behaviour in cats.
- What special investigations and measures are necessary when managing a case of feline house soiling in a multi-cat household?

# FURTHER READING

Crowell Davis SL, Murray T (2006) Veterinary Psychopharmacology. Ames, IA: Blackwell.

Frank D, Erb HN, Houpt KA (1999) Urine spraying in cats: presence of concurrent disease and effects of pheromone treatment. Applied Animal Behaviour Science 61: 263–272.

Herron ME (2010) Advances in understanding and treatment of feline inappropriate elimination. Topics in Companion Animal Medicine 25: 195–202.

Marder AR, Engel JM (2001) Long-term outcome after treatment of feline inappropriate elimination. Journal of Applied Animal Welfare Science 5: 299–308.

Mills DS, White J (2000) Long-term follow up on the spraying behaviour of cats with chronic non-sexual urine spraying treated with synthetic feline facial pheromone analogue. Veterinary Record 147: 746–747.

Mills DS, Redgate SE, Landsberg GM (2011) A meta analysis of studies of treatment for feline urine spraying. PloS ONE 6 e18448.

Seksel K, Coyle W, Chaseling S (2001) Stresses associated with moving house with pets. In: Overall KL, Mills DS, Heath SE, Horwitz D (eds) Proceedings of the Third International Congress on Veterinary Behavioural Medicine. Potters Bar: UFAW pp. 47–49.

# Chapter 8

# Separation-related Behaviour Problems in Dogs

## 8.1   INTRODUCTION

In this chapter we consider a range of problems that arise when a dog is left alone and how pheromonatherapy can help in their management. Specifically, we highlight:

- What actually makes up a separation-related behaviour problem, since a lot of confusing terminology is used in this field. For example, the term 'separation anxiety' is widely used in different ways by different individuals and should not be considered a diagnosis unless clearly defined as such, since, as we explain in this chapter, there may be different emotional responses underlying similar presenting complaints.
- How these separation-related problems can be prevented, as prevention is better than cure. Pheromonatherapy, together with some simple advice to owners, can help to prevent a lot of these problems from arising in the first place.
- How to differentiate underlying motivational–emotional factors. The behaviours that animals show when they are separated from their owner may superficially appear quite similar, but as illustrated in this chapter, a good history and careful examination of signs can help to identify significant differences in the emotional influences on the problem, which help guide the priorities of treatment.

## 8.2   SEPARATION-RELATED BEHAVIOUR PROBLEMS

### 8.2.1   PRESENTING SIGNS

Separation-related behaviour problems are extremely common, with 20–30% of dogs in some populations showing overt signs at some time and perhaps more than 40% showing mild signs of distress when alone. The risk is not equal between breeds and it seems that labradors are at a higher risk of showing signs of separation-related problems than breeds like the border collie.

*Stress and Pheromonatherapy in Small Animal Clinical Behaviour*, First Edition.
Daniel Mills, Maya Braem Dube and Helen Zulch.
© 2013 John Wiley & Sons, Ltd. Published 2013 by John Wiley & Sons, Ltd.

An initial evaluation should determine that the problem is genuinely an owner-absent problem and not a more general issue but the owner focuses on the problem when they are away. It is also very useful to determine the proportion of eliciting contexts (occasions when the problem can arise) which give rise to the problem. It is useful to go through the history and identify all of the eliciting contexts and the frequency or regularity with which they occur. An eliciting context might be that the owner goes to work; the frequency is how many times this happens. The problem might occur every time the owner goes to work, but often owners will say 'it happens every day' even when there is not 100% consistency, and so careful enquiry is required. This is where the skills of active listening and summarisation can be key. For example, we might respond by saying, 'If I have understood you correctly, the problem happened five times last week and five times every week since the problem began'. If it actually happens on only 4 days on average out of 5 in the week, we have 80% consistency, if they in fact go to work 5 days a week. These estimates are important measures when it comes to monitoring progress. So the proportion of eliciting contexts in which the problem occurs is calculated by dividing the number of times the dog shows distressed behaviour when left alone by the number of times it is left alone. It is better to get an owner to actually record these data each week than to rely on their retrospective recollection. This information, if gathered in the form of weekly summaries, is particularly useful when it comes to monitoring progress. In addition, access to a home camera or webcam can be very helpful in making a diagnosis, with the following signs being of most interest:

- *Destructiveness*: This can involve chewing or digging. It is worth differentiating between these, and also noting their location. This can help to differentiate destructiveness associated with an attempt to escape from less directed destruction (Figure 8.1).
- *Vocalisation*: This may be howling, barking or whining.
  - Barking is often used as an alarm signal and in order to try to elicit care and attention. It is used in defence and sometimes in isolation distress. It is also socially facilitated; that is, if one dog starts barking in the neighbourhood, another is more likely to start barking as well. It can be used in an invitation to play. So, barking can occur in almost any circumstance. Changes in pitch can be useful in identifying barking associated with social isolation, typically being of a fluctuating and higher pitch (see Chapter 3).
  - Howling is particularly associated with seeking contact and greeting, and is also socially facilitated. Howling is quite often associated with destructiveness in problem cases.
  - Whining is also a contact-seeking behaviour and is associated with distress. Occasionally, it can be used in a greeting or in social play, especially as a reinforced enticement behaviour directed towards owners.

Vocalisation, when associated with trying to establish social contact, may go on for a long time after the owner has departed, particularly if the owner tends to go for short trips as well as longer ones; this may be because on the short trips the animal howls until the owner returns, which it interprets as a result of its

(a)

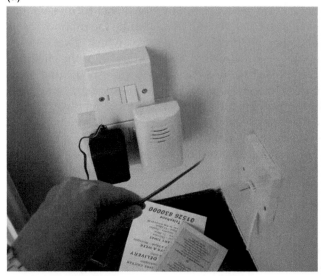

(b)

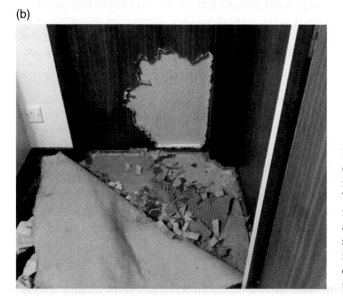

Fig. 8.1 The pattern of destructiveness can be informative in assessment. The damage shown in (a) is not specifically directed at an exit point, unlike that shown in (b). In the latter instance, the animal was clearly making an attempt to exit from the property.

howling, thereby learning that howling successfully brings its owner back. As a result, it howls for longer and longer periods. Video or just sound recordings can also be useful in evaluating the role of *social facilitation* in the problem when the primary complaint relates to vocalisation, addressing the question of whether there is any indication of another animal making a noise first.

• *Elimination*: This takes the form of urination or defecation when the owner is absent. Obviously, when dealing with house soiling it is important to differentiate the dog that is not properly house-trained from the dog that is actually distressed, for example through the presence of other signs of anxiety. If an animal eliminates as a consequence of some form of distress, this will occur completely independently of when the animal last went for a walk and evacuated its bladder and bowels. The reason for this is that the animal loses control when distressed. Taking up the water should not be considered a treatment option, treatment must focus on the primary cause of the problem.

- *Anorexia or 'depression'*: The owner may describe this as general apathy, inactivity or lethargy.
- *Overactivity*: Particularly when the owner returns. The dog may jump up at the owner when they return or pester the owner when they are around the house normally, constantly seeking attention.
- *Clinginess*: In which the owner says the dog never lets them out of its sight. The dog may not demand interaction, just the owner's presence.
- *Displacement behaviours*: That is, behaviours that appear out of context with the situation. An anxious dog, for example, may show a lot of lip-smacking, licking its lips, yawning or chewing-type behaviours without actually having anything in its mouth.
- *Repetitive behaviours*: Animals may circle or pace whether the owner is there or not and show a range of other repetitive behaviours, such as licking their paws – particularly the carpus and the hocks – to the point where they might actually make the skin quite sore and create open wounds.

In addition, a history of minor recurrent medical problems may be relevant, such as intermittent diarrhoea, vomiting and excessive self-licking. A number of drug trials that have investigated separation-related behaviour problems have noted how common vomiting is. This is not necessarily a reaction to the tablets but may actually be a sign of chronic or intense distress.

However, the identification of an animal in distress when left alone is not a diagnosis; rather, it is the starting point of a more complete evaluation.

## 8.2.2 PREVALENCE OF PRESENTING COMPLAINTS FOR SEPARATION PROBLEMS

Separation problems are very common and, as mentioned earlier, the signs dogs show vary, the most common being some form of vocalisation. However, this is not the most common complaint of owners, because it does not necessarily bother them so much. There are some cases in which it might bother the neighbour and the motivation to sort these cases out rests on the neighbour's complaint. These cases can pose particular challenges as far as motivating the owner to implement change is concerned (see Chapter 5).

The most common presenting sign is destructiveness as, clearly, the dog destroying the home is often a big problem for the owner. Nearly 20% of cases present with some form of elimination problem; that is, house soiling when the owner is absent. About a quarter of cases that are either destructive or vocalising show both of these signs. Independent of the actual behaviour the dog shows, the emotional problem for the dog may be considerable.

Another important feature of separation-related behaviour problems is that animals showing these problems are at a higher risk of a range of other problems as well. So it is important that these cases are carefully screened to obtain a full patient profile. The sorts of additional problem that these dogs will present with include:

- *Noise fears*: Dogs with noise fear are also at a higher risk of separation anxiety. So if a dog presents with one of these problems it is always worthwhile asking the owner if there is any evidence of the other problem as well. It is not surprising that these two problems are related. For example, a storm or some other loud, noisy event which scares the dog when the owner is absent can easily lead to a fear of being separated from the owner. However, this is a different type of emotional problem to one which relates to the type or level of attachment between dog and owner. This one relates to the emotional system of *anxiety–fear* rather than *panic–grief*.
- *Other attachment-related issues with the owner*: These dogs may engage in a range of attention-seeking behaviours in order to interact with the owner for more of the time, if they have an overdependence on the owner for security. So it is also worth screening these cases for attention-seeking behaviour problems.
- *High levels of activity*: In the authors' experience, the dogs that get presented typically appear to be quite outgoing individuals – more active rather than passive copers. It is therefore important that these animals get sufficient exercise and are not frustrated by their management.
- *Recurrent minor medical ailments*: Particularly diarrhoea and perhaps colitis and occasional vomiting. These may have been treated medically or simply accepted as a feature of the dog and so require some questioning to be revealed.

## 8.3   EMOTIONAL PROBLEMS RELATED TO SEPARATION (SEPARATION-RELATED PROBLEMS)

There is a growing interest in the causes of separation-related behaviour problems. Pageat (1995) proposed a role for hyperattachment to the owner in these conditions, which has since been developed further by Appleby & Pluijmakers (2003), who suggest three main types of emotional problem related to separation from the owner:

- *Type A*: A primary hyperattachment to the owner. This means that the dog transfers the attachment it has to its mother as a puppy to its owner and is not considered fully weaned.
- *Type B*: A secondary hyperattachment to an individual or possibly an inanimate object. This form of overattachment develops later in life, following a period of distress and the opportunity to seek comfort and safety, which causes a reopening of the bonding systems. It is possible for this to develop after a dog is rehomed.

- *Type C*: A conditioned fear of isolation. This includes cases where the animal has been scared by something such as a thunderstorm or a firework display when left alone.

## 8.3.1   *TYPE A – PRIMARY HYPERATTACHMENT*

The characteristic sign of this is an overattachment to a specific person. It starts in puppyhood, and it is suggested that these dogs may retain many puppy-like behavioural tendencies; for example, they may do a lot of oral exploration. Distress occurs when they are separated from their attachment figure or at signs of impending separation, and this relates to activation of the *panic–grief* system. For example, when an owner gets ready to go and puts on their shoes, picks up their keys and puts on their coat, the animal will show signs of acute distress. Characteristically, when the owner returns, the animal shows an excessive greeting and may jump all over the owner, bark, run around and so on.

The behaviours that an animal shows when it is isolated from the owner relate to attempts to try to reinstate contact. So it may be that the animal howls, digs, destroys doorways and so on. The signs are normally very consistent, occurring on a regular basis when the owner leaves.

An animal that has a primary hyperattachment is also at an increased risk of developing specific fears associated with isolation – that is, the Type C problem – as well. This means that it is important to screen these animals for both conditions and not assume that because one problem has been identified, another has been excluded.

As this problem is linked to a specific person, treatment is focused on reducing dependence on this person or individual, as well as on addressing the secondary problems. An important feature of hyperattachment is that the problem relates to the absence of a *specific figure* rather than isolation per se, and distress occurs even  when the animal is in the presence of other individuals. However, in some situations certain individuals may act as at least partial substitutes, and it is only when they all disappear that the overt problem behaviours arise.

## 8.3.2   *TYPE B – SECONDARY HYPERATTACHMENT*

This type of hyperattachment also relates to a dependent attachment, but this occurs after detachment from the mother has been successfully achieved, and may be to a wider range of stimuli, such as another animal or even an inanimate object. Like primary hyperattachment, it involves activation of the *panic–grief* system, but less consistently, although the problem itself is probably more common than primary hyperattachment. Onset is typically much later in life than with primary hyperattachment and coincides with a change in circumstances or the loss of an attachment object. A typical history might involve an owner who is off sick for an extended period of time, spends more time at home than usual and then has to return to work. The dog may have appeared fine with being left alone before this incident but now starts to show signs of struggling to cope without the owner present. When someone is laid off sick, they will often indulge their animal and may inadvertently encourage the dependence in a relatively short period of time.

Vocalisation seems to be particularly common in cases of secondary hyperattachment where there has been a change to the animal's routine. It has been found that if an animal is moved to a strange environment, the amount of distress vocalisation goes down. So if the owner says that they have tried moving the animal into another room and it seemed to solve the problem for a short period of time, this is not surprising.

Not only are the signs less consistent than in primary attachment, there is a greater potential to substitute one individual for another. This means that as long as somebody or something closely related to the attachment object and thereby acting as a substitute is present, it is likely that the animal will cope. In this case, something like a comfort blanket or one of the owner's sweaters may actually help the animal. The signs again often relate to attempts to regain contact but are also associated with comfort areas. The animal is seeking out stimuli that are associated with the attachment, so it may for example damage areas like the bed or sofa, which are strongly impregnated with the owner's scent.

As with Type A cases, these individuals are at increased risk of developing specific fears associated with isolation and so it is important to fully evaluate the case. The primary aim of treatment in these cases should be to focus on restoring comfort stimuli and things that actually help the animal to relax. Comfort stimuli are not simply resources, but rather are stimuli with a reassuring quality; thus a warm bed and reassuring chemical signals may be far preferable to a new toy. As substitutes are found, the animal becomes better able to cope with being left alone. Examples of inanimate objects that dogs can become attached to might be things like an indoor kennel or a crate. The owner removing this object or changing the bedding, for example, can act as a trigger for the problem. Something as simple as this might actually set off these sorts of problems, so, again, a careful history is necessary. Useful things to be aware of include the later onset and the coincidence with a change in the routine or housing of the animal.

### 8.3.3   TYPE C – CONDITIONED FEAR OF ISOLATION

The third group of distress-related problems that present in a similar way when the owner is absent relate to a 'conditioned fear of isolation'. In this case, the onset is associated with some unpleasant event when the animal was alone. Often this remains speculative, because we might not really know exactly what happened on the particular day the problem started. The owner may not remember what happened, because these cases are frequently presented quite late (but sometimes they can recall that there was a thunderstorm, a break-in, a lot of fireworks or something else distinctive).

According to Appleby & Pluijmakers (2003), about a third of these cases also show signs of high attachment. However, in their pure form, apart from when left alone, these animals appear to be generally well adapted in many other ways and show few signs of excessive attachment. As the onset of these problems is related to some unpleasant event, they can occur at any age. Some sort of distress is also apparent when the stimulus is delivered, even when the owner is present, because the problem relates partly to a primary aversion to the unpleasant event, which has become associated with the owner's absence. The clinical signs are typically less intense when the owner is present and sometimes the presence of the owner can completely calm the animal. Unlike the first two types of problem, the signs associated with this sort of condition often reflect less directed behaviour (Figure 8.1a) than an obvious attempt to reinstate contact with the owner (Figure 8.1b). Digging and destruction of immoveable objects, such as digging into the carpet or digging into the sofa, are typical signs.

Behaviour treatment obviously needs to focus on helping the animal cope with its underlying fear, rather than the attachment with the owner (unless there is also an attachment problem). As mentioned earlier, many cases present with a combination of conditions and it is important to tease them out.

## 8.3.4  OTHER COMMON EMOTIONAL CONSIDERATIONS

If an animal tries to reestablish contact with an attachment figure or tries to escape from an aversive environment to a safer area, it may be frustrated by its domestic enclosure (e.g. home or crate). This means the animal will be emotionally frustrated, and while this is usually secondary to the emotion encouraging escape, in some cases the problem might relate to a primary barrier frustration, not because the animal is avoiding an aversive, but because it is seeking an incentive outside the home. This might be simply the open space afforded outside the home, or it might be a specific stimulus such as the postman or refuse collector. The relative importance of *frustration* may therefore vary considerably between cases and be hard to determine, but consideration should perhaps be given to developing frustration tolerance skills (learning to tolerate the denial of rewards) as part of a treatment plan (especially in cases where the animal appears distressed when left alone but has not responded to the treatment measures aimed at attachment or fear of isolation).

## 8.4  PREVENTION OF SEPARATION-RELATED PROBLEMS

Clearly, prevention is better than cure in behaviour, and pheromonatherapy can play an important role in this regard, since dog-appeasing pheromone (DAP) can encourage the puppy or new dog to be more confident when left alone, even from a very early age. This, together with some simple management steps, can markedly reduce the stress involved with being alone and so prevent separation-related problems from occurring in the first instance. Key points are as follows:

• *Slowly introduce the dog to being left alone*: This is an important starting point, since it is essential that the animal does not learn that departures are always prolonged or intolerable. The stress of rehoming should be minimised, in order to help to reduce the risk of separation-related behaviour problems. It is acceptable to allow a new dog to stay in a crate in the owner's bedroom for the first night or two, but ideally it should be slowly moved away after this so it is not always with the owner (see Chapter 11).

- *Use DAP and offer reassuring things*: DAP, as the natural chemical produced by the mother which provides reassurance, may be very useful in helping to reduce attachment-related crying and development of an overdependence on an owner. Also, when a new dog is adopted, new owners should be advised to take a few things from the original home environment or rescue centre to give to the animal. For puppies, providing a hot water bottle with a blanket will often have an additional calming effect. A blanket the mother slept on, which can be sprayed with DAP, is likely to help as well, since the mother's scent may provide additional reassurance beyond the generic DAP signal. One study found that when DAP was used with young puppies, the puppies only cried for about three nights, compared to a week in the presence of a placebo. This effect was most marked in gun-dog breeds. Some cases, though, may not respond, and these should be managed as a high priority, being referred for specialist advice as necessary.
- There is a suspicion that rescue dogs are at higher risk of developing separation related problems after being rehomed, and so attention should be paid to the earliest signs of a problem in these cases. However, the following simple measures, which are adapted from a more detailed protocol available from the Royal Society for the Prevention of Cruelty to Animals (RSPCA), should be implemented as a precaution:
  - Gradually build up the amount of time the dog is left alone.
  - Reward relaxed, independent behaviour, and encourage the dog to have its own mat or bed on which it can settle.
  - Ensure the dog has things to do when left alone.
  - Make sure sufficient exercise is given consistently, according to the type of dog.
  - Do not punish the dog for anything it does while alone.

  This is sound advice for any new dog in the home and should not be limited to rescue animals. Unfortunately, even with implementation of all this advice cases of separation problems can still occur.

## 8.5   DIFFERENTIAL DIAGNOSIS

This includes the four differentials mentioned earlier, namely:

- Primary hyperattachment (*panic–grief*).
- Secondary hyperattachment (*panic–grief*).
- Conditioned fear of isolation (*anxiety–fear*).
- Barrier frustration (*frustration*), with or without a high level of attachment. For example, the dustman or others come to the house while the owner is at work

and the dog gets very excited, perhaps partly due to territorial tendencies or reinforcement of the response. The dog might jump up at the window and damage the curtains and furnishings around the area as a result. However, the owner simply notes that sometimes when the dog is left alone, destructiveness occurs. Another example involving the same emotional system, but which is contextually quite different, is the frustration that can occur as a result of being unable to reinstate contact with the owner. In this case, it is important to identify whether this is a primary or secondary problem (e.g. secondary to hyperattachment). Other emotional responses which may present as a similar behavioural complaint, and which need to be considered, include:

- Something happening which scares the dog when alone on a frequent basis (*fear–anxiety*). Although this involves the same emotional system as a conditioned fear of isolation, the trigger is not isolation but some other event, which typically happens when the dog is alone. This might be something like a backfiring car or noises from next door as new neighbours move in or do some DIY. Dogs may eliminate at this time, often leaving small puddles of urine or faeces where they have been excited. Generally, this type of problem is quite sporadic, and identifying both the occasions when and the locations where it occurs, as well as the regularity with which it occurs, will help eliminate an attachment-related problem or conditioned fear of isolation.

  ○ Playful or other investigation of the environment (*desire*). For example, with a puppy, if an owner does not provide appropriate outlets for chewing and train the animal to use them, it may start chewing on inappropriate items.

  ○ A coincidental event as a result of social play, such as two dogs playing together running around the house and displacing furnishings in the process (*social play*).

  ○ Relief of a primary need, for example the need to eliminate or to chew on something (*desire*). Quite surprisingly, many owners think that dogs naturally housetrain themselves. These owners may present an animal in early adulthood, saying that 'He has got separation anxiety' or 'He house soils when he is left alone'. When the history is closely examined, it becomes apparent that the animal has in fact never been housetrained. Some owners may also have unrealistic expectations of how long a dog can hold its bladder and bowels. They may feed it in the morning and then leave it for 10–12 hours, expecting it to cope. This is unrealistic and in such situations it is essential that the owner not only changes the feeding patterns so that the dog is fed when they get home but also provides the dog with human company during the day, or at the very least someone to let it out. Also *desire* related, it is also possible to include marking behaviour that is not sexually directed. In scent marking we typically expect to find the elimination has occurred against the wall rather than directly on the floor, although both bitches and dogs may mark directly on to horizontal surfaces too. This can become an owner-absent problem if it has been punished in the owner's presence. It is important to distinguish pools of saliva from pools of urine. Often owners will assume that a liquid is urine but some animals who are very distressed will actually produce a lot of saliva, so a sample may need to be tested.

## 8.6   TREATMENT

### 8.6.1   *MONITORING*

Because improvement often takes time, it is important that the owner keeps good records and that cases are carefully monitored. We need to identify the range of eliciting contexts: that is, when do any of the signs (not just the presenting complaint) happen? It is important to try to identify with the client as many different eliciting contexts as possible.

The second step is to record the frequency in each of these eliciting contexts. They might occur every time the owner goes to work but only every other time the owner goes shopping. Monitoring both the range of eliciting contexts and the frequency of each individually can be a very useful guide, because there may only be a slow reduction over time. Even if the problem has not disappeared completely, it is important to be able to demonstrate to the owner that they are making progress, in order to encourage them to continue. This can be done by plotting a graph of the proportion of eliciting contexts in which the problem was displayed against the week.

### 8.6.2   *RISK ASSESSMENT*

As previously mentioned, a risk assessment is an integral part of case management (Chapter 4). If in the history we identify episodes of aggression or of injury not caused by aggression, such as the overexuberant dog that scratches its owner, these are serious cases which call for specialist assistance.

In terms of the risks for the actual patient, many of these cases represent a welfare concern because they have a negative psychological impact. However, in some cases the animals may harm themselves (e.g. Figure 8.2). Some dogs can break their teeth; others may lick themselves excessively and make themselves sore.

Finally, the risk of recurrence needs to be considered. It should be recognised that certain individuals will be more predisposed to this than others. For example, animals that are temperamentally more anxious are going to be at a higher risk of relapse of fears in the owner's absence than animals that are less anxious. Dogs are highly social animals, so being left alone is stressful for many of them. The job of the counsellor is to try to minimise that distress when separation is inevitable, as well as advocate realistic expectations on behalf of the pet's interests.

### 8.6.3   *RESTRICTION OF THE PROBLEM*

Restriction of the problem does not typically focus on addressing the underlying concerns about the animal's motivational–emotional state, but this may be necessary in the short term, especially regarding the minimisation of the previously mentioned risks. In the case of an animal that suffers separation-related problems, the owner may need to kennel the animal for a short period of time, but a dog-sitter or doggy daycare is preferable. In some cases, using a commercial

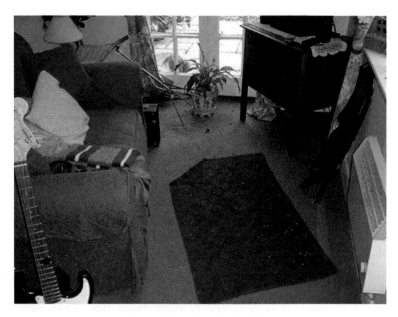

**Fig. 8.2** Damage caused by a dog with a fear of isolation. The dog has not made an obvious attempt to escape, but has knocked over the music stand. The red staining on the carpet nearby is from the bleeding that occurred as it scratched at the carpet in a frantic bout of activity.

kennel may be far preferable to using a cage in the house, but either of these cases can cause the animal a lot of distress (see Figure 1.2).

Punishment is unlikely to be productive and may actually exacerbate the problem, so as a general rule *all* punishment of the behaviour should stop. Other restrictive measures which might be used in the short term include feeding the dog a low-residue diet and feeding only after the owner has returned, if the problem relates to defecation. Owners should also clean up any mess away from the dog in order to minimise the risk of bringing attention to the problem (stimulus or local enhancement).

## 8.6.4   RESOLUTION OF THE PROBLEM

In order to resolve the problem, we must consider factors predisposing the animal to show the problem behaviour, since it is not normally possible to eliminate the trigger (owner absence). This might mean trying to reduce dependence on the owner or some other object of attachment in cases involving hyperattachment, so that the animal can cope with being left alone, and/or deconstructing learned associations with isolation or owner absence.

Pheromonatherapy can be particularly useful in helping the dog develop a safe haven within the home, as well as other associations that lead to greater detachment in cases where this is appropriate. It is also believed to be useful in the management of sound sensitivities, which often co-occur with this problem (sound sensitivity is discussed in detail in Chapter 9, so we will not explore it in detail here). In these cases it is also important to decide whether or not there are background stressors such as uncertainty in the home that are likely to exacerbate the problem too. A stress audit should therefore be undertaken, and any significant factors treated, if success is to be maximised (see Chapter 2). Consistent interactions between the owner and their pet may be particularly important in this regard. Any contributory medical problem (e.g. cognitive dysfunction or focus of pain when lying for a prolonged period) must also be addressed before purely behavioural measures are implemented. As in all cases, we can consider options relating to all four of the available techniques for behaviour modification:

- Environmental manipulation.
- Chemical manipulation.
- Physical manipulation.
- Psychological manipulation.

A range of common recommendations are summarised in Table 8.1, alongside an indication of the associated motivational–emotional states for which we believe they are most relevant. It is generally recommended that these measures be continued until 4–6 weeks after a stable state has been achieved; that is, until there is no further change. This may be more than 6–8 weeks after the owner expresses satisfaction, and the importance of this should be explained at the outset of treatment. It is also another reason why keeping good records is so important, as easing up on the measures too soon can increase the risk of relapse.

In the rest of this section, we discuss in more detail the use of drugs and pheromonatherapy, since this problem is often a significant welfare issue and there is often a need on the part of the owner for it to be completely resolved as soon as possible, with minimal risk of relapse. Both of these elements may be important in this regard.

## 8.6.5   THE USE OF PSYCHOPHARMACOLOGY

Separation-related problems are one of the few conditions for which there have been a good number of well-controlled studies using drugs, in particular the serotonergic agents clomipramine (Clomicalm®) and fluoxetine (Reconcile®). But before we discuss these, it is worth considering some general guidance on the use of drugs in the management of behaviour problems, since this is an area in which there can be some considerable misunderstanding, resulting in unnecessary animal suffering.

### 8.6.5.1   GENERAL PRINCIPLES

Some individuals use the rejection of drugs as a marketing point, and this perhaps reflects a failure to appreciate their potential importance in specific cases. If an animal is experiencing extreme suffering as a result of, for example, being left alone, we would argue that we have a duty to consider all available options to

**Table 8.1** Some measures to help resolve separation-related problems according to their putative motivational–emotional basis. Note all treatments must be calibrated according to the case and not all measures are recommended is a given case.

| Intervention | Panic–grief primary | Panic–grief secondary | Anxiety–fear isolation | Anxiety–fear event | Frustration | Desire investigation | Desire relief | Play |
|---|---|---|---|---|---|---|---|---|
| **Chemical** | | | | | | | | |
| High-residue diet to increase satiety | | | | | x | x | | x |
| Benzodiazepines | | x | x | x | ?x | | | |
| S/NSRIs | x | x | x | | | | | |
| Calming diet and supplements | x | x | x | x | | | | |
| **Environmental** | | | | | | | | |
| Environmental enrichment, e.g. Stuffed Kongs around the house for dog to find while owner is absent (hide-and-seek game) – enrichments need to be relevant | | | | x | x | x | | x |
| Blocking access to triggers | | | | x | x | x | | |
| DAP close to dog's resting place | x | | x | x | | | | |
| **Physical** | | | | | | | | |
| Massage/touch therapy to encourage relaxation and reduce risks of peeks | ?x | x | x | | x | x | | x |
| **Psychological** | | | | | | | | |
| *Departure and return* | | | | | | | | |
| Incremental habituation to predictive leaving rituals | x | x | x | | | | | |
| Feeding before owner leaves to decrease arousal | | | | | x | x | | x |
| Increasing exercise prior to departure to encourage sleeping etc. | | | | | x | x | | x |
| Changing location of dog when owner leaves so as to form a new and positive association | x | ?x | x | | x | | | |

(continued)

Table (cont'd).

| Intervention | Panic–grief primary | Panic–grief secondary | Anxiety–fear isolation | Anxiety–fear event | Frustration | Desire investigation | Desire relief | Play |
|---|---|---|---|---|---|---|---|---|
| Calm departures | | | | | | | | |
| Ignoring dog until it is calm for a short while after coming home | × | × | × | | × | | | |
| *Dog–owner relationship* | | | | | | | | |
| Stopping owner reinforcement of attention-seeking/needy behaviour (emotional check-in) | × | × | × | | | | | |
| Discouraging owner from indulging the dog and creating a dependence on themselves | × | × | | | | | | |
| Reducing the dog's dependence on its attachment figure by encouraging autonomy | × | × | × | | | | | |
| Rewarding spontaneous independent behaviour | × | × | | | | | | |
| Providing regular signalled sessions of attention at predictable times, so the animal learns not to expect attention at other times | × | × | | | | | | |
| Teaching the dog to lie still away from the owner | × | | × | | × | | | |
| Signalled period of nonattention | × | | | | | | | |
| Owner choosing when interaction occurs | × | | × | | | | | |
| *Safety and relaxation* | | | | | | | | |
| Reinforcing calm behaviours | × | × | × | | × | | | |
| Creating a safe haven | × | × | × | | × | | | |
| Providing comfort cues, such as owner-scented items | | × | × | | | | | |
| Redirecting behaviour, e.g. a sandpit for elimination or scratching | | | | | × | × | × | |
| Counterconditioning and response substitution | × | × | × | × | × | × | | |
| Learn-to-earn programme to teach frustration tolerance | × | | | | × | | | |

Table 8.2 General functions of some biogenic amine and amino acid neurotransmitters in the central nervous system (CNS).

| Neurotransmitter | Function |
| --- | --- |
| *Biogenic amines* | |
| Serotonin | Restrains threshold variables, facilitating sensory filtering, sensory streamlining and motor output |
| Noradrenaline/norepinephrine | Increases arousal and attention by increasing signal–noise ratio |
| Acetylcholine | Mediates psychobehavioural action and helps sustain information processing and gating of threshold stimuli for attention |
| Dopamine | Encodes positive motivational significance (*'desire'*) and structured motor arousal |
| *Amino acids* | |
| Glutamate | Promotes learning, memory and consciousness |
| Glycine | Provides motor inhibition and some glutamate regulation associated with cognition |
| GABA | Inhibits homeostatic circuits |

alleviate that suffering. This means that drugs may need to be considered, if only as a temporary measure, to help improve the animal's well-being. Medication, like pheromonatherapy, is not a substitute for poor husbandry or poor behaviour-management skills, but used correctly it can be a tool that directly safeguards the welfare of patients and increases the potential for owner compliance with a behaviour-management programme. However, its use is not without risks, and these need to be carefully evaluated against the predicted benefits in any given case. When using psychopharmacology, the aim is to alter a complex balance of neurochemicals in the brain in order to bring about a desirable change in an inferred mental state. Tables 8.2 and 8.3 list the general biological functions of some of the main neurotransmitters in the brain and the common drug classes affecting these.

It is not uncommon to have treatment failures, because of either a misdiagnosis, the wrong drug being prescribed for the condition or the drug being used without a concurrent behaviour-modification plan.

A vast array of drugs are available for use and there is no shortage of opinions about when certain ones may be more effective, but the evidence for this is more limited. In the human field it is advised that nonspecialist doctors develop a list of 'preferred' drugs about which they are quite knowledgeable in order to rationalise treatment, rather than try to learn a little about a wider range of drugs, and the same approach seems sensible in the field of clinical animal behaviour. It is important to cover the different chemical classes, since these will typically work through quite different routes. Many drugs are metabolised by the liver (which may result in active secondary compounds) and excreted from the body in the bile or via the kidneys. It is therefore important to establish that the liver and kidney

Table 8.3 Common transmitter types and related, frequently used drug groups.

| Neurotransmitter | Class of drug |
|---|---|
| *Amines* | (Specific and nonspecific) serotonin reuptake |
| 5HT/serotonin | inhibitors (S/N)SRIs |
| Noradrenaline/norepinephrine | |
| Adrenaline/epinephrine | |
| Acetylcholine | |
| Dopamine | Monoamine-oxidase inhibitors |
| *Amino acids* | Benzodiazepines |
| Glutamate | |
| Gamma-amino butyric acid (GABA) | |
| *Opiates* | |
| Endorphins | |

are functioning well before drugs are prescribed; otherwise the risk of a toxic overdose is greatly increased. It is also important to appreciate that the metabolism of one drug may alter the metabolism of another, so prescription needs to be done with care and with full knowledge of both the animal's health and its medical status. In addition, some drugs are contraindicated in combination with specific supplements or nutraceuticals as their risk of toxicity may increase. This is why, in the UK and many other countries, the ability to prescribe is limited to veterinarians. Prescription should be based on the available evidence and not marketing material or the blind recommendation of others, since only in this way can individual choice be justified.

In order to individualise an effective treatment, the following questions need to be answered:

- Is the drug appropriate?
- Is the form appropriate?
- Is the dosing regime appropriate?
- Is the duration of treatment appropriate?

In this context, 'appropriate' refers to the efficacy, indication, convenience and safety of the choice for the given patient (which recognises their position in a much larger interactive system – see Chapter 1), while taking account of any contraindications and possible interactions with other drugs, herbal products, dietary supplements and so on.

## 8.6.5.2  *PSYCHOPHARMACY AND SEPARATION ANXIETY*

In cases of separation-related behaviour problems, the recommended drugs typically speed up the rate of response to behaviour modification while safeguarding immediate welfare concerns. The drugs licensed for use in this sort of problem are either serotonergic (clomipramine and fluoxetine) or dopaminegic (selegiline) agents, with directly relevant published clinical trial results only available for the former. The serotonergic agents may be useful in attachment-related problems, since attachment is mediated through the opiate system and these drugs can help blunt the psychologically painful effects of the opiate withdrawal response that occurs when the animal is left alone. Recent work suggests that fluoxetine, at least, does not simply inhibit the behaviour but actually elevates mood too. There are other drugs of the same groups, mainly SSRIs such as sertraline or fluvoxamine, that are being used in pets worldwide but are not registered for these species, and so their indication must be carefully evaluated by an experienced professional.

The evidence to date suggests that using a drug does not increase the proportion of animals with separation-related problems that respond to treatment – that is, it does not make an animal get better that was not going to get better anyway – but it does increase the rate of response to the behaviour-therapy programme. It is essential that the owner appreciates both this and the importance of concomitant behaviour therapy strategies. Perhaps 60% of separation-related cases respond to medication within a couple of weeks, but it may take up to 6 weeks to determine whether an animal is going to respond or not. Various studies suggest that perhaps around 80% of animals respond to this sort of intervention.

## 8.6.6   THE USE OF PHEROMONATHERAPY IN SEPARATION-RELATED BEHAVIOUR PROBLEMS

There is one published study on the use of pheromones with separation-related behaviour problems. It was a blinded comparative study of dogs involving both DAP and clomipramine over a 28-day period. Each owner was provided with both a diffuser and tablets to give to the animal. In some cases, the diffuser was active (verum) and the tablets were blanks (placebo), and in others the tablets were active (verum) and the diffuser was blank (placebo). This study focused on three signs: house soiling, vocalisation and destructiveness. In this section, we examine the results as they relate to DAP, before comparing DAP to clomipramine.

Patients were not diagnosed in the way described earlier in this chapter, but in a less specific way (which is a common feature of all of the published clinical studies to date). It is therefore worth considering a few details of the study: in order for dogs to be included, they had to show at least one of the signs of destructiveness, vocalisation or house soiling in the absence of the owner, as well as three signs of overattachment. These could include: the dog following its owners around the house incessantly and attempting to maintain physical contact when they were at home; the dog showing signs of distress when the distance between it and its owners increased, for example when the owners went into another room and shut the door; and the dog showing signs of distress when the owners left it in the house and giving them a very exuberant greeting on their return. These results thus relate to animals that do not just show certain signs when they are left alone but also signs of overattachment. The dogs also had to be physically healthy.

Twenty dogs presented with destructiveness, and there was a 30% reduction within the first 7 days; by the end of 4 weeks, 85% of the dogs were considered improved or 'cured'. In the case of destructiveness, the DAP seems to have had a rapid effect and became increasingly effective with time. Slightly fewer dogs presented with vocalisation, but they would vocalise very frequently. As with destructiveness, a decrease was seen within the first week, but in only about a quarter of cases; for nearly three-quarters of cases, this sign improved or had disappeared within 28 days. House soiling was much less frequently presented, with only 12 dogs showing this problem, although those that presented with this sign would house soil quite frequently. Interestingly, the effect of DAP in this group seems to be more delayed, with only a very slight drop in the first week. So, if DAP is to be recommended for a presenting complaint that relates to house soiling, the owner should be advised not to expect much change for the first couple of weeks. Also, the level of response to treatment was not quite as great, with only about two-thirds of subjects actually responding at the end of the 4 weeks. These treatment-outcome values are quite important when advising owners as to what they can actually expect with pheromone treatment.

The interpretation of the DAP results in comparison with clomipramine requires some caution. As the sample size in this study was relatively small, it is not surprising that no significant differences were found, but this does not mean the two interventions are equivalent. Typically, in a study in which you are comparing one treatment with another you require several hundred subjects in order to be confident that the treatments are equivalent. From a practical perspective, and in the absence of any further evidence to guide us, there are some interesting trends to consider. In the case of destructiveness, it seems that DAP might be more effective than clomipramine, but in the case of house soiling it seems that clomipramine is more effective. This latter suggestion seems understandable, as a recognised potential side effect of clomipramine when used in other studies is a reduction in elimination. However, it should also be remembered that the use of the two products does not have to be exclusive, as there is no contraindication for combining DAP with clomipramin, so it is not a case of having to decide which to use in place of the other. A final decision must be made in respect of the individual patient and their individual circumstances.

## 8.7  PROGNOSIS

With an individualised programme, nearly all cases can be expected to improve, but that does not mean the problem will stop altogether. So, while generic handouts can be useful, it is also important to try to tailor the treatment programme to the individual patient. One study suggests that near-complete resolution may occur in almost half of cases, although this might be a conservative estimate as it was carried out before the more specific diagnoses discussed in this chapter were recognised. If the problem is left untreated, more than half of cases are reported to get worse or remain unchanged, but it has been suggested that about a third of them will actually resolve on their own. This does not mean that these cases should be left untreated (as this would mean leaving the animals' well-being to chance) but it shows that spontaneous recovery is possible.

## 8.8   CONCLUSION

In conclusion, separation-related problems are relatively common, particularly in dogs. The risk of their development can be minimised with sound management practice, including pheromonatherapy. Much of the time, clinical cases can be managed effectively with relatively straightforward advice. Behaviour therapy is essential and the use of pheromones may help to speed up the rate of response. This can be a lifesaver, since many owners need a quick response due to the amount of damage or misery that these animals are causing them – some owners become effectively housebound as they are too worried to leave their dog alone. An apparent relapse may be expected in about 10% of cases, but if an animal should appear to relapse, the case needs to be systematically re-evaluated: it should not be assumed that the animal is showing the same separation-related problem again. It may well be that there has been a change in the environment or circumstances that is eliciting one of the other motivational–emotional forms of the problem.

## REVIEW ACTIVITIES

- Consider the features which will help you differentiate the possible reasons why a dog might show destructive behaviour in the absence of its owner.
- It is thought that DAP provides a sense of safety in the environment. Consider the implications of this; that is, when the use of DAP is and is not indicated for the management of a separation-related problem and how you would determine this.
- An owner reports an unsatisfying response to a basic treatment programme using DAP for their dog, which house soils when left alone. What is your plan of action?
- You are running a puppy socialisation class: think of the general advice you would give the puppy owners in order to avoid separation-related problems with their dogs.
- Discuss the implications for treatment of the different possible emotional states that can be associated with separation-related problems in the dog.
- What special investigations and measures are necessary when managing a case of separation-related problems in a multi-dog household?

## REFERENCES

Appleby D, Pluijmakers J (2003) Separation anxiety in dogs. The function of homeostasis in its development and treatment. Veterinary Clinics of North America Small Animal Practice 33: 321–344.

Blackwell E, Casey RA, Bradshaw JWS (2006) Controlled trial of behaviour therapy for separation-related disorders in dogs. Veterinary Record 158: 551–554.

Gaultier E, Bonnafous L, Vienet Legue D, Falewee C, Bougrat L, Lafont-Lecuelle C, Pageat P (2009) Efficacy of dog-appeasing pheromone in reducing behaviours associated with fear of unfamiliar people and new surroundings in newly adopted puppies. Veterinary Record 164: 708–714.

Pageat P (1995) Pathologie du Comportement du Chien. Maisons-Alfort, Cedex: Editions du Point Vétérinaire.

RSPCA. Separation related behaviour. Available from http://www.rspca.org.uk/allabout-animals/pets/dogs/company/separationrelatedbehaviour.

## FURTHER READING

Takeuchi Y, Houpt KA, Scarlett JM (2000) Evaluation of treatments for separation anxiety in dogs. Journal of the American Veterinary Medical Association 217: 342–345.

# Chapter 9

# Sound Sensitivity

## 9.1   INTRODUCTION

A few surveys have looked at how frequently sound sensitivities occur. These show that the prevalence of the problem ranges between 20 and 50% of dogs attending veterinary clinics, though in some breeds, such as the bearded collie, the prevalence has been reported to be as high as nearly 75%. Our own data suggest that in the UK the most common sound sensitivity in dogs is a fear of fireworks, followed by thunder and loud bangs, gun shots, party poppers, vacuum cleaners, bird scarers, engines and the sound of people arguing; all other sensitivities occur in less than 20% of affected dogs. However, a review of the caseload of the Association of Pet Behaviour Counsellors indicates that noise fears in pets make up less than 5% of their case load. Clearly, while these problems are common, they are perhaps not readily being referred for specialist treatment, and so there is enormous potential for their management in general practice. When asked, just under a third of owners said they would actually seek advice for the treatment of a noise fear and about 15% said they would seek help from their vet. This means that for every three cases that are seen in practice, seventeen go unmentioned. Our own data also suggest that typically the problem goes on for about 4 years before owners seek advice, although there is an enormous range.

A recent report by the People's Dispensary for Sick Animals (PDSA) suggests that around 45% of cats are afraid of loud noises, including fireworks, with the figure rising to 56% if vacuum cleaners are included.

Sound sensitivities also occur in other companion-animal species, such as rabbits, but there are no data available for this, probably for a mixture of reasons: owners may have difficulty recognising fear in rabbits, the sorts of reaction that rabbits might show to noise fears may not be problematic for the owner and these animals may live outside in a hutch, meaning their behaviour goes unseen. However, the failure to recognise the welfare problem does not mean that it should go unmanaged or that owners should be left unaware of their responsibility to help their pet.

*Stress and Pheromonatherapy in Small Animal Clinical Behaviour*, First Edition.
Daniel Mills, Maya Braem Dube and Helen Zulch.
© 2013 John Wiley & Sons, Ltd. Published 2013 by John Wiley & Sons, Ltd.

Clearly, there is not only a large potential case load but also a large, largely untreated welfare problem here. This chapter will focus on the problem in dogs, as this is the area in which there has been most research, but the principles can and should be applied to any species affected in a similar way.

## 9.2   THE NATURE OF SOUND SENSITIVITY

The term 'sound sensitivity' is used here, as this is often the simplest way to capture the presenting complaint without making too much of an inference about the underlying motivational–emotional state. It is for the clinician to determine exactly what form the sensitivity takes and whether it should be considered a fear, a phobia, perhaps a learned attention-seeking response (pseudophobia) or some other issue. The term 'sound sensitivity' also allows for recognition of the fact that there are at least three elements to the response to a sound, any of which may form the basis of a complaint from an owner (Figure 9.1). There is the initial perception of the sound, which may result in a startle response such as jumping, especially if the sound is sudden or unexpected in some way; and there are two strategic elements following the processing of the sound: the possible decision to monitor the situation, which may result in behaviours like hypervigilance, and the possible adoption of an attempted coping strategy with certain consequences, such as hiding. It is useful to identify within this process where the signs of most concern to the owner originate, so that management strategies can be prioritised accordingly.

Across species, sudden loud noises (and other intense unexpected sensory stimulations) are a common trigger for a startle response, but loud noises are not the only type of sound that animals are scared of, and not all sound sensitivities relate to loudness. Different species show differences in the sorts of things they readily become scared of in the longer term (i.e. they are biologically prepared to become scared of different types of stimulus), and current genetic work suggests that differences in more general cognitive processes (i.e. processes involved in more than the processing of sound) are at the heart of many sound sensitivities. Both of these findings reinforce the importance of distinguishing between a condition that relates to an unexpected event (surprise) and one that relates to more complex sensory processing. While fireworks, thunderstorms and gun shots are all clearly very loud sounds, and indeed the volume from a rifle being fired may be so loud (160 dB) as to be perceived as painful, vacuum cleaners might be no louder than normal conversation (60 dB) and yet the higher pitch or some other perceived aspect of the stimulus can still be found aversive. In some cases, the sound sensitivity is a learned association with some other aversive event, such as the beep of a smoke detector – and similar sounds like the beep of a microwave oven – after there has been a fire in the home. A recent survey in Spain suggested that the types of noise which dogs become scared of can be grouped into three categories, which tend to co-occur: everyday sudden brief noises like bangs, slamming doors, traffic and so on; more specific stressors such as fireworks, thunder and gun shots; and familiar household noises such as the vacuum cleaner, cooking appliances and the TV or radio.

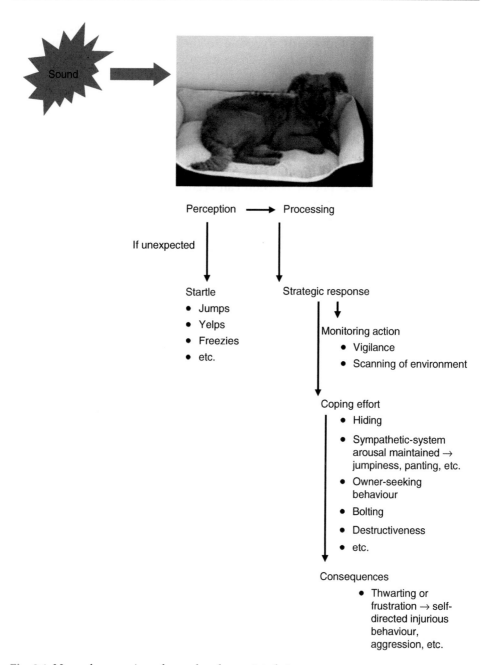

**Fig. 9.1** Normal processing of sound and associated signs.

A startle response does not necessarily mean the animal has a clinical fear or phobia, only that it is surprised, and it is important for owners to recognise that when treating a sound sensitivity the animal may continue to startle at sudden or unexpected noises. This should not be a cause for concern unless extreme or accompanied by signs associated with the further processing of the sound as something significantly aversive to the individual, which may be indicated by a high priority being given to monitoring of the environment at the expense of attending to possible available incentives (extreme vigilance behaviour) or by persistent effort being made to try to cope (hiding or restlessness).

The terms 'fear' and 'phobia' are often used interchangeably, or else the term 'phobia' is used simply to describe a more severe fear, but we believe it is worth making a distinction between them. A fear is typically an adaptive response that helps to protect the animal from unpleasant events. However, a phobia is a maladaptive response. A phobic reaction can occur even when there is nothing unpleasant happening to the animal and the animal is simply anticipating the situation. A phobic response is often ungraded or poorly graded; this means the magnitude of the response is unrelated to the potential threat. It is typically extreme every time the animal is exposed to the trigger stimuli, even if they are at a very low intensity. So while fear is a normal protective response (even if inappropriate in the current environment), phobias are maladaptive in virtually all contexts. In a phobic response we see:

- A reduction in behavioural variation or plasticity, which leads to the behaviour no longer being adaptive to the circumstances.
- Interference with day-to-day functioning because the animal becomes socially withdrawn.
- Hypervigilance and hyperreactivity, due to a change in the baseline level of activity in a part of the brain known as the *locus coeruleus*.
- Broad attempts to avoid what is going on in the environment.

Animals suffering from a phobia in this sense have more than just a severe fear and are much more challenging to treat. They typically need psychopharmacological support in the short-term to help them have a reasonable quality of life while a behaviour-modification plan is instigated.

## 9.3   EVALUATION OF NOISE FEARS

### 9.3.1   *DESCRIPTION OF PRESENTING SIGNS*

The most common signs that a dog shows when it is scared of noise include: panting, trembling, hiding, restlessness and cowering. Dogs also occasionally drool a lot, but this is rarely a problem for the owner. Other signs are less common but more likely to be of concern: destructiveness, elimination and vocalisation. While being less common, these feature very frequently in referred cases, simply because they pose a problem to the owner and not because they indicate a more severe problem for the animal. This may in part explain the disparity between the occurrence of sound sensitivities and their referral for treatment described in Section 9.1. In the studies we have undertaken into sound sensitivities, we have tended to ask owners about 18 categories of sign (see Appendix B):

1  Running around.
2  Drooling saliva.
3  Hiding: under furniture, behind the owner and so on. Indicate where.
4  Destructiveness: of furniture, doors, carpets and so on. Indicate which items tend to be damaged.
5  Cowering: tucks tail, flattens ears and so on.
6  Restlessness or pacing.
7  Aggression: growling, snapping or biting.
8  Freezing to the spot.
9  Barking, whining or howling. Indicate which.
10  Panting.
11  Vomiting, defecating, urinating and/or diarrhoea. Indicate which.
12  Owner-seeking behaviour.
13  Vigilance or scanning of the environment.
14  Bolting.
15  An exaggerated startle response.
16  Shaking or trembling.
17  Self-harm.
18  Other reactions not covered in the above.

Typically, animals show about eight of these signs. In addition, each is scored for both frequency and intensity over a period of time. Scoring allows us to monitor progress more objectively, since cases do not suddenly get completely better. The frequency score has a range from 0 to 3.

* An animal scores 0 if it never shows the sign.
* 1 if it rarely shows it.
* 2 if it frequently shows it.
* 3 if it shows it every time.

The intensity score ranges from 0 to 5 and depends on the specific sign. For example, for a sign like running around an intensity score of 0 means that the individual does not show this behaviour, while a score of 5 is given if it shows it an extensive amount, continuously running around when scared. The full questionnaire is given in Appendix B.

A global score for the problem over the given time period can be calculated by multiplying the frequency of each sign by its individual severity and summing the scores for all signs. Typically the cases we see have an initial global score of around 20.

This scoring system is aimed at increasing the objectivity of the data obtained from owners, by asking them to focus separately on the frequency and the intensity, and owners have been found to be quite reliable in their personal use of the scale from one situation to another. This makes it particularly useful for trying to monitor progress. It is also important with some signs, like destructiveness, to identify the targets of the behaviour, because one of the indications of change may be a reduction in the number of targets that are being destroyed. For example, when asking about destructiveness, we might ask owners to indicate what the animal is destroying: furniture, doors, carpets and so on. They will be asked to score both the frequency of damage of each of these targets (never–rarely–frequently–every time) and the intensity of the behaviour towards each target (ranging from 1 (for a small amount of damage, such as a few scratches) to 5 (for an extensive amount of damage, such as holes in the wall)). For some behaviours, owners may need help in clarifying what information is being sought. For example, some clients are not familiar with the term 'cowering', so we describe it as the animal tucking its tail and flattening its ears. By doing so, we can get a consistent picture of the owner's evaluation of the animal's behaviour in response to sound, alternatively they may be shown videos.

## 9.3.2   *DEVELOPMENTAL BIOLOGY*

A developmental evaluation focuses on the extent to which the emergence of the fear was learned or spontaneous. Learning plays an important role in the instigation of many sound sensitivities. Clearly, exposure to some noises is traumatic for an animal and as a consequence the animal learns to avoid them: this is the typical 'learned fear'. A very loud bang, for example, might scare the animal, who in future may become scared of similar situations. However, some owners believe their pet has learned its fear from another dog. We therefore have at least two mechanisms:

- Traumatic association.
- Observational learning.

Learning may also be important in the development of a phenomenon known as a 'pseudofear', which is an important differential from a welfare perspective. In a pseudofear an animal which has shown a mild, fearful response to an unpleasant event learns from the owner's response that is an effective attention-getting behaviour. Thus the animal learns to show this response in order to gain its owner's attention in a wide range of situations, including when sounds like the original trigger are heard. Exposure tests may be necessary in order to differentiate a pseudofear from a noise fear; these might involve playing noise recordings to the animal and monitoring its heart-rate response and pulse, with and without the owner present. If the response is limited to when the owner is present or if the heart-rate response and pulse do not rise very much in response to the sound, this might suggest that the animal is showing a pseudofear. However, it is important to appreciate that for some animals heart rate and pulse will go up when they are scared and for others, often those with long-standing problems, they can actually slow down, due to dysregulation of the hypothalamic–pituitary–adrenal (HPA) axis in response to chronic exposure to stressors (see Chapter 1). It is the lack of change that is suggestive of an animal having a pseudofear rather than a true fear. Clearly, animals showing pseudofear will not respond to interventions like drugs designed to treat a fear, as they are not actually scared. Any case that does not respond to treatment and in which the owner is being compliant with the treatment should be carefully re-evaluated in this context; that is, whether the problem may be an attention-seeking activity. Animals with pseudofears will be less likely to show signs in the absence of the owner, but their response in a veterinary clinic may be very different to their response at home, so it may be necessary to instruct the owner to set up a camera to view the animal's response at home when they are not there. The concept of the pseudofear suggests that owners can play an important role in the learning process associated with fears, and this is important when we consider the basics of problem management. If such a condition is suspected, it is important to counsel the owners carefully so that they do not feel they are being deliberately 'duped' by their pet, but rather that it is natural and normal for animals to do what works for them.

Clearly, some fears relate to stimuli that we might expect an animal to be bio-logically predisposed to perceive as aversive, and these can be expected to occur unless the animal has been habituated to them. Other fears develop in response to specific traumatic associations. However, in some instances fear develops as a result of cumulative aversive experiences, none of which alone would be great enough to produce a learned association with noise. *Sensitisation* is the process by which an animal is exposed to something mildly unpleasant which on its own would not evoke a significant fear response but which on repeat exposure over a relatively short period of time comes to be perceived as significantly aversive. We believe this may be quite a common occurrence in certain noise fears, such as a fear of fireworks. It is not a single specific traumatic event that sets the animal off, but the exposure to the same stimulus repeatedly over a period of time.

Another way in which cumulative stressors can provoke the emergence of a fearful response relates to a process known as *stress-induced dishabituation*. Stressors in the form of either a singular traumatic event, such as the experience of a car accident, or a series of events over a longer period of time (see Chapter 1) may precipitate this phenomenon. When an animal is highly stressed it can forget some of the things that it has learned; for example, a puppy that has been habituated to loud noises may come to be afraid of these as an adult. We are only just beginning to realise how common this may be, but the more we examine it in relation to stress auditing (see Chapter 1), the more apparent it appears. In these cases, it is obviously essential to treat the underlying stress load of the animal and not just focus on the noise fear. Specialist referral may be required and pheromonatherapy clearly has an important role to play in these cases.

Finally, in some cases dogs will present with fears in later life as a result of a lack of earlier *habituation* to the relevant stimuli. If an animal is not exposed to noises when it is very young, it does not have the chance to create the episodic memories that form a reference database of things that are 'safe'. Younger animals are generally more accepting of unusual and novel events, so if unfamiliar noises are encountered for the first time later in life, an animal is more likely to become scared of them. This appears to be particularly true for engine noises and loud bangs. However, it is not a question of playing loud bangs to puppies, as this might scare them and induce a traumatic fear; instead, quieter noises should be played to them in acoustically complex environments, and the volume steadily increased in order to make them tolerant of louder sounds and unfamiliar sounds.

### 9.3.3   THE EFFECT OF OWNER RESPONSE

The description of a fear as learned or not focuses on the initial development of the response. However, it is worth emphasising the role of learning in the subsequent development of that response. In the case of both true and pseudofears, owner attempts at reassurance or consolation may provide relief and negatively reinforce the behaviour, thereby making it more intense. In the case of a true fear, the owner may additionally become a conditioned safety signal, in which case the animal can cope better when they are present but has no way of coping when they are absent. As a result, the problem may present as an owner-absent problem (see Chapter 8). In either case, we need the animal to be more confident, as opposed to just seeking the owner. Therefore the involvement of the owner in these situations has to be evaluated for every individual case, and encouragement of behaviour that signals an apparent lack of interest by the owner in the animal's response is often a key element to the management of many of these cases.

Another common way owners react to their pet being scared is to try to punish it verbally, if not physically, by scolding, in a misguided attempt to tell it that there is nothing to worry about. This is only likely to make matters worse, since the animal will learn that the sound is now predictive of the owner punishing it. This not only intensifies the fear but also undermines the owner–pet bond and can lead to aggressive behaviour towards the owner. As a consequence of such a situation, the animal is also more likely to become generally more scared and develop other problems.

Although one study looking at thunderstorm-anxious dogs found that in this particular case the owner's reactions had very little influence on the dog's behaviour (Dreschel & Granger, 2005), it is unclear to what degree this finding can be generalised. We believe it is important to identify what owners do in response to an animal's behaviour and to correct any misconceptions. This is important because even if punishment is not making matters worse, the owner needs to be educated that their response is not in the animal's interests. This study also found that the owner's mood affected their behavioural response to their dog; for example, if the owner was angry, they were far more likely to punish the animal. This reminds us that we must do more than tell owners not to punish their animals; we need to let them know that, while we understand that they might want to punish their dog when they get angry or frustrated with it, it is not the dog's fault that it gets scared and they should try not to get angry in the first place. The aim is to try to increase the owner's understanding of their pet's problem in order to bring about a change in their behaviour, which will help the dog.

### 9.3.4 OTHER ASSESSMENTS OF THE SOUND-SENSITIVE PATIENT

Other assessments that can help us to form a fuller picture include the following:

- *Screening the animal for other behaviour problems*: For example, separation-related problems.
- *Assessing the animal's general health*: A veterinarian should look over the animal to check that there are no underlying physical issues which might be exacerbating the problem. For example, pain can occur when an animal tenses its muscles if it has arthritis, and older animals may be suffering a more general change in *anxiety–fear* reactivity.
- *Reflection on the age of onset*: Clearly, animals with a late age of onset are less likely to be suffering from a lack of habituation – they are more likely to be suffering from dishabituation or a problem related to cognitive decline.
- *Review of any ongoing or associated medication or therapy*: These may not be related to the noise fears, but might still be of relevance; for example, if a medication increases blood pressure, it can predispose an animal to a fearful response. Concomitant treatment with corticosteroids, for example due to itchy skin, also seems to predispose animals to the development of fear responses.
- *Clinical tests*: It is often quite useful to evaluate an animal's responses in the presence of the fear stimulus. In some cases we can get this information from the owner; in others we can play a recording to the animal and measure its response. This has to be done with sensitivity and care. Important evaluations are:
  ○ How much will the animal play with and without the noise in the background?
  ○ Will the animal eat with and without the noise?
  ○ How long does it take the animal to return to normal when the noise stops?
  ○ How does the animal behave with and without the owner present? A marked improvement in the absence of the owner may suggest that the behaviour has a large component of attention-seeking.
  However, a big challenge with the use of recordings is the tendency for many animals not to respond to them with anything like the same degree of response they exhibit for the spontaneous noise. This might also limit their value as a potential treatment recommendation. In our research studies, we have found little evidence to suggest that the quality of the sound system or recording has much effect on the likelihood of an animal responding in the normal way.
- *Identification and classification of predictive stimuli*: It is important to identify all the stimuli that trigger the problem, not just the one that set it off initially. In some cases, a noise fear may be associated with fears linked to other sensory channels; for example, an animal that is afraid of fireworks may also be afraid of the smoke from a fire and become scared of the fireplace at home. A distinction should be made between primary and secondary stimuli: *primary stimuli* are those that the animal first becomes scared of and *secondary stimuli* are those that the animal has learned through association to become scared of. When it comes to treatment, it is often

easier to address the secondary stimuli first. If the fear has started to generalise into a more complex problem or a phobia, there will clearly be secondary stimuli.`

## 9.4   DIFFERENTIAL DIAGNOSIS

The main emotional differentials to consider in relation to sound sensitivity are:

- Activation of the *anxiety–fear* system in the case of a true fear or phobia. The posture and response of the animal to sounds both with and without the owner may be useful in reaching a definitive diagnosis, together with a clearly relevant history of onset.
- Activation of the *desire* system, as occurs in a pseudofear.
- Activation of the *desire* system, as occurs when an animal is trying to play with a noise-producing object, such as a vacuum cleaner, but the owner misinterprets this as fear. The body posture here does not normally involve fearfulness, unless the animal has been punished, in which case there are signs of mixed motivational–emotional arousal.
- Activation of the *frustration* system, as occurs when an animal seeks to interact with a sound-producing object but is denied access. As with object-directed play, the animal may be highly aroused, and in the case of dogs this, together with barking, may be misinterpreted as fear by an owner. In this case, the behaviour only occurs in the context of denied access to the physical stimulus and the animal will become less aroused if given access to the focal resource. The animal may also be more likely to show redirected and conflict behaviours during the response, without obvious signs of fear, unless it has been punished by its owner.

## 9.5   MANAGEMENT OF NOISE FEARS

As with any behaviour problem, the preferred element of management is prevention, and this is one area in which pheromonatherapy may be very useful. However, we must also obviously consider intervention treatment. This follows the 'three Rs' principle: we must assess the Risks involved, Restrict the problem and Resolve the problem.

### 9.5.1   *PREVENTION*

Habituation of animals to a wide variety of sounds is clearly key to the prevention of a range of noise fears, and there are many good texts on this topic. In the largest survey of its kind, we have reviewed the data from dogs with noise fears and matched controls; we found that if the dogs were not exposed to engine noises when they were very young (less than 6 months old), they were much more likely to develop a noise fear later in life. Interestingly, other work by Appleby *et al.* (2002) has suggested that puppies who are not exposed to an urban environment are also in danger of developing a wider range of fears later in life. It might be that these two findings are linked. At the very least, we should consider it important for clients who live in rural areas to be encouraged to take their animals into towns and cities when it is safe to do so, in order to expose their pets to a wide variety of sights, sounds and smells and to help the animals develop appropriate responses for later in life. However, it is important to do this in a managed way, in order not to overwhelm the puppy. Carefully observing the puppy's body language is important for judging the right amount of stimulation at a given point in time. The animal should ideally be able to create positive associations with these stimuli, rather than simply habituate to them. In addition, there are now a large number of CDs and recordings available to play to animals when they are young in order to help them develop appropriately. There may be an important role for pheromonatherapy in this context, as we would expect that the provision of signals which encourage a sense of safety should encourage and speed up the acceptance of novel stimuli, including sounds, although no specific study has sought to confirm or refute this to date. Getting the animal out and about and carefully exposed to sights and sounds may be preferable, as it allows a greater range of associations to be made with all senses, which might serve to create a greater acceptance of novelty in general. However, a potential disadvantage of this is the reduced level of control over the intensity of the stimuli compared to recordings, which can be started at a very low volume so that we can be confident that the animal is not going to be scared. While out on a walk, for example, a car might suddenly backfire and potentially cause a problem, if not managed appropriately. It is therefore important for owners to be made aware of how to handle such an eventuality. In general, they should not draw attention to the event and should themselves show a lack of interest in the stimulus, although they should ensure the animal is safe. If they have something that the animal likes then the owner should draw attention to this and show them how good it is, so that the animal chooses to express a more positive motivational–emotional priority (see Section 9.5.3). It must not be forced on the puppy though, as this could be perceived as intimidating. If the animal appears particularly traumatised, the owner should be encouraged to seek immediate veterinary assistance, since in some cases benzodiazepine drugs can be used to try to block the memory of an event, if they are administered shortly afterwards (a couple of hours at most).

## 9.5.2   RISK ASSESSMENT

As with any case evaluation, the following need to be examined before intervention recommendations can be made:

- The risk to immediate contacts.
- The risk to the patient.
- The risk to others.

The risk of recurrence should also be considered.

Animals that are scared can pose a number of risks to owners and other individuals in the family. They can become aggressive and can cause damage to property in their attempts to escape. Quite apart from the obvious risk to the patient's well-being caused by the existence of a specific fear, patients can also harm themselves as they try to escape. They may also be a significant risk to others: animals afraid of traffic noises can run across a road and cause a traffic accident. In all of these situations, specific control measures may need to be put in place.

Specific restrictive control measures may be required to limit the risk in the short term – including avoidance of exposure where possible – while the problem is resolved.

In relation to the risk of recurrence, neither the duration nor the severity of the problem has been shown to be predictive of treatment success, and so these factors alone are not of value when trying to predict risk or relapse, although they may reflect current threats to welfare. The risk of recurrence is obviously high if we do not address the specific triggers of the response. Likewise, animals that have developed a fear as a result of stress-induced dishabituation are at a higher risk of relapse if the wider underlying stressors are not addressed. Individuals that are temperamentally predisposed to *anxiety–fear* are also at a much higher risk of recurrence, and the outlook in such cases has to be much more guarded than in those who have more emotionally balanced characters.

## 9.5.3   *RESTRICTION OF THE PROBLEM*

Restriction of the problem focuses on immediate control in order to minimise risk. Some of these measures also lay a foundation for longer-term resolution of the problem. Many methods of problem restriction are described in the literature, and a few of the more common ones are discussed below. Their appropriateness will vary from case to case; in extreme cases, containment to limit damage and self-harm may be required in the short term:

- *Avoidance of exposure*: Until the problem has been brought under control, it is important to try to avoid exposure to problem sounds, if possible. This might mean keeping the animal in a quiet room or allowing it access to a cupboard with plenty of cushions, in order to soundproof the area. Earplugs and doggy ear defenders are also a possibility. These can be home made by carefully placing cotton wool in the animal's ears, perhaps together with a head stocking to hold things in place. Although many dogs will resist this initially, often they can be trained to accept it with time, patience and positive reinforcement. Another technique is to use noise masks. The idea here is to play music, which can be tolerated, to mask (and thus avoid exposure to) other noises that the animal is scared of. For example, if the animal can cope with some classical music, this could be played quite loud while there are fireworks going on outside so that the actual sounds of the bangs are masked to a degree.
- *Blunting of physiological and behavioural responses*: In the case of fears, an animal's physiological and behavioural responses can have feedback effects; that is, an animal that shows a very marked physiological response is likely to become even more scared the next time. Therefore, controlling the physiological and behavioural responses can be quite important in trying to reduce the intensity

of the behaviour in the short term. Nonsedating but tranquilising drugs, food supplements and pheromonatherapy may be very useful in this regard. In severe cases, and those with temperamental traits which exacerbate the problem, the use of drugs is also warranted on welfare grounds, since such animals are suffering to an unacceptable degree. However, medication should not be used as a long-term solution to a problem that can be managed with effective psychological behavioural intervention. Drugs like acepromazine should also be avoided because it is believed that they may actually worsen the sound sensitivity in the longer term, as the animal loses all control over the fearful event when it is sedated. It is essential that a veterinarian be consulted if it is thought that drugs may be necessary, in order to ensure that the risks are fully explained. Not being a veterinarian is not a reason to exclude using drugs in favour of supplements or other interventions – the welfare of the patient must come first. It is also important to distinguish between long-term and short-term medicinal strategies. Short-term strategies focus on helping the animal through the immediate crisis, such as the use of benzodiazepines to control the response to specific events. Longer-term strategies aim at broader mood control, such as the use of serotonergic agents (e.g. clomipramine or fluoxetine), in the control of underlying anxiousness, in cases of a seasonal nature (e.g. around the new year).

- *Changes in owner behaviour*: There are simple things that the owner can do to try to restrict the problem and not make it worse. The owner should stop any punishment that they are giving. Similarly, they should stop any inadvertent reinforcement, for example by personally trying to comfort a scared animal (our data suggest 70% of owners do this). The ideal response of an owner when there is noise of which their pet is scared is to signal to the animal that the sound does not bother them. This might involve carrying on as if nothing has happened or showing an intense interest in something else. This could be a favourite toy or treat, but it should not be offered directly to the animal; that is, the owner should not overtly try to engage their pet in a new activity, but rather focus their own attention on something of potential interest and sees if the animal wants to engage as well (Figure 9.2). If it willingly chooses to engage, without being prompted by the owner, then there is a greater chance that the negative emotion will have been replaced by a more positive one, since the animal is not joining in simply because it has been told to do so. If the pet does choose to join them, the owner can then play with, give treats to or otherwise engage with the pet, thus reinforcing the choice to engage in positive rather than negative emotional behaviour.

- *Provision of a safe haven*: When animals have a noise fear, they need to be trained to the site of a safe haven (see Chapter 1). This is an area where the animal is in control and which has become a conditioned place of safety outside of times when there are problematic sounds. Thus, when the stressful situation does occur, the animal can retreat to this area and should feel relatively safe. This often helps to reduce panicky reactions. It is important that the animal is trained to this area when it is not scared and that the area is not simply provided as a bolthole but rather is a place where the animal has only positive experiences: its toys are there and its favourite treats are often placed there for it to find. The use

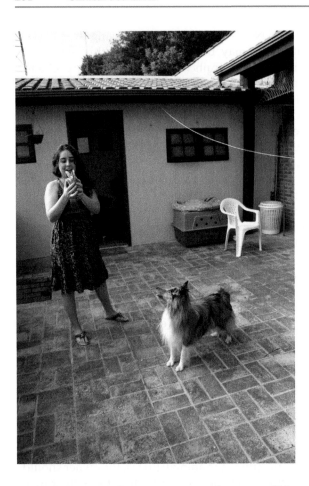

Fig. 9.2 When trying to use a distracting stimulus to interrupt a negative emotional state, it is important to find something which interests the animal and to enhance its value by paying attention to it, rather than try to force the object on the animal. Notice how the owner's attention is focused on playing with this toy, rather than on the dog, who is now choosing to engage in the new activity. In this way, problem behaviour is not reinforced.

of pheromonatherapy to provide unconditioned safety signals can be very helpful in this regard. Once this positive association with a number of signals of safety is made, the animal's decision to retire to this area in situations when it is uncertain and stressed should be respected, as this will help it to cope. It may be useful to introduce a fearless companion. However, it has to be certain that this animal is truly fearless and not likely to develop the fear as a result of being in the company of the noise-phobic or noise-scared animal.

These are all measures that might help restrict the problem and stop it from getting worse, but in the longer term we must try to resolve the problem through the use of some additional measures.

### 9.5.4   RESOLUTION OF THE PROBLEM

It is important that the client appreciates the importance of long-term resolution over simple containment or convenience management of the problem. To this end, it is worth spending some time explaining the animal's needs and interests first, and agreeing with them how important these are to the animal's well-being. In this way, the client recognises and acknowledges the longer-term commitment that they will need to make at the outset; otherwise there is a much greater risk that they will only want to restrict the problem if it is easier for them. If we are to resolve the problem, it is important that we are fully aware of any other underlying problems which might also need management, such as stressors in the home. Even if the reaction to noise is not related to stress-induced dishabituation, a chronic stress load in the home will make treatment much more difficult as the animal is unlikely to have anywhere that it feels safe. As already mentioned, many animals with noise fears might also suffer from separation-related problems, which must be kept in mind.

Since the sense of safety is so important in sound-sensitivity cases, it is not surprising that pheromonatherapy is thought to be very useful in the management of these, although it does not treat the sound sensitivity directly and so should not be used alone but rather as part of an overall strategy. In our experience, we think it helps to improve both the rate of response to related behaviour therapy and the creation of a safe haven. Details of a range of interventions described in the literature are given in Table 9.1. In this section we will focus discussion on two particular elements of importance: the effective implementation of sound-desensitisation procedures and pheromonatherapy.

It is worth emphasising at this point the importance of monitoring progress, since these problems do not suddenly go away. Treatment can take a long time and it is only by monitoring progress that owners can be encouraged that they are on the right track and specific additional needs can be identified.

## 9.5.4.1  BEHAVIOUR THERAPY

Behaviour therapy is key to the resolution of sound sensitivities. This typically involves *habituation* and/or *systematic desensitisation* techniques, together with *counterconditioning*. In essence, the animal is exposed to noises at levels with which it can cope and the volume is gradually increased using a structured programme. When using these techniques, short and frequent sessions are preferable to longer ones. There are many commercially available CD training programmes that can be used for this purpose, but some CD products are designed to be used quite differently (e.g. as noise masks). It is therefore important to be familiar with specific products so that specific recommendations can be made with confidence. Even among those designed for desensitisation, there may be some variability in the way the sounds are put together and how the CD is supposed to be used. In this section we will highlight some important principles and common errors in the use of these programmes, since the detail is not always clear.

In general it is worth using a prescribed system, with owners taken through the instructions for the given CD programme, with emphasis given to key points.

It is also important to ensure that an appropriate recording is used, and this may vary from patient to patient. Obviously the animal must respond to the recording, but it must also be recognised that some animals can show signs of sensitisation to

Table 9.1 Some measures for helping to resolve apparent sound sensitivity in dogs, according to their putative motivational–emotional basis. Note that all treatments must be calibrated and adapted according to the case, and not all measures are recommended in every case.

| Management procedure | Anxiety–fear | Frustration | Desire – stimulus play | Desire – pseudofear attention-seeking |
|---|---|---|---|---|
| **Chemical** | | | | |
| Nutraceuticals based on magnesium, alpha-casozepine, tryptophan, l-theanine etc. | x | | | |
| Herbal supplements – skullcap, valerian, St John's wort, lavender, chamomile | x | | | |
| Benzodiazepines | x | | | |
| N/S SRIs fluoxetine, clompramine etc. | x | | | |
| MAOIB: selegiline | x | ?x | | |
| Trazadone | x | | | |
| Clonidine | x | | | |
| Phenobarbitone and propranolol | x | | | |
| **Environmental** | | | | |
| Safe haven (note that a large percentage of owners have a difficult time understanding this concept. It is worth reviewing and checking understanding) | x | | | |
| Dog-appeasing pheromone (DAP): tailor format (diffuser, spray, collar) to the dog's situation. | x | | | |
| Music therapy: such as classical music (low-frequency) to calm the dog | x | | | |
| **Physical** | | | | |
| Thundershirt/Anxiety Wrap® | x | | | |
| Antistatic cape for thunderstorm fears (dogs who seek out bathroom/discharging objects) | x | | | |
| **Psychological** | | | | |
| Behavioural control exercises (e.g. shhh on command) | | x | x | x |
| Signal of no reward | | x | x | x |
| Increase in interaction with the owner when the dog is not showing problem behaviour | | | x | x |
| 'Enough' cue to stop activity | | | x | x |

Table 9.1  (cont'd).

| Management procedure | Anxiety–fear | Frustration | Desire – stimulus play | Desire – pseudofear attention-seeking |
|---|---|---|---|---|
| Training of frustration tolerance | | x | | x |
| Respondent counterconditioning | x | | | x |
| Negative punishment of attention-seeking and positive reinforcement of incompatible behaviour | | | | x |
| Reducing the dog's dependence on the owner | | | | x |
| Behavioural control exercises (leave, wait) | | x | | |
| Desensitisation and counterconditioning | x | x | x | x |
| Signal to refocus animal (nose touch/watch me on verbal cue, recall training?) | x | x | x | x |

these recordings. This means that when the owner starts to play the CD, the animal's reaction gets worse on repeat occasions, even when used at a low volume. In these cases, the owner should stop all treatment immediately and seek further specialist help. It is likely in these cases that supplementary medication will be required to help the animal.

The following points regarding the training programme should be kept in mind:

- *Keep a diary*: Owners need to be encouraged to keep records, and it is worth providing them with a daily diary for this purpose.
- *Ensure the animal has a safe haven (rather than bolt hole)*: This is one of the most common misunderstandings on the part of owners. Pheromonatherapy in the form of dog-appeasing pheromone (DAP) sprays applied to the area or a nearby diffuser can be very useful in helping to facilitate this.
- *Train away from high-risk situations*: Often owners will seek help during or a week or two before a big firework event if their pet is scared of such sounds. At this time, steps aimed at resolving the problem are limited, and attempting desensitisation is not advised, as the animal is likely to be exposed to severe and uncontrollable events which can undermine any training put in beforehand. It needs to be explained to the owner at this time that, in the longer term, they will need to address the root of the problem, although short-term containment is possible.
- *Work on secondary stimuli first*: There is some evidence to suggest that greater progress can be made by working first on stimuli which do not provoke too great a response or on secondary stimuli; that is, stimuli which have been

learned by association. Secondary stimuli might include the smell of bonfires in an animal who is scared of fireworks. The animal was not scared of bonfires in the first instance but because bonfires have been associated with the fireworks it is now scared of the smell of burning wood. Alternatively, the secondary stimuli might be other noise stimuli, so that the animal who is scared of fireworks is now also showing signs of being scared of other banging or high-pitched noises. By working on these stimuli, which the animal responds to less, we can start to make progress sooner. As the animal starts to improve, we stand a better chance of making improvements with the more intense stimuli as well, as it learns to cope with previous aversions. While these secondary stimuli might not be the primary focus of the owner, the owner is more likely to buy in to a longer-term treatment strategy if the need for these initial measures is explained and they see quick progress in these peripheral concerns.

- *Train little and often*: Training should be done on a little-and-often basis and should not be too monotonous. Our own research suggests that the frequency rather than the duration of a typical training session is a better predictor of the success of the programme.
- *Use powerful rewards*: The idea is to provide the animal with strong signals of pleasure in order to counteract any tendency to feel scared. Possible incentives need to be identified in advance and ranked accordingly.
- *Exercise*: It can be useful to advise the owner to exercise their pet before every training bout. This will encourage it to relax.
- *Reliability*: It is important to give clear instructions as to what is meant by 'reliable' when considering moving on to the next stage of training. This will need to be adapted for individual cases. With animals that are very anxious, a higher level of reliability and a greater duration are often needed in every phase before moving on.
- *Pheromonatherapy to help facilitate training*: Both DAP in dogs and F3 in cats have been used in this context. Although there are no published trials, there are sound reasons to believe that by creating a greater sense of security in the home, learning will proceed more smoothly and rapidly, with less risk of relapse. This effect is additional to the value of pheromonatherapy in helping create a safe haven.

## Systematic desensitisation

*Systematic desensitisation* basically means raising the threshold at which an animal responds to a given stimulus, through controlled incremental exposure. If an animal reacts to a noise at a certain level, after systematic desensitisation it should not react to the noise at that or at any other level.

In order to carry out systematic desensitisation we must try to reduce the impact of the problem situation at a number of levels, in preparation for controlled exposure:

- *Intensity*: We might want to reduce the perceived intensity of the stimulus. In the case of noise fears, this is relatively easy – it can be done by reducing the volume in the majority of cases.

- *Context*: Changing the context might help. For example, if the animal tends to be in one particular room when it gets scared, training it in a different room might help it to make progress, as it does not have the same associations with the new room. However, it is also important to recognise that learning may be context-specific and so at least some training will be required in the other rooms if the animal is to generalise its learning effectively.
- *Stimulus complexity*: If there are a number of components to the problem, for example flashing lights and noises in the case of fireworks, then getting the animal used to flashing lights in the first instance (which can be done by using a flashgun and a range of filters at night) may help it when it comes to getting used to noises.

Several authors have suggested that before a systematic desensitisation programme is started, the animal should be habituated to levels of sound that can be readily tolerated. This means playing recordings for prolonged periods of time at a very quiet level, while the animal goes about its normal business. In the early stages it might be worth playing them at a very low level when the animal is about to be fed. A 'very low level' is one at which the animal does not show any extended change in its behaviour, beyond perhaps an initial pricking of the ear towards the sound. It is important to clearly define an acceptable level of response. The aim is for the animal to show some recognition of the stimulus (but not a significant startle response) and to rapidly accept it, returning to its other activity within a few seconds of exposure.

Not only should the deconstruction of the problem be defined for initiation of treatment, but so should its reconstruction for progress and consolidation of the associated learning. Key elements to consider concerning progress within a systematic desensitisation programme are:

- *Stimulus gradient*: This refers to the definition and sequencing of intensity of individual component stimuli to which the animal needs to be desensitised. The intensity of events needs to be defined both within a stimulus category and between stimulus categories, in order to produce a sequence of events that ranges from those that are most readily accepted to those that are the most challenging. Each element that the animal is scared of is introduced in turn, at the lowest acceptable level of intensity for that stimulus. If necessary, pretraining to cotton-wool earplugs may be required, not only to reduce volume but also to muffle the suddenness of the sound. As the animal's behaviour improves, less cotton wool can be used – but obviously not pieces so small that they might be lost or difficult to remove.
- *Criteria for climbing the gradient*: While the principle of gradually increasing the intensity is fairly simple to understand, in practice it helps to define the criteria for climbing the gradient. For example, it is preferable to say, 'When you have played the track five times while the dog behaves perfectly normally, you can start turning the volume up by one notch,' rather than just, 'As the dog seems to adapt you can turn the volume up'. The latter explanation leaves a lot of room for error and misunderstanding. This measured change is what we mean by 'climbing the gradient'.

- *Combining stimuli*: The animal should be systematically desensitised to one stimulus at a time. It may be that it gets desensitised to one type of sound, such as bangs, before it gets desensitised to another, such as the whizzing noises of fireworks. Once it has become desensitised to these two types of noise, they can be combined. This should, however, be done at a lower volume than the dog can tolerate when each sounds is played individually, as the fact that it can accept the individual noises does not mean that it will be able to adapt to the combined noises at the same volume.
- *Maintenance schedule*: Once the animal has become desensitised, it is important to remember that the change achieved is a learned response. So the animal should occasionally be reminded that it can cope with the sounds, and not just left alone for a year until the next firework season comes along and it has forgotten that it can cope. Playing the CD or sound recording on an occasional basis throughout the year and checking that the animal can cope is important to maintaining success.

## Counterconditioning

*Counterconditioning* means eliciting a behaviour that is not compatible with the problem behaviour: 'conditioning' describes a type of learning and 'counter' means 'against'. There are two forms of counterconditioning:

- *Respondent counterconditioning*: In this case, an unconditioned response is used. For example, the arrival of food is associated with noises. If the animal accepts the food, this is not compatible with being scared.
- *Operant counterconditioning*: In this case, the animal is trained to carry out a specific behaviour for a reward. For example, it might sit or lie down to receive treats.

In either case, the principles are the same. What is important is to find something that the animal is highly motivated to do, whether this is a trained or a natural response. When using counterconditioning, a clear stimulus should be used which signals that the animal is about to get rewarded. This signal should trigger the desired emotional response, which is counter to fear. For example, teaching the animal 'now we are going to play' and getting it excited before the recording is turned on may reduce the tendency for the animal to react with fear to the recording (especially if the recording can be switched on remotely). Generally speaking, counterconditioning is used in combination with systematic desensitisation; that is, the animal is trained to express a particular motivational–emotional state in a given way, which it is then asked to do while it is exposed over time to gradually increasing intensities of the noise that it was originally scared of.

The following are some general guidelines regarding the effective use of counterconditioning in practice:

- Do not try to evoke the counter response in the actual problem setting before the animal has properly learned it. If an owner is training an animal to play and there are noises that the animal might otherwise be scared of, the owner should not try to encourage the animal to continue to play with the specific cue used in training. They might have a number of other signals for play which they can try, but they should protect the conditioned signal. For this reason, it may be worth training several cues for play at the outset, and so reduce the danger that all the hard work be undone by a single bad experience and an error on the owner's part.

- Use a powerful unconditional stimulus or train an operant response until it becomes a habitual stimulus response association. If the animal is very highly motivated by food or play, these can be excellent responses to use. However, if the animal has to be trained to do something, it is important that it is very consistent in its response to the command request before this is combined with the problem stimulus. It is not sufficient to have an animal that sits seven times out of ten. The animal must sit ten times out of ten, and do so very quickly. This may be too difficult for some owners, in which case additional training support should be provided.

- Introduce the problem scenario in accordance with an agreed schedule. Before the technique is combined with a systematic desensitisation gradient, it is useful to check the robustness of the counterconditioned response in the presence of a range of increasingly complex, but not too emotionally arousing, distractions. Only when a very reliable response has been established in these contexts should we consider combining the counterconditioning with the systematic-desensitisation part of the programme. It is normal for the animal's response to deteriorate slightly and temporarily as more challenging scenarios are faced, and it should be supported to make the right decision at such times; if this is not successful (i.e. the desired response is not restored within five repetitions), the owner will have to go back a stage and repeat the earlier training.

- *Intermittent refreshers*: Once training is complete, it is important that the animal has occasional refreshers to make sure that it does not forget its learning and that its response remains sharp. The focus of reinforcement should be on a short latency of response to the cue.

## 9.5.4.2   *ADJUNCTS TO TRAINING*

While training is the mainstay and the individual programme will vary from case to case, there are adjuncts to training which can be essential for success, such as addressing underlying anxiety and stress-related problems. This not only improves the welfare of the patient but also improves the learning process by helping the animal to pay attention to the training and helping it to consolidate its memory. In our opinion, pheromonatherapy can help to speed up the rate of response. Medication may also be used for this purpose, but a danger with this is that owners become less compliant with the behaviour-therapy elements of the programme. This is perhaps a good reason to consider using pheromonatherapy in preference to medication for milder cases. However, if necessary the two can be combined. Supplements can be used in a similar way, although there is at least a theoretical risk from combining tryptophan and certain herbal extracts, such as St John's wort, with serotonergic drugs.

### 9.5.5 *PHEROMONATHERAPY AND SOUND SENSITIVITIES*

Both F3 (in cats) and DAP (in dogs) have been recommended for use as an aid in the management of sound sensitivities at a number of levels: prevention, management of the immediate problematic response and as part of the longer-term resolution of the problem. All of these effects are based around the idea that the chemical message creates an emotional bias in favour of perceived safety. In the context of prevention, this means certain sound stimuli never develop an aversive quality. In the context of immediate exposure, it means the animal is less likely to perceive the current stimuli as threatening. Finally in the context of resolution, the signal encourages a more positive emotional bias during training, speeding progression up the stimulus gradient. The products may also have broader background effects that are no less important, helping to reduce background stress and aiding in the creation of a specific safe haven. However, it is also important to appreciate their limitations. These products are not anxiolytics and so their effect is somewhat contextually limited. Also, if an animal is panicking at the slightest instance of the noise, the chances of successfully using pheromonatherapy without a structured desensitisation programme are much lower. In these sorts of cases, it is worth combining the pheromonatherapy with medication; this must only be done under veterinary supervision.

DAP seems to have little effect, at least initially, on owner-seeking behaviour, and so it is not indicated for use with pseudofear. The lack of an effect in clinical studies on this aspect of the problem is not surprising as most owners have a history of giving their animal a lot of attention and the withdrawal of this attention is part of the standard management protocol. As a result, any behaviour that was previously reinforced and which no longer receives a reward may be expected to get worse before it gets better (an *extinction burst*). It is thus not surprising to see that such behaviours do not reduce significantly at first. It is, however, important to counsel owners that this is the case.

Another important feature to note when using pheromonatherapy is that the animal is not sedated. It will still quite often be vigilant and may startle in response to the noise but then go back to doing what it was doing before. This type of response is quite different to the traditional response seen when sedatives are used. Since many animals will have been treated with sedatives previously and most owners are quite happy to see their animal appear to sleep through the noisy event, it is important to address this expectation, otherwise owners may be disappointed by the effect of pheromonatherapy. It is important to counsel the owners beforehand on what to expect and ensure that realistic expectations are set. The fact that the animal does not sleep through the event is actually a good sign and indicates that it is getting better; the startle indicates it is still alert and processing the information in a much healthier way.

## 9.6   PROGNOSIS

In those studies in which the outcome of treatment was specifically examined, no significant relationship between any measures of severity and reported treatment success was found, meaning that just because a problem is long-standing does not mean that the chances of treatment are reduced; that is, it is never too late to start.

In a study in which clients' use of a systematic desensitisation programme with DAP but no medication was closely monitored, around 90% of owners reported some improvement after treatment, and so this seems a reasonable expectation if clients can commit to the necessary training. Typically, there was a 60% reduction in signs, but this varied with the particular signs. Most improvement – that is, more than a 70% reduction – was seen in the signs of destructiveness, drooling, freezing, bolting and startling. By contrast, the least improvement was seen in owner-seeking, panting and vigilance. If destructiveness is a problem for the owner, the outlook is very good. In fact, every individual in this study stopped being destructive. Owners saw a significant response to the training within the first month.

Curiously, in another study, we have found that where animals have a fear of fireworks and a fear of thunder, treatment with a desensitisation programme seems to be more successful than in those who have just one of these fears. The possible reasons for this are unclear, and it may simply reflect a more committed owner or an increased ability to generalise experience by the dogs concerned. In our experience, we have consistently found that when using DAP the behavioural signs more typical of fearful arousal and extreme coping effort tend to disappear more readily than the signs of monitoring, including vigilance and anxiety.

In a long-term follow-up study in which owners were asked to systematically desensitise their animals using a CD and DAP, it was found that there was little evidence of any relapse 2 or 12 months after cessation of the formal training period.

A number of case reports suggest that F3 can help cats adjust to noise fears in the same way that DAP does for dogs. However, to date there are no fully documented cases in the scientific literature.

## 9.7   CONCLUSION

In conclusion, noise fears are a very common problem that can be successfully treated in the majority of cases through the use of behaviour therapy and phero-monatherapy. The severity of the signs and the duration of the problem do not predict the likelihood of treatment success; that is, even the most severe case stands a reasonable chance of improvement with careful management. The positive message that it is never too late and that no case is too bad for it to be worth attempting treatment needs to be given to owners. Finally, it is worth emphasising that while we want to keep things simple for clients in order to ensure good compliance, we must be careful about making them lazy. Pheromonatherapy, by addressing some of the stress-related issues but not sedating the animal, may help encourage owners to persist with the behaviour programme, to the benefit of their pet. In addition, pheromonatherapy can be very important in addressing other stress-related issues that can exacerbate sound sensitivities.

## REVIEW ACTIVITIES

- Design a handout for clients on how to prevent sound sensitivities. Include advice on what to do in a case of inadvertent traumatic exposure.
- What are the key features that allow the differentiation of a pseudofear from an aversive perception of sound? How would you explain this condition to a client who believes their dog is terrified of certain sounds?
- Make a suggested treatment plan for a dog who reacts to the doorbell ringing by running up to the door and barking and who will not calm for several minutes afterwards.
- Consider the possible reasons why an owner might report the failure of a desensitisation and counterconditioning programme with a noise CD.
- An owner reports an unsatisfying response to a basic containment programme based around the use of DAP by their dog, who is scared of fireworks. What is your plan of action?

## REFERENCES

Appleby DL, Bradshaw JWS, Casey RA (2002) Relationship between aggressive and avoidance behaviour by dogs and their experience in the first six months of life. Veterinary Record 150: 434–438.

Dreschel NA, Granger DA (2005) Physiological and behavioral reactivity to stress in thunderstorm-phobic dogs and their caregivers. Applied Animal Behaviour Science 95: 153–168.

PDSA (2011) The State of our Pet Nation. PDSA Animal Wellbeing Report. Available from http://www.pdsa.org.uk/pet-health-advice/pdsa-animal-wellbeing-report.

## FURTHER READING

Animal Behaviour Clinic of the University of Lincoln. Resources available from http://www.lincoln.ac.uk/dbs/abc/.

Levine ED, Ramos D, Mills DS (2007) A prospective study of two self-help CD based desensitization and counterconditioning programmes with the use of DAP for the treatment of firework fears in dogs. Applied Animal Behaviour Science 105: 311–329.

Mills D (2005) Management of noise fears and phobias in pets. In Practice 27: 248–255.

Sheppard G, Mills DS (2003) Evaluation of dog-appeasing pheromone as a potential treatment for dogs fearful of fireworks 152: 432–436.

# Chapter 10

# Travel-related Problems in Pets

## 10.1   INTRODUCTION

Travelling with a pet can be difficult for many reasons: the behaviour shown by the animal can distract the driver or may be a sign of compromised welfare. Dogs can show a wide range of unwanted behaviours when travelling, including barking, whining, jumping, running around, salivating, vomiting, cowering and general restlessness. All of these behaviours can be perceived as problematic by the dog's owner, but not all are indicative of a negative emotional state in the dog. However, if the behaviour *is* indicative of the dog not feeling comfortable in the car, over time it may result in the dog not wanting to get into the car at all.

Travel-related problems are very common in dogs. A few years ago, the University of Lincoln conducted a survey of several hundred dogs in the UK and found that nearly a quarter of them were reported to be restless when travelling in the car. Another study in the USA suggests that between 10 and 15% of dogs seen in a general practice may suffer from motion sickness, and a more recent survey found that just over a third of travelling dogs have experienced travel sickness at some time. Indeed, it has been reported that about half of the vets in the UK see at least one case of travel sickness in a dog each month. It is important to recognise that motion sickness is not the only factor that can cause travel-related problems. Indeed, far from feeling sick or anxious, some dogs are simply overexcited by the car, as they are looking forward to a walk in the park or are overstimulated by the abundance of visual, acoustic and olfactory information available to them. Travel sickness typically starts when the animal is a puppy, but other travel problems can start at any age.

A review of cases seen at two established behaviour-referral practices in the UK suggests that less than 1% of the cases seen present as travel-related problems. This indicates that many animals who have problems with travelling are not being referred to specialists. There is therefore a significant role for those in general practice to assist with the management of this problem, but first we need to understand the nature of the problem being encountered. Although this chapter focuses primarily on dogs, because most research has been performed on this species, cats will be

*Stress and Pheromonatherapy in Small Animal Clinical Behaviour*, First Edition.
Daniel Mills, Maya Braem Dube and Helen Zulch.

considered briefly at the end (in Section 10.4), since they too can exhibit travel-related problems. It is believed that pheromonatherapy may help in some of these cases, too.

## 10.2   THE NATURE OF TRAVEL-RELATED PROBLEMS

As already mentioned, problems can arise for a range of reasons, but the link between behaviour and motivational–emotional state is not always very clear: for example, restlessness may be a sign that an animal is excited (*desire* or *frustration*), anxious (*anxiety–fear*) or feeling nauseous. In order to offer specific advice, it is necessary to determine the pattern of signs associated with different underlying problems. Historically this has tended to be done using individual clinical judgement alone, but it is possible to do it more objectively by using mathematical models to describe the collection of signs that tend to cooccur. This was done in a study by Gandia Estelles & Mills (2006), who evaluated the potential value of pheromonatherapy in the management of the different conditions revealed by statistical analysis. This study will be discussed in some detail, but the results of any study should only be generalised as far as is indicated by the nature of the population studied, so we will first examine the subjects recruited in this case. *Inclusion criteria* are the criteria that the animal must meet in order to be included in the study and *exclusion criteria* are criteria which, if present in the animal, exclude it from participation.

In order to be included in this particular study, dogs had to be aged between 6 months and 12 years, had to routinely travel in the car at least twice weekly and had to show at least one of the following signs:

- Running around in the car.
- Incessant vocalisation, e.g. barking, whining, howling.
- Trying to get closer to people in the car.
- Jumping up and down in the car.
- Vomiting.

However, if any of the following held true they could not join the study:

- They had any other significant behaviour problems.
- There were any anticipated changes to their management over the 2 months of the study.
- They were bitches currently suckling or in season, because the hormonal changes might interfere with our understanding of what was going on.
- The problem had only very recently developed, because then it might relate to a specific incident rather than a more general change in the dog.
- They had a history of reaction to collars or unwillingness to wear a collar, because treatment would involve the use of a pheromonatherapy collar.

Many more males (14 entire, 29 neutered) than females (5 entire, 11 neutered) were recruited, which may be of clinical significance. Urinating in the car was the least frequent sign, whereas panting, restlessness and failure to respond to commands were the most common signs. Figure 10.1 shows how often a given sign occurred in the population.

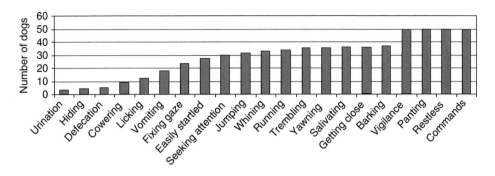

Fig. 10.1 Prevalence of different behaviours shown by 59 dogs with travel-related problems. Note, 'commands' refers to a failure to respond to commands.

However, just because a sign commonly occurs in a dog does not mean it commonly occurs during every car journey for that dog. Some signs tend to occur more consistently than others. For example, when barking was reported, it normally occurred every time, as did salivating, panting, running, hiding, vigilance, restlessness, a failure to respond to commands, getting close to the owner and seeking attention. Urination, licking and easy startling, on the other hand, tended to occur quite rarely. The other signs were expressed quite often.

When these data were subjected to factor analysis (a statistical data-reduction technique to define groups of signs which tend to go together), three relatively well-defined problems appeared from the signs that tended to be associated together:

- Excitability.
- Nausea.
- Tension/anxiety.

A fourth category existed for those showing other signs such as specific learned behaviours, including attention-seeking actions or other routines.

An important point to note is that these problems were not defined by any *single* behaviour alone, but by a profile of signs/features, some or all of which tended to co-occur in a given patient; that is, no feature of the patient was sufficient on its own for a diagnosis, although certain features were more typical of a given problem. This is not surprising, since, as discussed in Chapter 2, a given behaviour may occur in association with a diversity of motivational–emotional states, even if it is more typically associated with only one of these. Likewise, nonbehavioural features, such as breed, are also risk factors affecting the probability of a given diagnosis, although they should not be used alone. In order to assess the value of using the mathematically defined behavioural profiles to help build a clinical consensus, each case was reviewed by two veterinary behaviourists, who assigned it to a group based on the presenting signs. Diagnostic agreement between the two behaviourists was very high (93%), suggesting that these conditions can be reliably identified if sufficient attention is given to the range of signs being expressed. Details of the diagnostic groups and their characteristic signs are given in Table 10.1.

Table 10.1 Overview of the four groups based on the prevalence of behavioural signs shown by dogs with car travel-related problems.

| Group | Gender | Breeds | Defining signs |
|---|---|---|---|
| Excitable group $n = 30$ | 25 males 5 females | 10 pastorals 7 gundogs 5 crossbreeds 3 utility breeds 2 hounds 2 terriers 1 working-dog breed | Running Barking Whining Jumping Restlessness Vigilance Failure to respond to commands |
| Nausea group $n = 13$ | 6 males 7 females | 4 gundogs 3 crossbreeds 2 toy breeds 1 hound 1 pastoral 1 terrier 1 utility breed | Vomiting Salivation Hiding Cowering |
| Anxious–tense group $n = 8$ | 7 males 1 female | 2 gundogs 2 crossbreeds 1 pastoral 1 terrier 1 utility breed 1 working-dog breed | Getting close to owner in the car Trembling Licking Yawning Easily startled Panting |
| Others $n = 8$ | 5 males 3 females | 2 gundogs 2 crossbreeds 1 pastoral 1 terrier 1 toy breed 1 utility breed | Attention-seeking Elimination Unclassified behaviours |

Associated with these groupings are some interesting demographic features. In the 'excitable group' there were five times as many males as females, which suggests that excitability is much more common in male dogs. The most common breeds with this problem were the pastoral breeds, followed by the gundogs and the crossbreeds. Excitability appears to be quite uncommon in terriers and working dogs. By contrast, there were roughly equal numbers of males and females suffering from nausea ('nausea group'), and very few pastoral breeds, but a larger number of gundogs and crossbreeds. Anxiety (*anxiety–fear* – 'anxious–tense group') was again more common among males, with seven times as many compared to females suffering from this problem, but with a relatively even distribution between the different breeds. Within the 'others' group the clinical case review suggested there might be at least another two conditions to consider, but these occurred quite rarely. A few animals seemed to simply engage in attention-seeking behaviour – associated with a variant of activation of the *desire* system – and a small number of others just eliminated, with few other signs to clarify the underlying motivational–emotional predisposition leading to this behaviour. Finally, there were a few animals who did not neatly fit into any group, and obviously these cases would need much more extensive evaluation. Numbers in these latter groups were too small to make any confident statement about their breed or sex distribution.

Although no single sign may be diagnostic, certain behaviours appear to be more useful than others in guiding the assessment of the patient. A behaviour such as 'getting close to the owner' is not a very diagnostic sign, since it features in all conditions with some regularity. However, signs like 'restlessness' and 'barking' are much more commonly associated with excitable animals (but it must be borne in mind that they can occur in the other conditions as well). Thus, as stated earlier, individual signs should not be used to make the diagnosis; instead the whole cluster of behaviour signs should be considered. In summary, the primary differentials to consider for travel-related problems in animals are:

- Excitability (a combination of *desire* and *frustration*).
- Nausea (medical causes must be eliminated first with a health check).
- Anxiety (*anxiety–fear*).
- Attention-seeking (*desire*).
- Elimination problems.

In our experience, a proportion of excitable dogs appear to have visual impairments and so a careful veterinary examination of the eye is recommended as part of the initial health screen.

## 10.3   TREATMENT OF TRAVEL-RELATED PROBLEMS

### 10.3.1   *RISK ASSESSMENT*

The main risk to others from travel-related problems is associated with the driver becoming distracted and causing an accident. For this reason alone, the problem should be taken very seriously. Animals do not typically harm themselves when travelling, but if they are nauseous or anxious their welfare is obviously compromised. Depending on the cause, the risk of recurrence varies, but it is important that owners do not inadvertently reinforce or reinstate the behaviour by interacting much with the dog when in the car. A casual disinterest in the journey is the best general advice. As will be seen in Section 10.3.3, the long-term outlook for many cases is generally excellent.

### 10.3.2   *RESTRICTION OF THE PROBLEM*

The following general advice can help to immediately contain the problem:

- All punishment should cease as it is unlikely to be helpful and is likely to increase arousal or anxiety and thereby exacerbate the problem.
- Similarly, owners should not try to reassure the dog if they think it is distressed because this might teach it to engage in the same behaviours to get attention.

It is best to try to ignore the dog. Owners should be advised to intervene only if there is a good reason to do so; for example, if the dog is about to be sick then they will have to attend to it accordingly.

- If safe to do so, the owner should reward the dog with gentle praise if it is calm, although this is not relevant to nauseous animals and has to be used with caution in easily excitable dogs, as the sound of the owner's voice may be enough to excite them anew.
- The recommended degree of restraint of the dog will vary according to the assessment:
  - If restraint is indicated, it is preferable to secure the dog in the car using either a carrier or a harness behind a grill. In some cases, tying the dog below the level of the window on a relatively short lead is advised in order to stop it from looking outside; this can be particularly useful in excitable dogs.
  - However, in the case of dogs suffering from car sickness, giving them the opportunity to see objects far in front of the car can be helpful, if it can be safely arranged. Opening the windows may also produce air-pressure changes that help to reduce motion sickness.
- If the presenting complaint relates to a prediction of where the journey is going, an attempt can be made to make car journeys unpredictable. This may be relevant to excitable or anxious dogs. Even if the location must be the same, it is preferable to use a variety of routes to get there. If the animal gets very aroused, it is worth pulling over when safe to do so and waiting until it has calmed before moving on. In some cases, focusing on reinforcing calm behaviour while the car is on the driveway for a gradually increasing period of time can be all that is required to break the animal out of the cycle of excitable behaviour.
- Pheromonatherapy, in the form of the application of a dog-appeasing pheromone (DAP) spray to a travel blanket 10 minutes before putting the dog in the car, can be useful for the immediate control of some of the problematic signs. One double-blind randomised placebo-controlled study found that even without further behaviour modification, DAP rapidly reduced somatic signs such as salivating, vomiting and eliminating in the car, though it was less effective on more overt behavioural signs, such as barking.
- Drugs may be used in the short term to manage the problem. Traditionally, sedatives like ACP have been used, but recently a specific antiemetic for dogs (maropitant) has been developed. This drug is a neurokinin receptor antagonist that blocks the effect of substance P in the brain. It is therefore only available from vets and is not available in all countries. Although it is generally safe, unfortunately in about 1 in 20 cases the drug can itself cause vomiting, and in a small proportion of subjects it can increase anxiety. Nonetheless it can be very useful for the immediate control of problem vomiting.

## 10.3.3   RESOLUTION OF THE PROBLEM

If a dog has developed an aversion to the car due to any kind of negative association (e.g. nausea or anxiety), behaviour-modification interventions will be needed to retrain the animal to accept travelling. Similarly, if it has become overly excited in the car, desensitisation and counterconditioning can be used to help alleviate this response. In principle, this involves initially getting the dog to reliably settle for a prolonged period on command at home, and then transferring this command to the car, initially when stationary, but later when moving. An assistant is required to monitor the dog's behaviour and reward appropriate responses, so that the driver can concentrate on the road. The assistant should instruct the dog to stay settled and reward it frequently, without overexciting it. The driver should make frequent stops so the exercise does not go on for longer than the dog can cope with. This is where an assistant who can read the dog's body language is very important, allowing the driver to stop before the dog breaks the down stay. When the car is stopped, the dog can be taken out, but it must settle before being allowed to leave the vehicle. If the dog suffers from nausea, anxiety or some other aversive association with travelling, it may be allowed to sniff around and relax for a short while before returning to the car; but if it is an excitable dog, it should not go for a walk or be excited in any way. However, it might be asked to do some exercises calmly. This is potentially a time-consuming procedure and requires a lot of commitment from the owner, but if combined with pheromonatherapy the results can be very rapid. It is believed that the DAP alters the dog's perception of the car so that it is less likely to get aroused in a problematic way. It then rapidly learns appropriate behaviour. However, research suggests that the effect of DAP on the different problems is not equal, and so we undertake a closer analysis of the use of pheromonatherapy in this context, so that realistic expectations can be generated.

In the study by Gandia Estelles & Mills (2006), after categorisation, dogs were managed with the use of a DAP-impregnated collar for a period of 6 weeks. The use of DAP was supplemented with behavioural advice similar to that described in Section 10.3.2 (which was subsequently found to be implemented inconsistently by owners).

The behaviour of the animals was assessed by questionnaire and using selected video samples at baseline, then weekly for the next 4 weeks and finally at the end of the study after 6 weeks of treatment. Follow-up surveys were undertaken at 3 weeks and between 3 and 5 months after DAP treatment stopped. After the programme, owners were offered advice on how to desensitise animals to travelling excitement or aversion (however, very few felt the need to follow this advice).

In order to evaluate the effect of the intervention, a global score was used, which was an overall assessment of the severity of the problem and a list of the primary target signs of interest. These were based on the signs which were typically of most concern to owners:

- Running around.
- Barking.
- Whining.
- Getting close to the owner in the car.
- Jumping.
- Vomiting.

In addition, the typical signs of each diagnostic condition (see Table 10.1) were evaluated.

Although overall improvement in global score (a proxy for owner satisfaction) was high, the results suggest that the value of this intervention may vary with the diagnosis.

- *Excitability (desire/frustration)*: 30 dogs appeared to have a problem with excitability in the car. This was the largest clinical group, representing just over 50% of the total study population. There was a decline in all of the signs, with little evidence of relapse. Although statistically significant, the decline was not very great for any of the behaviours, even though it appears from the owner reports that it was sufficient for many of them to be happy with the results. On the basis of these results, we continue to recommend the use of DAP, but particular attention should be paid to the behaviour-modification elements relating to inadvertent owner reinforcement of the behaviour and the predictability of the journey when offering advice on this problem. In addition, we would assess the dog's general level of impulsivity and frustration tolerance and implement training games for these as necessary (see Zulch & Mills, 2012). It is worth noting that there was no evidence of significant relapse to baseline levels in any of the target or defining signs at follow-up. This indicates that improvements are sustained.
- *Nausea/travel sickness*: This occurred in just over 20% of subjects presented with travel-related problems. The treatment programme was associated with a marked and significant decline in virtually all important signs, with the exception of 'hiding'. Improvements in behaviour in the car seemed to occur quickly, although a reluctance to enter the car took longer to resolve. This is unsurprising as there is undoubtedly a largely learned component to this aspect in the majority of cases, and it is unlikely to change much until the dog is confident that it is not going to feel sick in the car as a result of a consistent series of nonaversive experiences. This would suggest that pheromonatherapy offers a useful alternative to medication for car sickness. There was no evidence of significant relapse in any of the signs, suggesting that these animals got better and that they stayed better even without continued DAP treatment.
- *Anxiety–fear*: This occurred in just under 15% of subjects, but again it responded rapidly to the treatment programme. However, improvement appears to have been less sustained for some signs once treatment with DAP was discontinued. Trembling and panting seem to be in danger of resurfacing after 3 or more months, and this may be the early sign of a more general relapse in the problem. In light of this, we suggest a longer period of treatment with DAP, for at least 4–6 weeks after the reduction in all signs has stabilised. The take-home message must be that it is worth considering DAP treatment in these cases and that perhaps DAP treatment for tense animals needs to go on for a little bit longer.
- *Other problems*: It is difficult to comment on the value of pheromonatherapy in other conditions that cause travel-related problems in dogs as there are so few documented cases. However, what data are available suggest that the programme described above may produce steady improvement, with little evidence of relapse. Further work is necessary before we can be more confident

about its value in this context, but anecdotally DAP may help in some attention-seeking behaviours, perhaps by creating some form of safe base for an animal, reducing the need for contact with the owner.

## 10.4   TRAVEL-RELATED PROBLEMS IN CATS

Cats are less likely than dogs to cause a serious accident or be attention-seeking when travelling. However, it is quite clear that travelling is stressful for many cats, and pheromonatherapy may be very useful in the management of this problem.

There has been one study on the use of Feliway® to help cats that are being transported. This was a blinded placebo-controlled study involving 58 cats. Either F3 or placebo was applied eight times, half an hour before the animal was transported in its basket. The behaviour of the animal was then recorded during travelling and an overall assessment of its responses made. The results showed that cats treated with Feliway® appeared to cope significantly better than cats in the placebo group.

We will consider the potential use of pheromonatherapy in cages and other containment systems again when we review the use of pheromonatherapy in the veterinary practice in Chapter 12.

## 10.5   CONCLUSION

Travel-related problems are very common in both cats and dogs and are perhaps under-recognised in both species. They can arise from a range of motivational–emotional states, but pheromonatherapy can ease the distress triggered by these conditions. However, different conditions should receive specific management recommendations focused around the underlying cause and should be treated with 'pheromones' for different periods of time. In general, treatment should continue for several weeks after the problem has disappeared or has reached a stable and acceptable level. Independent of the use of pheromonatherapy, owners should always restrain their animals in a safe and comfortable way in order to minimise risks and avoid accidents. Finally, it is also important to remember that any animal that is showing organic signs like vomiting must be checked to establish that it is otherwise healthy before a behaviour-management programme is begun.

## REVIEW ACTIVITIES

• Consider the key differentials for a dog whose owner complains of travel-related problems. What are the important questions to ask in order to differentiate these, and how might you tailor your management recommendations accordingly?
• Develop a fact sheet for clients, illustrating the key points to remember when travelling with their pet in order to keep it happy and safe.

• How would you manage a case in which the client reports that their pet 'knew he was coming to the vet's, because of the journey'? What simple measures can be taken to prevent this problem from arising in the first place?

## REFERENCES

Gandia Estelles M, Mills DS (2006) Signs of travel related problems in dogs and their response to treatment with dog appeasing pheromone. Veterinary Record 159: 143–148.
Zulch H, Mills D (2012) Life Skills for Puppies: Laying the Foundation for a Loving, Lasting Relationship. Dorchester: Veloce Publishing Ltd.

## FURTHER READING

DEFRA (2006) Protecting the welfare of pet dogs and cats during journeys – advice for owners. Available from http://www.defra.gov.uk/publications/files/pb10308-dogs-cats-welfare-060215.pdf.
Gaultier E, Pageat P (1998) Effect of feline facial pheromone analogue on manifestations of stress in cats during transport. Proceedings of the 32nd Congress of the International Society for Applied Ethology. France: Clermont Ferrand. p. 198.
Happy to Travel. An international Web site on travel sickness in dogs. http://www.dog-car-sickness.co.uk.
Mills DS, Mills CB (2003) A survey of the behaviour of UK household dogs. In: Fourth International Veterinary Behaviour Meeting Proceedings No. 352. Post Graduate Foundation in Veterinary Science. Sydney: University of Sydney. pp. 93–98.

# Chapter 11

# Introducing the New Dog or Cat into the Home

## 11.1 INTRODUCTION

The introduction of a new pet into the family is an exciting event, but also potentially difficult for both the pet and existing family members, be they human, conspecifics or of other species. There are a variety of approaches and techniques that can ease this transition period, and this chapter will examine some of these, and additionally will discuss how pheromonatherapy can assist in the process of adaptation to the new environment. The chapter covers general advice for owners of new pets, but it is crucial to bear in mind that every situation has individual requirements. As has been stressed in previous chapters, we aim to treat the individual rather than give blanket instructions. Most of the advice will apply equally appropriately to pets adopted into the home as puppies or kittens and those adopted as adults, but there are specific requirements relating to different ages that will need to be borne in mind.

This chapter's aim is to assist the behaviour-management team in:

- Recognising potential problem areas.
- Assisting in the implementation of measures aimed at preventing problem development.
- Easing the transition of the new pet into the home, in order to minimise stress.
- Understanding the process of young-animal education for problem prevention, including socialisation and habituation.

We will not deal with the provision of health care or the meeting of basic physiological needs, such as nutritional requirements. Instead, we focus on the meeting of psychological – including emotional – needs, such as the provision of toys suitable for not just the species but also the individual, as individual dogs and cats vary in the type of toy they prefer. We will also look at the need to aid appropriate development through early-life education classes and the role of pheromonatherapy in this. It is important to realise that this area has relatively little published research on which to base recommendations. What is presented here is a distillation of what we believe is the best advice currently available from numerous sources.

*Stress and Pheromonatherapy in Small Animal Clinical Behaviour*, First Edition.
Daniel Mills, Maya Braem Dube and Helen Zulch.
© 2013 John Wiley & Sons, Ltd. Published 2013 by John Wiley & Sons, Ltd.

### 11.1.1   *THE TEEME APPROACH TO PET COMMITMENT*

It may be useful for owners to remember the acronym TEEME when planning for a new pet, as it summarises the commitments involved in taking one on:

- Committing **T**ime.
- Investing in an appropriate **E**nvironment.
- Investing in appropriate **E**quipment.
- Investing **M**oney, not only in equipment and the environment but also in care and education.
- Making an **E**motional investment in the new relationship, which requires a willingness to commit to trying to resolve things when they are not meeting expectations.

Many owners might consider the initial investment of the purchase price of the pet and any legal requirements (depending on the country of residence), but do not actually prepare the home or make sure that they have appropriate facilities in place. Perhaps one of the things that is most commonly overlooked is how much time and effort it can take to help a new puppy, kitten or adult animal to settle in and ensure that its education is appropriate in order to minimise the risk of problem development.

## 11.2   POTENTIAL STRESSORS IN THE INITIAL SETTLING IN PERIOD

We should consider the introduction into its new home from the pet's perspective. It has been taken away from its mother – or another attachment figure, in the case of adults – and must integrate into a new family unit. This means that established bonds will need to be broken and new ones forged. There are many risks associated with this process. Unfortunately, interaction with the new social group may be forced in some situations; this is a particular danger when there are young children in the house who want to play with the new pet as children are generally even less able than adults to read the signals that an animal displays when it wants to avoid interaction. Other pets may also attempt (or be encouraged by owners) to interact at a level with which the new pet is not comfortable, or else they may not accept the arrival of the new pet. The new environment is going to be unfamiliar: both the new home and also the type of people the animal is encountering. Again, the presence of children may be a novelty, but so might the presence of a person who uses a walking aid, or even a man with a beard or a person who laughs loudly. The pet will need to adapt to all this. Pheromonatherapy can help, but it is not a substitute for good management practice. *Hazard management* means taking all reasonable steps to reduce the risk of harm from a process.

It is very important when very young animals encounter new things that the first encounter is pleasant, so that they build up a database of pleasant experiences and learn to accept novelty as something positive rather than something to be avoided or overwhelmed by. For this reason, bearing in mind past experiences (where known) and the likelihood of novelty within the new environment, owners need to be prepared for carefully considered introductions.

Looking at the introduction of the new pet from the owner's perspective, often they may not have chosen the right pet for their lifestyle, which can be an unforeseen problem. If they work long hours then a dog might not be appropriate: it may be that a cat or rabbit is better suited to their schedule. However, these species too will need interaction and have needs which must be met, and they too may be overlooked. Additionally, the owner needs to be aware of the differences in behaviour not only between species – they should not expect their cat to have the same needs as a dog or vice versa – but also between individuals. This might sound obvious but it is frequently overlooked by owners. Many owners choose a dog to accompany them in an activity that they wish to participate in on an occasional basis, such as agility training, rather than as a companion for all the other hours in the day. Others choose a dog on the basis of its appearance alone. Encouraging owners to remember that, first and foremost, their pet will be a family companion may help them when choosing a breed and an individual.

Other owners might adopt the same breed or even type of individual as their previous pet, expecting it to behave in the same way. This often results in unmet expectations, and owners need to be willing to accept the individual they take in for who it is and must try not to compare it with former pets.

In addition, the owner may not have prepared properly for the change that a new pet will bring to their life. A new addition to the household is always going to provoke a marked change, which may require changes to routine and can cause tension between individuals.

It is also important for owners to recognise that a pet is a different species to them, with its own species-specific needs, which may come into conflict with their own wishes from time to time. This means they should not anthropomorphise their pet's behaviour, nor indulge it like a child, and must be prepared to make compromises to ensure a healthy relationship. Only in this way can the animal fulfil its potential within the family.

## 11.2.1  *MAKING THE TRANSITION LESS STRESSFUL*

The easiest way to reduce long-term stress in the owner–pet relationship and help adaptation occur more quickly and easily is to start off right in the first place. Encourage clients to only buy their pets from reputable breeders or a reputable rescue centre and to take time to select the individual that is best for their situation. If they are considering acquiring a puppy or kitten, they should see or get details of both parents, if it is possible, and make their decision in light of this information. This can give them an idea of how large the pet is likely to grow and its possible behavioural tendencies, for example. Information about other family members, particularly pups or kittens from previous litters of the same breeding, can also be useful. People should not be rushed when selecting the individual puppy or kitten. Although there is little evidence to show that behaviours seen in puppy tests, other than those associated with fearfulness, are very predictive of long-term behavioural responses, certain tendencies towards behavioural reactions and styles are likely to be detectable through careful observation and provide a basis for future management priorities. Therefore, owners should spend time watching the whole litter interact and should not just pick a puppy or a kitten because they feel sorry for it, because it seems to hide away in a corner or look very sad or because it runs up to them first. In the former cases, they may be picking an individual that has tendencies towards developing problems associated with lower confidence and, unless they are experienced in raising animals, this can be challenging. When watching the litter interact, the following two features are important to note (not as predictors of future behaviour, but to derive information regarding what input the pup or kitten will benefit from in minimising the risk of long-term behaviour problems):

• The reactions of the animals to novel situations and objects.
• Their responses to being handled. Does a puppy or kitten relax or does it struggle a lot of the time?

It is just as important to watch adult dogs and cats, if the animal is being taken from a rescue, to see how they get on with conspecifics and members of other species. In addition, owners should ask the rescue for as much information as possible regarding the individual they are considering. Most rescues are honest about the behaviour of the animals in their care and will tell you everything that they know based on the previous owner and their own experience in the shelter. It is not in the interests of a well-established charity to hand over animals under false pretences.

Having decided on the individual that they wish to adopt, the new owner needs to consider at what time they want to pick up their pet. It is probably best to collect it in the morning and at a weekend. By picking it up in the morning, the animal has more time to settle by the evening, and by picking it up at the weekend (or during a holiday) the owner will have more time to spend with it and help it adapt in those first few very important days. It is also important to remember that this in itself can lead to problems, however, such as when a pet is never alone for the first few days or weeks in the new home and then is left for a whole working day once the holiday comes to an end. From the outset, management must look to prepare the pet for what can be predicted about the future. See Section 11.4.1 for advice on how to avoid problems associated with this situation.

Owners should be encouraged to minimise the number of new routines that their pet is expected to cope with in the first few days. For example, they should keep the pet on the same diet as before it came to the new home. It may be that they change the diet later on, but this should be done gradually after the pet has settled, in order to minimise the total stress load at any given time. There are also positive measures the owner can take in order to help the environment feel more familiar to the pet: they can bring a little bit of the animal's old home with it into the new environment, such as a blanket, or in the case of a cat perhaps a cardboard box that it has rubbed up against and which has its scent on it. In many cases a pet will not be adopted at first meeting and therefore, if the rescue or the breeder does not have anything to send with the pet, the new owner can take a blanket, a box or a toy and leave it with the pet in its current environment for a few days before taking it home. In addition, or as an alternative, pheromone products may be used:

dog-appeasing pheromone (DAP) for dogs and F3 for cats. These seem to help reassure the animal when it comes into the new environment (see Section 11.2.2).

Finally, the golden rule for success is to *start as you mean to go on*. Owners need to be aware that their pet is learning from all experiences and that therefore they are *always* training their pet – learning does not only occur in 'training sessions'. Every time they interact with their pet, the animal learns something about them and also about the wider environment. It is very tempting to give new pets, especially small, cute puppies and kittens, leeway for behaviours that will be considered undesirable in the long term, such as mouthing. This, however, is more likely to lead to stress and long-term problems than will setting house rules from day one and enforcing them fairly and consistently (Figure 11.1).

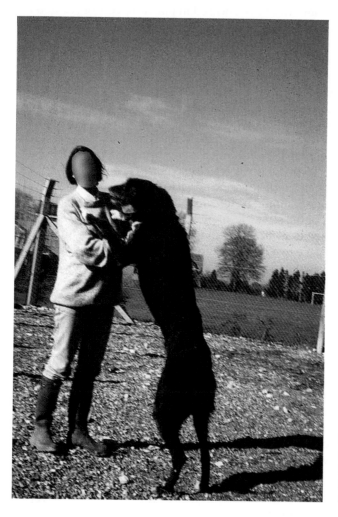

Fig. 11.1 Jumping up may seem cute in a puppy, but it can develop into a serious problem as the animal grows.

## 11.2.2   *PREPARING THE ENVIRONMENT*

It is important to make sure that the home is properly prepared for the arrival of a new pet. The following are a few things to consider:

- The home should be safe, from the perspective of exploratory pets:
  - Owners should make sure that all ingestible items are inaccessible. Small toys and little trinkets can easily be swallowed and can cause serious problems.
  - Cleaning products should be safely stored in locked cupboards.
  - Wastepaper bins and kitchen waste bins should be carefully secured.
  - Owners need to be aware of whether or not any plants in the house are dangerous to animals. It is easy for an animal to chew on a leaf and be poisoned. Web sites exist which describe the toxicity of various household plants and other items for dogs and cats (see the Further Reading section at the end of the Chapter).
  - If there are exposed wires in the house, for example from the backs of TVs, stereos and computers, they should be encased in plastic covers or secured in such a way that the animal is not tempted to chew them. Flexes should not be left dangling from table lamps or irons on ironing boards either, as these can be very tempting to grab with teeth or claws.
  - Food should be kept locked away, so as not to tempt the animal to learn how to steal from counter tops, tables and so on.
- It is important that the pet is provided with a safe haven from day one. This is an area where the pet can go to get away from it all and take control of its situation (see Chapter 1). You can use a dog pen or caged area, or, for a cat, even a bed under a table or on top of a shelf. It must never be used as a punishment area and must never be associated with negative experiences; rather, it is a place where pleasant things happen. Some toys and some food can be provided there, and when the animal is there it should be left alone. DAP or F3 can be beneficial in assisting in the creation of the sense of safety in this area.
- The home environment needs to be interesting, particularly for animals like cats. We tend to think of space in a house in terms of the floor area, but for cats it is far more three-dimensional and owners can afford to be quite imaginative in how to make use of this (see Section 11.2.2.1 and Further Reading).
- Opportunities to dig and chew (in the case of dogs) or to scratch (in the case of cats) must be provided. For dogs, a child's sandpit can be provided as a place where it can dig safely, and appropriate objects/chew toys can be hidden there for it to discover. For cats, a range of scratching posts should be provided in appropriate locations, and training them to use these is essential. Chemical signals based on those deposited by a cat when it scratches can be used to encourage scratching on the right surfaces from the outset.
- A suitable designated toilet area (or areas) needs to be available. Animals develop substrate preferences at quite a young age, so the toilet area needs to be where the owner would like it to remain for the fully grown animal. Use adult cat litter from the outset and allow puppies to eliminate on grass areas when out.

In addition, should there be spaces to which an owner does not want their new pet to have access, ensuring that these are blocked by closing doors or installing pet gates will prevent pets from making mistakes.

## 11.2.2.1 *ENVIRONMENTAL ENRICHMENT IN THE HOME*

Environmental enrichment does not involve simply providing items with which the pet may or may not interact, but rather meeting the psychological needs of the animal – their motivational–emotional predispositions. In other words, we should think in terms of psychological space rather than physical space. For space to be beneficial to an animal, particularly if it is confined to that space at all times (e.g. an indoors-only cat), it needs to encourage emotionally positive activity. For example, a room in which an animal can sit in the corner and see the whole space without having to move is not very interesting and does not encourage exploration (*desire*). If the room is divided up by partitions and furniture, it has to be patrolled in order to monitor what is going on and is therefore psychologically far more enriching. However, environmental enrichment is not just about increasing the stimulation of the animal, but also involves providing it with an appropriate level of predictability and control so as to reduce the stress load. Both extremes – having things that are too predictable and having things be completely unpredictable – can be distressing for an animal, but giving it, for example, a safe haven or access to specific areas through a pet-controlled door can help it retain a degree of control.

Predictability with respect to owner interactions is also important, and this may be one of the mechanisms by which 'nothing in life is free' protocols exert change on behaviour: the pet has a predictable consequence for specific actions. However, there is a danger when using such protocols that the animal's opportunities to communicate with its owner are ignored, as there is a focus on total obedience to the owner, rather than on a less stressful relationship which respects the needs of both but has clear boundaries. Training the animal can itself be an enrichment, and both dogs and cats can benefit from training. The predictable structuring of rewards and interactions that this delivers can be enriching for both the pet and the owner.

There are a multitude of excellent enrichment-feeding devices and other appropriate enrichment toys on the market, and discussing them is beyond the scope of this text. We recommend that a selection should be provided and their presentation to the pet rotated so as to retain its interest. Some pets learn to use toys quite quickly, while others need more training; the approach must be adapted to the individual. Additionally, providing a range of safe-to-eat plants, such as kitty grass, can be beneficial, as can the provision of catnip for cats that have a response to it. However, some cats get overexcited when chewing catnip, so owners need to be careful.

## 11.2.3 *THE JOURNEY HOME*

For newly adopted puppies and kittens, the journey to their new home may be the first time they experience travel, and this can be a very distressing experience for them. Their distress can be minimised by planning ahead. The use of pheromona-therapy in this context was discussed in Chapter 10, but in summary, it is important that the pet is safely restrained for travel. The appropriate product should be sprayed on to a blanket 10–20 minutes ahead of travel and the blanket should then be placed in the pet carrier, or where the animal will travel if it is to be restrained by a harness. For particularly long journeys, the spray may need to be topped up along the way, but it is important that the pet be removed from the carrier or blanket when the bedding is sprayed and that the alcohol be given time to evaporate before the pet is put back.

Other important points to remember when transporting a pet by car for the first time include closing the doors gently so as not to scare it by slamming and to drive considerately. For this reason too, pets should not be transported just after they have had a large meal. Ensure that there is a good supply of towels in the car, in case the pet is sick or eliminates during the journey. If it does, it is important to clean the mess up quickly, but without making an issue of it or reprimanding the pet, as this may negatively affect how the pet views car travel in the future.

## 11.2.4   INITIAL ARRIVAL AT THE NEW HOME

As already mentioned, pheromonatherapy in the new home can help with adjustment, and it should be put in place in advance. On arrival in the new home, the first thing that should be done is to take the pet to the toilet area. In the case of a kitten, it should be placed in the litter tray, and in the case of a puppy, it should be taken outside to the designated toilet area and given some space and time in its new environment. The owner might have to be patient, as the animal is likely to take some time to habituate to the new surroundings and may not choose to eliminate immediately. Obviously, the owner will want to watch their new pet at this time, but they should not stare at it. By giving the animal both time and space and resisting the urge to immediately interact, examine, handle and stroke it, the owner will help the pet to adapt and to see the new environment as nonthreatening. Interaction should be rationed and structured over the first couple of days so that the new pet can gradually gain confidence in the new physical and social environment without feeling overwhelmed. The owner must remember that everything is new for the pet – everything is a first encounter – and first impressions are very important. They should be made as positive and agreeable as possible. Because everything is new, it is also important to allow the pet enough rest.

## 11.2.5   THE FIRST FEW NIGHTS

The first few nights in the new home are critical in assisting the new pet to adapt and minimising the risk of later problems. A puppy or a kitten will have been separated from its initial family group for the first time. Previously, it was probably sleeping with littermates, and now it is in a new house with a new social group that it is unlikely to have such a close relationship with at first. In most cases, it is not recommended that the kitten or puppy routinely be allowed to sleep in a bed with the owner, although psychological comforts may be just as important as physical comforts at this time, and so company over the first few nights may be important, it needs to be carefully managed. Providing the animal with a warm water bottle – not too hot and wrapped in something soft – or a heat mat over the first few nights may also be useful. The plan for the bedtime routine needs to be clearly defined and not varied according to the demands of the pet. For example, placing a puppy in a crate alongside the owner's bed to sleep, from where contact can be made, can be useful in helping it to settle quickly. However, if the pup is taking time to settle and the owner lifts it out of its bed and into their own, it has immediately learned how to avoid sleeping in its own bed, which may cause problems later. Placing a pheromone diffuser next to the pet's bed can help it to settle and may provide a useful substitute for a conspecific. There is good evidence to show that using DAP markedly reduces whining and crying in puppies at night. Typically, this may occur for a week or so, but when DAP is used it is typically reduced to just one or two nights. It is likely that F3 will help cats to adapt as well.

Other approaches to helping a pet to settle include a routine which keeps it active for a few hours prior to bedtime, feeding it a late meal and ensuring that it has an opportunity to go to the toilet just before it goes to bed. If a puppy is being kept in a crate overnight, it should be big enough for it to be able to eliminate away from its sleeping area. Should a puppy wake in the night and cry, a calm trip to the toilet area and a return to bed with minimal interaction can help it to learn that play and interaction will not be forthcoming in the middle of the night, but that its needs will be met and it does not need to soil its bed. For owners who do not want a puppy to sleep in their bedroom long-term, after the pup has settled and night routines have been established the cage can gradually be moved out of the room to the place where the pup's final bed will be. The provision of a pheromone diffuser at the new sleeping site is recommended to help ease this transition.

## 11.3   DOS AND DON'TS FOR FIRST ENCOUNTERS WITH A NEW PET

### 11.3.1   *PEOPLE AND PETS*

Any pet entering a new home will meet a range of new people and the following should be borne in mind in order to help ensure that these introductions are successful and do not predispose future problems:

- Ideally, the pet should be allowed to approach people rather than be approached by them, so that it can meet them in its own time and in a manner which puts it in control of the situation and therefore makes it more comfortable.
- When somebody approaches or interacts with the pet, they should carefully observe the animal's behaviour so that they can respond appropriately to any signals the pet gives that it is uneasy with the interaction.
- A competent adult should always supervise interactions between pets and children so that they can advise on appropriate behaviour and monitor the pet for signs that it is not coping with the situation, and step in should a potentially problematic situation occur.

- Anybody approaching a new pet should do so slowly and gently, using a quiet tone of voice and a nonthreatening body posture.
- All family members, but children in particular, need to know the rules and should be instructed in how to act around the pet. Their excitement at meeting a new pet, particularly a puppy or kitten, may mean that they talk loudly or wave their arms around or want to cuddle or hug it, any of which can scare it. It is important not to rush, hug or scream at the animal or to startle it, tease it or play too roughly with it. Sudden movements of the arm can trigger an undesirable defensive response.
- Owners should not expect their pet to know instinctively what it is and is not allowed to do. They will need to guide its behaviour during these initial encounters so that it learns appropriate responses.
- Finally, everyone needs to remember that the first encounter counts for a lot. If it goes badly, the animal may very quickly learn that it wants to avoid a particular person. If it goes well, the relationship is off to a good start.

Pheromonatherapy may be particularly helpful in easing initial meetings with people. Using F4 or DAP on a person's clothing may encourage a cat or a dog, respectively, to make the initial approach. Care must be taken if a person has known allergies as the products are not licensed for use on human skin.

## 11.3.2   INTRODUCTION TO RESIDENT PETS

If an owner already has animals in the home, some familiarity with their body language can be expected. This can help in structuring and managing introductions to minimise the risk of conflict. Two unfamiliar animals should never be forced together and, particularly if these animals are adults, very structured meetings, possibly in a neutral area in the case of dogs and potentially with the assistance of a suitably qualified behaviour practitioner, are advised. Although not licensed for use directly on animals, in the author's experience the application of F4 to a cloth which is then rubbed on to the animals being introduced can help in the introduction of a new cat to other pets (cats or dogs). DAP is not recommended by the authors for use in this way, although a DAP or F3 diffuser may be used as described for initial settling-in according to the species involved.

   In all cases, it can be beneficial to first introduce the animals to each other's odours, for example by crossing over their blankets at night or allowing them to lie on each other's blankets, before they meet physically. However, once again this should not be forced: the blankets should be placed in the environment and the pets given an opportunity to approach as they choose. This scent familiarisation may need to take place over a few days in some cases, particularly in cats. Initial physical introductions must be supervised and should be relatively short, ideally in a non-core territory area of the house in the case of cats or an outdoor area for dogs. One pet should not be encouraged to approach another in its bed. It is recommended that precautions be taken so that the animals can be restrained should the introduction prove problematic, so for example dogs might wear house lines attached to an appropriate collar or harness and held loosely by competent adults. The lines are simply there as an emergency aid and must not be used to manipulate the animals in any way, as they need to make their own decisions regarding speed, trajectory and proximity of approach. Most cats have not been trained to wear a harness and so having another means of interrupting the introduction, such as blankets to throw over them, is a good idea. However, in cats even more structured introductions are usually recommended (see Section 11.3.2.1), which should avoid the need to intervene in this manner.

If there are several pets already resident in the home, the new pet should be introduced to each in turn, rather than to the whole group at once. Lots of praise should be given to both the new and the resident pet on their first introduction. If the animals wish to avoid each other, the owner should allow them to do so and should make sure they have escape routes they can use without getting harmed. It is not uncommon for there to be an initial hiss or growl, but owners should be encouraged to look for earlier signs of uneasiness and reduce proximity as they are detected. For example, cats will tend to look away, while dogs may look away, yawn, lick their lips, sniff or turn their whole body away. In the presence of these low-level signs of unease at the introduction, the situation should be deescalated by increasing the distance between the animals, blocking their view of one another or removing one or both pets. It may take some time to introduce the animals to each other and special time should be set aside for these supervised and carefully monitored introductions. Time spent at this point may avoid conflict later. Indeed, one study suggests that initial conflict upon introduction is one of the strongest predictors of later intercat problems in the home; therefore, it cannot be overemphasised how important it is to proceed at a pace with which the individuals can cope.

At all times, owners need to be aware of the risk of inadvertent injury to themselves, for example through redirected aggression, when introducing animals to one another. For this reason, and to reduce the risk of frustration in the pets, animals should not be held in the owner's arms or sat on a lap during introductions.

Signs that pets are relaxing in one another's company should be noted, as at this point supervision can be relaxed and the pets allowed together for longer periods. Signs to look out for include cats rubbing against each other and dogs initiating play, or at least exploring the environment together. If the introductions do not seem to be going well, the owner should be encouraged to seek early help from a professional.

## 11.3.2.1   *INTRODUCING A NEW CAT TO A CAT HOUSEHOLD*

As already mentioned, the introduction of a new cat to a household with a resident cat or cats requires particular attention. Ideally, before bringing the new cat home, a separate core-territory area should be prepared for it, and initially the cats should be kept totally separate, with the resident cats able to access their established core territory and the new cat confined to its new area. Access to non-core areas should be time-shared initially, to aid in the scent swapping, which should also be done in a structured manner, as described earlier. After a few days the cats can be gradually introduced, initially through a barrier, which ideally should allow olfactory as well as visual access, and through which the sight of the other cat is paired with that of food treats or similar. Even at this point, however, the cats should not be encouraged to get close to one another through the use of food, but should rather be allowed to choose their own proximity at their own pace.

In a study examining the introduction of new cats into a household, it was found that the majority of owners did not follow advice similar to that given in this section when it was provided to them on advice sheets, highlighting the importance of discussing these issues in detail with clients rather than simply handing them a sheet.

## 11.4   PROBLEM PREVENTION THROUGH EDUCATION

### 11.4.1   *LEAVING A PUPPY ALONE*

Teaching puppies to feel safe when left alone is a very important lesson. Although separation-related problems are described in cats, it is much less common and most cats adapt to periods alone. When leaving a puppy alone for the first time, it is important that it is in a safe and secure area with access to its safe haven and that it is not left for a long time. DAP can be used to help the pup feel reassured, either as a diffuser near the safe haven or sprayed on to a blanket placed within it. All the pup's needs should be catered for when it is left, with a separate bed and toilet area provided. Ensure that the toilet area – newspaper or puppy pads – is placed at a distance from the sleeping place or the pup might not use it. Ensure that water is left for the pup, as well as a variety of safe toys and chewable items.

Initially, pups should only be left alone for very short periods of time. These should be structured into the days that the owner spends at home after acquiring the pup so that by the time of the owner's return to work the pup has adapted to being alone. In the initial stages it is best to leave the pup when it is less likely to miss the owner in any case. Ensure that it has had a game, been fed and had an opportunity to go to the toilet. Ideally, it should be ready to settle for a nap. When leaving, it is important that the owner does not make a big fuss, as this will make the contrast between their presence and their absence more marked. Ignoring the pet for a short while before actually going can be a useful strategy. Similarly, when the owner returns they should not make a big fuss of the pet, as once again this highlights the contrast between the owner's presence and their absence.

It is important for the owner to try not to return to the pup if it cries when they leave, but rather to wait until it settles, so as not to reinforce unwanted behaviour. However, as with all things, this advice must be adapted to the situation and if a pup is becoming very distressed then the owner will need to return and implement a different strategy, possibly with the help of professional advice. This situation is unusual for puppies, as long as initial departures are kept short, but may be more of a problem in rehomed rescue dogs, where the same approach should be taken as described here.

Helping a pup to learn to amuse itself independently of its owner, even when the owner is at home – for example by playing with food-dispensing toys or chewing on a chew – can also teach it that it can occupy itself and thus is not dependent on the owner's attention or presence.

## 11.4.2   EARLY-LIFE EDUCATION

Experiences during the first few months of a puppy or a kitten's life are key in shaping its long-term behaviour, and this is what makes *early-life education* so important. By using this term, as opposed to the traditional reference to socialisation or training classes, we aim to make it clear that all aspects of experience need to be considered. Puppies and kittens need to be appropriately socialised with their own and other species, they need to habituate to their environment (in all aspects: car, house etc.), they need to be trained so that they learn to respond to cues designed to protect them or those around them and they need to be taught *life skills* such as self-control, good manners and frustration tolerance.

Initial basic education within the home will include some of the aspects already covered – such as learning where to go to the toilet and learning to tolerate being alone – but it will also include learning to inhibit their biting or clawing actions when in contact with people and to restrict them to appropriate toys. To aid puppies and kittens in learning these things, the family should decide on a set of house rules before the pet enters the home. These house rules should be consistently applied by all members of the family, in order to ensure that they are clear and can be complied with. We suggest writing them down and putting them in a prominent place for all to see, such as the refrigerator door.

Training, which most owners find easier to implement with the aid of a structured training class, includes teaching obedience-type behaviours: to come when called, walk nicely on a lead, wait when asked to, let go of something in the mouth, cope with novelty and socialise with other puppies. A number of different types of class exist and selecting an appropriate one is essential to problem prevention. Owners need to be counselled on how to make these choices: refer to the handout in Horwitz & Mills (2009) for advice to assist clients.

It is important for clients to appreciate the difference between puppy parties and puppy classes.

## 11.4.2.1   PUPPY PARTIES AND PUPPY CLASSES: THE DIFFERENCE

*Puppy classes* and *puppy parties* are often referred to as if they are one and the same thing, but there are differences of which owners should be aware. A party is usually a single event that is organised in a veterinary clinic and involves a little bit of socialisation and general information. Classes are a much more structured series of events. They may be based in a veterinary clinic or at a specific training venue.

Different countries have different schemes that accredit or regulate classes to a greater or lesser degree, and becoming familiar with these and what quality assurance they offer owners is advisable. Poorly run classes or parties can do far more harm than good. Most classes involve basic training, management advice and opportunities for a puppy to socialise with other puppies and people and habituate to novel objects. Contrary to some popular promotions, puppy education should be the domain of the experienced rather than the novice trainer.

Most puppy training classes will cover a similar curriculum, relating to exercises such as:

- Handling the pup, including examining it and grooming it.
- Teaching basic obedience, such as sit, stay, lie down and recall.
- Teaching loose lead walking.
- Habituating the puppy to novel objects.
- Socialising the puppy with other puppies and people, and occasionally other species.

The aim is to develop a puppy that is well adapted, gets on well with a whole range of different people and animals and is accepting of the objects and other stimuli (such as noises) that it will meet in daily life.

A good puppy class will have a limited number of puppies, typically a maximum of six per instructor, to ensure that adequate time and attention can be given to each. Many puppy classes will accept puppies for registration in the first 20 weeks of life and ideally owners should be encouraged to begin the process as early as realistically possible.

Studies investigating the use of DAP in puppy training classes suggest that it can help in a variety of ways when used either in a diffuser at the venue or in collars on the puppies. One study found that when puppies wore a DAP-impregnated collar they were much less excitable and their owners were more satisfied with them. DAP may help puppies to be more socially competent, learn more efficiently and habituate to novelty better, and these effects may continue to be evident up to a year after the classes have ended. For kitten parties, using an F3 diffuser may help the animals to accept the novel environment, but to date this has not been investigated experimentally and increasingly many are suggesting kitten-owner information evenings may be a more efficient way of ensuring kittens are handled well from the outset and develop appropriate behaviours (focusing on providing owner education rather than a particular experience for the kittens).

## 11.4.2.2   SOME ADDITIONAL POINTS REGARDING WHAT PUPPIES NEED TO LEARN

The window of opportunity for learning to accept novelty is relatively small, so the experiences that a puppy has within its breeder and home environment are very important, since its vaccination status may preclude attending classes for a while. An owner can expose it to stimuli and situations in the home to maximise appropriate learning.

When considering how to socialise or habituate an animal, it is important to *minimise risk but maximise opportunity*. Everyday occurrences such as the use of a vacuum cleaner can be an opportunity for learning: the puppy should be occupied with a desirable food toy or chew in a safe place away from the vacuum as it is turned on, and it should initially be used for only short periods in order to help the pup learn that it is not dangerous and can be ignored. It is important that owners never push or move a vacuum cleaner, hairdryer or similar towards a puppy as this can lead to long-term fear-related problems. First experiences should ideally be good, or at least acceptable. Most puppy classes will expose puppies to day-to-day objects as well as some items that they may never have previously seen, such as crutches, a pushchair or bike, an umbrella and so on. Again, a good puppy class will make sure that puppies can cope with these exposures and are never frightened by the introduction of new things.

Additional things to which puppies should be habituated but which can be forgotten include travelling and the veterinary surgery (see Chapters 10 and 12). Owners should be encouraged to bring their new pet to the veterinary surgery for a series of check-ups, so that the first times it goes are pleasant experiences.

In addition, the concept of life skills is one that two of the present authors (Zulch & Mills, 2012) have developed to assist in preventing some of the common problems seen in behaviour referral practice (see Further Reading). The main aim of the 'life skills' approach is to develop resilience and encourage the pup to remain in control by showing appropriate behaviour when faced with a challenge, encouraging good behaviour as opposed to simple obedience. While puppies do need to be responsive to their owners' cues, it is also less stressful for both owner and dog if the dog learns to think for itself and understand the correct choices in specific situations. This reduces the need for constant vigilance and instruction or correction by the owner.

## 11.4.2.3   KITTEN EDUCATION

In the case of cats, initial training may focus on the use of the litter box and scratch post. If the owner is to have a cat flap, the cat may also need to be trained to use this. It is often advantageous to use a see-through cat flap, at least initially, to assist the cat in learning. Many cats do not like pushing with their face and this can lead to problems in the use of a cat flap, hence the importance of training.

Additional skills training for cats can be very similar to some of the life skills developed for dogs, but adapted for species-specific tendencies. This may sound counterintuitive as they are such different species, but sharing the same environment means that there are similarities in what is expected of them. Cats need to be taught to accept being handled and groomed by strangers as well as their owners. Many cats will turn and bite a person if they are handled too much or inappropriately, and therefore it is recommended that they be desensitised to this type of handling in case they ever need veterinary treatment. Cats can be taught to respond to cues, and teaching cats to come when called and to wait in a specific place can make their day-to-day management much easier. In addition, cats need to accept car travel and household appliances and to be socialised to members of their own and other species. Although the concept of kitten training classes is not well established in most countries, and they would in any case differ markedly from those run for puppies, owner education as to the amount of education required for good welfare should not be neglected. It should also be remembered that the sensitive phase in which kittens are most able to learn to accept many aspects of novelty often ends at around 9 weeks of age, significantly earlier than in dogs.

## 11.5   CONCLUSION

By following the guidance above, owners can greatly reduce the potential for initial distress by the dog or cat newly introduced into their home. Additionally, they can help it adapt to the new environment and develop into a well-socialised, stable individual. Pheromonatherapy seems to be particularly useful in helping pets accept the many novel stimuli they encounter when going to a new home, as well as impacting positively on some aspects of puppy training classes and assisting in reducing travel-related problems. Indeed, it might be argued that its value in terms of improving welfare is greater in helping prevent problems than in managing them once they have arisen. Encouraging owners to plan carefully for the integration of a new pet into their home is key to making the process more reliable and a positive experience for all involved: both owners and their pets.

## REVIEW ACTIVITIES

- Cats and dogs are different species, and even though they may encounter the same stimuli, they have different needs. Consider how the approach used for the introduction of a new cat differs from that used for a new dog.
- Make a list of possible challenges a new dog coming into a household might encounter and how their impact can be minimised.
- Consider the potential problems that might arise in a puppy class. How can their risk be minimised and how should each be managed should it arise?
- Collect video sequences from available resources to educate clients about the body language to observe in their new pet and how they should respond if it occurs.
- Develop a handout advising clients how to recognise the early signs that a new introduction is not working and what to do in these circumstances.

## REFERENCES

Zulch H, Mills D (2012) Life Skills for Puppies: Laying the Foundation for a Loving, Lasting Relationship. Dorchester: Veloce Publishing Ltd.

## FURTHER READING

ASPCA. Toxic and non-toxic plants. Available from http://www.aspca.org/pet-care/poison-control/plants/.

Denenberg S, Landsberg G (2008) Effects of dog appeasing pheromone (DAP) on anxiety and fear in puppies during training and on long term socialisation. *Journal of the American Veterinary Medical Association* 233: 1874–1882.

Ellis S (2009) Environmental enrichment: practical strategies for improving feline welfare. *Journal of Feline Medicine and Surgery* 11: 901–912. Available from http://www.fabcats.org/behaviour/cat_friendly_home/Environmental_enrichment_JFMS%20article%20for%20website.pdf.

Horwitz DF, Mills DS (2009) BSAVA Manual of Canine and Feline Behavioural Medicine. Gloucester: BSAVA.

Levine E, Perry P, Scarlett J, Houpt KA (2005) Intercat aggression in households following the introduction of a new cat. *Applied Animal Behaviour Science* 90: 325–336.

Pet Poison Helpline. http://www.petpoisonhelpline.com/.

Taylor K, Mills DS (2007) A placebo-controlled study to investigate the effect of dog appeasing pheromone (DAP) and other environmental and management factors on reports of disturbance and house soiling during the night in recently adopted puppies. *Applied Animal Behaviour Science* 105: 358–368.

# Chapter 12

# Stress and Pheromonatherapy in the Veterinary Clinic

## 12.1 INTRODUCTION

This chapter will discusses situations that both pet owners and professionals working in veterinary clinics encounter regularly. Some of the behaviours shown in a clinic can make the veterinarian's job difficult, impede evaluation of the patient or be quite dangerous for all involved.

In the early 1980s, Stanford undertook a review of dogs coming into the veterinary clinic and, quite worryingly, over 80% of the animals appeared to be frightened: 60% of them were clearly anxious, 18% showed signs of fear biting and 5% showed other active defensive behaviours (these might include various forms of aggression but also escape behaviours) (Stanford, 1982). A more recent study found similar results, with 78.5% of dogs showing fearful behaviour, especially on the examination table (Döring *et al.*, 2009). Clearly, for the majority of dogs, it seems that veterinary clinics are an extremely stressful place. Comparative studies in cats do not exist, but many clinicians and owners will tell us that cats do not tend to like to enter the carrier at home but usually (sometimes to the surprise of the owner) have no problem getting back into it at the veterinary clinic, indicating that the cage shifts from being something aversive in the home to a preferred place in the context of the clinic, which suggests that the clinical environment is an even worse alternative.

Being aware of the challenges faced by a visit to the veterinary clinic and implementing some relatively straightforward measures can help make the situation less stressful for everybody and ensure that future visits are easier for all concerned. In the same way that we would not find it acceptable for a pet to go to the vet's and return with an additional physical wound from poorly designed facilities or management, it is unacceptable for an animal to return with a psychological wound. We therefore begin by taking a broad look at stress within the context of the veterinary practice and examination, and how it might be expressed, before considering techniques and procedures that can be used to minimise handling and management problems in the veterinary clinic.

*Stress and Pheromonatherapy in Small Animal Clinical Behaviour*, First Edition.
Daniel Mills, Maya Braem Dube and Helen Zulch.
© 2013 John Wiley & Sons, Ltd. Published 2013 by John Wiley & Sons, Ltd.

## 12.2   THE VETERINARY VISIT

### 12.2.1   *IDENTIFYING POTENTIAL STRESSORS*

Many owners report that their pets do not like a trip to the vet's, but the reasons for this are diverse. The perception of stressors and the resulting response varies greatly from individual to individual. In many cases there is some pathophysiological process in the body which is biasing the animal's perception negatively or influencing its strategic choices (e.g. painful joints may lead to a preference for an aggressive display as a way of avoiding contact, since fleeing is a difficult option given the pain). Pain, sickness behaviour and possibly the feeling of something 'different' in the body may also reduce the level of control an animal perceives itself as having over a situation and change its priorities as a consequence, with an increased irritability being perhaps one of the most obvious manifestations of this. So, the pet's health status at the time of the veterinary visit influences the degree of stress it perceives and also its capacity to cope with stressful events. Additionally, previous experiences at the vet's – from which the animal has learned – will influence how it approaches this situation. What must not be forgotten is that problems can build up over time, and with every additional stressor the capacity to cope gradually approaches its limit. This is often not noticed by the people involved, as the behavioural signs shown by animals can be quite subtle at first (see Chapter 3).

Apart from ill health and the resulting challenge to the body, there are many other potential stressors which may confront an animal on a trip to the veterinary clinic:

- The owner is likely to be distressed and worried themselves (and their pets are generally very good at picking up even slight changes in body language).
- The animal has to be prepared for transport to the veterinary practice (we often hear that the cat 'just knows' when it is to be taken to the vet's and disappears as soon as the transport cage appears).
- The transport itself (which can be stressful whether by car, foot or public transportation).
- The animal enters a new or a known environment (possibly associated with past unpleasant events) filled with information and impressions.
- The animal may have to wait in the waiting room. There are other living beings around: both people, some of whom will interact with it (potentially in a quite threatening way: looking it directly in the eye, bending over it, attempting to pet it etc.) and other distressed animals, which it can see, hear and smell.
- The animal will be confronted with a plethora of information to assess, and this will be psychologically very demanding. This may mean attentional resources are at their limit, which will encourage a sensitivity to anything which can even vaguely be perceived as aversive, since there is no time to fully process the details of the situation.
- The animal will be handled and examined by a person most likely unfamiliar to it or possibly associated with past unpleasant experiences. Even if it is just a

routine physical examination, it is likely to involve at least some potentially unpleasant, if not overtly painful, elements. The degree to which this is stressful to the animal will vary according to its predispositions as well as prior learning, including the amount of time the owner has spent habituating or counterconditioning it to invasive touch.

- On top of all of this, the animal generally has no control over the situation; that is, its confidence and ability to cope are likely to be decreased. At this time it will probably turn to its owner for social support and signs of safety, which may not help matters. The people surrounding the animal most often will not respond to its more subtle attempts to communicate its distress and may reinforce the distress or punish overt attempts at avoidance, escape or self-defence.

These are not all of the possible stressors that an animal might be confronted with, but the list serves to illustrate that we should recognise that by the time the animal enters the actual consultation room it will have had to cope with many issues already and, depending on its psychological and physical predisposition, may have reached its tipping point.

It is worth emphasising at this point that the relationship and the quality of communication shared between a pet and its owner both have an impact on how and how well the animal (and the owner) copes with the situation. A pet within an owner–animal partnership that has a good bond and an efficient way of communicating may be much less distressed than one who is left to cope on its own or who feels threatened or is made insecure by its owner – an owner who may be uncertain as to how to handle the situation or intolerant of an animal they believe is 'misbehaving'. Supportive actions from a sensitive owner might be as simple as recognising that their cat feels stressed being placed right next to another cat or a dog in the waiting room and therefore changes seats, places a towel over the cage or takes the cat back out into the car in order to allow it to relax until it is called for a consultation, or understands that their dog feels threatened on the examination table and asking the veterinarian whether it can be examined on the floor instead. Some animals are calmer when their owner is present, whereas others seem to be more distressed – often, the owner is not capable of deciding this on their own and it is up to the practice team to make suggestions and explain to the owner in a supportive way how the animal can be helped to feel safer.

Possibly the most threatening aspect of the consultation for the animal is being shut in a (usually relatively confined) environment with unknown people who approach it in a potentially threatening way, place it in locations where it feels unsafe and touch or prod it in ways that might be uncomfortable or even painful. Unfortunately, the veterinarian and technicians often do not have any choice but to inflict a level of discomfort in order to derive the information they need. In spite of this, it is however possible to be sensitive to the signals being emitted and adapt human behaviour accordingly. In order to convey this information, the normal behaviour and communication of the species treated must be known and understood (this will be discussed further in Section 12.2.2).

At times, animals are left at the veterinary practice for further tests or surgery. Again, they are confronted with unknown surroundings full of different smells, sounds, people and animals. Other animals might be howling or have secreted alarm pheromones into the environment. Depending on the practice layout, there might be a lot of movement going on, with people and animals coming and going past the holding area. The animal is experiencing all of this without the potential security of its owner; that is, one of its coping mechanisms (provided there is a healthy bond between owner and pet) is not in place. Pheromonatherapy may provide one way of ameliorating the inevitable impact of some of the novel stimuli in this context. We can also help to reduce the impact of all the potential stressors by reflecting upon the range of features which affect the intensity of perceived stress (see Chapter 1) and developing appropriate management policies as a result:

- *The type and number of stressors*: The number of contacts encountered can be reduced by having an appointment system and a well-designed waiting area (see e.g. FAB, 2006).
- *The intensity of the stressor*: The intensity of an individual stressor will vary according to the type of stressor, but simple measures like controlling the proximity to unknown conspecifics can alter the intensity of exposure.
- *The duration of the stressor*: Minimising the length of the trip to the veterinary clinic will help the animal cope, so long as it is not rushed: the longer the waiting period, the longer the examination and testing and so the greater the stress. It is important that consultation times are realistic and animals discharged as soon as is feasible.
- *The predictability of the stressor*: In the context of a veterinary practice, some of the potential stressors, such as being restrained, might be predictable, and if an animal is taught that it can cope with this, for example by the owner practising the routines at home and rewarding the pet accordingly, it will be more able to cope when the cue is given in the clinic. Some unpredictable stressors such as a staff member rushing by can also be managed by practice policies relating to staff behaviour in the clinic and the interruption of clinical procedures.
- *The level of control*: Animals can be given more control in the clinic by, for example, giving them time to habituate before they are examined, or in the case of a cat by giving it a 'hide' of some description in its hospital cage.
- *Novelty*: This can be reduced by ensuring animals have items from home with them, whether that be in the consultation room or for longer hospitalisation, and possibly by the use of pheromonatherapy.
- *The previous consequences of the potential stressor*: This is where the effect of learning comes into play and why prevention is such an important factor in reducing the stress of veterinary visits. The more positive experiences the animal has during its initial veterinary visits, the greater the probability that it will come back without fear. Pheromonatherapy may again help in reversing the effects of previous adverse experiences (see Section 12.3.3), but it should not be used as a substitute for good management practice.

It is also worth mentioning the domestic stress level of the animal at this point, and consideration should be given to a 'stress audit' (see Chapter 1). Problems with interpersonal relationships within a family can lead to poor communication and inconsistent responses to pets (by humans and other animals), environments that are too stimulating or unpredictable or which lack sufficient stimulation, changes in family dynamics or moving home, over- or under-exercise, pain or sickness, can all lead to a significant 'subclinical' stress problem. This may not only reduce the animal's ability to cope at other times but, over the longer term, contributes to certain diseases (see Chapter 1). The significance of this chronic stress might only become apparent when an additional acute stressor, such as a veterinary visit, is added.

## 12.2.2   RECOGNISING EMOTIONAL AND ASSOCIATED STRATEGIC RESPONSES IN THE VETERINARY CLINIC

Given the range of potential aversives encountered in the clinic, the significance of *anxiety–fear* arousal is obvious, but there may be other significant negative emotional states too, such as *pain* (it is important to distinguish the impact on behaviour of the affective component of *pain*, which may increase the tendency to show aggressive displays, from its sensory component, which may manifest as lameness and so on), *frustration* associated with restraint and the denial of opportunities to move to safety (when it may be combined with elements of *anxiety–fear)* and *panic–grief* associated with separation from the owner. We must thus know about these predispositions as part of an animal's clinical record.

To counteract these emotions we need to not only minimise the occurrence or intensity of triggers (for example by using minimal-restraint measures to reduce *frustration* or being aware of our body language so as not to induce *anxiety–fear* by looming over the animal or moving suddenly) but also positively encourage more appropriate motivational–emotional predispositions (Figure 12.1). For example, stimulus-bound appetitive behaviour (*desire*) in the form of curiosity and willingness to explore the environment must be encouraged and rewarded with the discovery of valuable incentives, such as treats. However, some positive motivational–emotional arousal needs to be carefully managed. One dog may want to socially interact with another in the waiting room or want to approach a dog passing it while leaving the examination room, for example, but this can lead to frustration when it is not obtained, or else it may not be tolerated (perhaps for good reason) by the other dog or its owner, leading to a significant aversive experience. The line between excited arousal and dangerous loss of control can be very fine and needs careful consideration.

Arousal can be associated with specific negative or positive emotions but may not be attributable to any specific emotion. The type of autonomic arousal reflects the predicted effort required by a subject rather than the subject's perceived level of control and therefore, level of arousal, on its own, does not reliably correlate with how the animal might behave. A supposedly calm animal may show only very subtle signs of discomfort and threat and then suddenly strike, such as the cat who sits on the table allowing a physical examination to be done seemingly calmly and then attacks, or the dog who is fine and happy until something is done which it finds very aversive and then channels this arousal into a furious response. The importance of looking at the whole situation

(a)

(b)

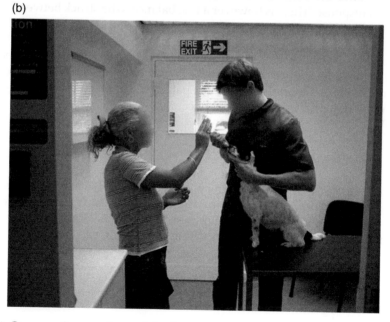

Fig. 12.1 Compare the experience of the dog receiving intranasal vaccination in these two images. In (a) the dog is heavily restrained and is likely to find the experience aversive, while in (b) it is being lured to show supportive behaviour and given more choice, so is more likely to accept the procedure both this time and in future (both images courtesy of K Shepherd).

(animal, owner and other people involved) should not be underestimated, and it is worth training oneself to observe the animal at all times out of the corner of one's eye, even while talking with the owner or performing a physical examination.

Individuals will tend to use the same strategy in similar situations of distress, if it has a history of success (negative reinforcement of behaviour and associated inflexibility or response – see Chapter 2); for example, a dog who shows aggressive defensive behaviour when uncertain outside the clinic may do the same inside the clinic. The animal's behaviour in the clinic should therefore be seen as a mirror of its broader response style under certain types of stress. This may warrant the need for more extensive behavioural intervention, to prevent a potentially serious incident in wider society. The problem should not be seen as a 'vet-only' issue, even if the animal does discriminate the vet from others, but rather as a strategic preference associated with arousal of a wider motivational–emotional predisposition which might be encountered elsewhere.

If the examining veterinarian ignores the (more or less) subtle signs the animal is giving to communicate that it would rather be left alone, in order to treat an immediate problem, then there is a risk that the animal might escalate its response to one including overtly harmful behaviour, or escalate the expression of aggressive threats until the veterinarian desists, in which case it is reinforced for this higher level response. There is however a fine balance to be struck between getting the job done and not making things worse for the next occasion the animal needs treatment. Being able to do more to help the animal requiring veterinary attention is another important benefit of a preventative approach. When this is too late, remedial desensitisation and counterconditioning to the clinic and veterinary procedures should be considered for some patients, and this should be flagged up as soon as the first problematic response occurs.

## 12.3   MANAGEMENT OF CLINIC-RELATED PROBLEMS

The aim of management is to target the potential stressors so as to minimise their impact on animals coming to the clinic. We therefore focus on prevention in both the long and the short term, beginning with the animal's development, before considering preventative management within the clinic itself.

### 12.3.1   PREVENTION THROUGH APPROPRIATE PREPARATION IN THE HOME

The best way to address possible problems is to prevent them from occurring in the first place. With knowledge of the importance of factors like socialisation and habituation during the first few months of life on the subjective perceptual biases of an individual and the development of its behavioural biases, it makes sense to put as much effort as possible into prevention, especially with young animals. Habituation and emotional counterconditioning to as many potential stressors as possible form one element of this process, as they decrease the number and intensity of potential stressors encountered and make the ability to cope more reliable and predictable as a consequence. Training a specific coping strategy such as 'turn to my carer' for situations in which an animal is unsure, increases the animal's perceived level of control over its environment, increasing resilience as a result. These are important skills for animals to learn and should not be left to chance. Details about how to develop broader strategies for building resilience and appropriate behavioural tendencies are beyond the scope of this book, although some aspects, especially in relation to the use of pheromonatherapy, have been covered in the previous chapter and can be sourced from some of the reading material referenced at the end of this chapter (see especially Zulch & Mills, 2012 for a specific programme developed for dogs).

## 12.3.1.1   COLLABORATION WITH THE VETERINARIAN FROM AN EARLY AGE

Ideally, owners and veterinarians would collaborate from the very beginning, arranging 'fun' visits to the clinic with young animals, where nothing aversive happens and the animal gets to investigate and to play and receives treats. This is, of course, not always possible due to the time constraints of both veterinary staff and the owner and the fact that not all pets are adopted at a young age. However, if it can be done, this may help to address many of the issues discussed: it can help the animal to learn to cope in new environments and with the veterinary practice in particular and it will allow it to perceive the veterinary clinic in a positive way, thereby learning that it should not be afraid the next time. There is the additional benefit of the owner most likely being more relaxed as well, knowing that their pet is able to cope with the situation. This of course does not guarantee that the animal will not be distressed, especially if it undergoes a painful procedure; it does, however, decrease the risk, and allow any problem that does develop to be more efficiently rectified with remedial training as necessary.

## 12.3.1.2   TRANSPORT PROCEDURES

As mentioned previously, the animal is confronted with possible stressors even before it leaves its home. Problems with travelling have been covered in Chapter 10, but there is more to transport than the car. Cats need to learn to perceive the carrier as a safe place. This will not happen if the carrier is only brought into the house immediately before the cat is taken someplace. Instead, it should be a normal part of the cat's environment, a place in which it might sleep or eat in its everyday life, and which from time to time is also used to transport it from one room to the another, where there are favourite treats waiting for it. Or perhaps the cat can be taken for a drive around the block inside its carrier and then brought back home. Using pheromonatherapy in this context can greatly enhance the positive perception of the carrier. If it is then used once in a while to take the cat to the

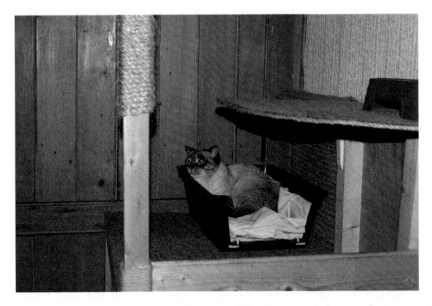

**Fig. 12.2** Using a cat's carrier as part of its normal furniture can help to make transport less stressful. Carriers from which the top can be completely removed are preferable for this purpose.

veterinary practice, the presence of the cage and being locked into it are not additional stressors. In order to help to extend this sense of well-being into the clinic, it is preferable to use a carrier whose top half can be removed, so that the cat can easily be accessed and remain on its safe bed while being examined (Figure 12.2).

### 12.3.1.3   *MUZZLE TRAINING*

Even the most friendly of dogs, if in pain, can bite in anticipation of pain when being approached or as a reflex when a painful area is being manipulated. Every dog should be trained to enjoy being muzzled irrespective of the current need for it (details of how to achieve this are available in the Further Reading section at the end of the chapter). This is as important as training a dog to walk on a lead: it could save its life. Willing acceptance of the muzzle is one less potential stressor in the clinic. Training should be gradual and always associated with something positive (most frequently food). It should not be left to when the dog needs to go to the clinic, but rather should be part of its early training.

### 12.3.1.4   *BEING HANDLED WITH INTENT*

If an animal is not used to being handled or touched with intent, this alone can be quite stressful. If there is additional pain, discomfort or confusion, the animal will be even more challenged. If the animal is used to being touched in a more invasive manner than simply petting or stroking, however – that is, it is used to having its ears and eyes looked at, its mouth opened, its body palpated, its temperature taken – then the number and intensity of stressors is diminished, making it easier for the animal to cope. It is important for veterinarians, dog trainers and puppy-class trainers to emphasise the relevance of practising this to owners; but it is equally important to give the owners clear instructions on how to practise this so as not to hurt or overwhelm the animal, building positive associations instead.

### 12.3.1.5   *TEACHING CLIENTS TO READ THEIR PETS*

Giving owners guidance on how to correctly read their animals and how to appropriately react to them when they are showing signs of distress is important. If owners are aware of the need to both avoid and prepare for the potential stressors discussed in this chapter, they are likely to want to learn what they can do to minimise them. Awareness-raising is therefore as important as offering advice.

### 12.3.2   *PREVENTION IN THE CLINIC*

If good-quality information has been communicated to clients then they are responsible for ensuring that journeys to and from the veterinary clinic are as stress-free as possible (see Section 12.3.1.2 and Chapter 10). The veterinary staff is responsible for ensuring the same within the clinic environment. We will look at the different aspects of this more closely, from the waiting process, through the consultation room to the hospital area.

### 12.3.2.1   *THE WAITING ROOM AND CONSULTATION ROOM*

Although there is some evidence to suggest that for certain dogs spending more time in a waiting room can help them adapt and therefore enter the consultation room feeling more relaxed, for most dogs and perhaps all cats this is unlikely to be the case. Ideally there should be a separate waiting area for dogs and cats, but where this is not possible it helps to have at least two parts to the waiting area, which are visually separated, and to ensure that there are shelves high up on which owners can rest their cat carriers, away from dogs and others. Another consideration is flooring: this should not be slippery, so that walking is easy, especially for older and sick animals.

Using pheromonatherapy in the waiting room area can be very helpful too. Diffusers which produce the feline facial fraction F3 should be used to create a greater chemical sense of security, without risk of cross-reaction. A double-blind within-subjects placebo-controlled study found that dogs with a history of problems at the clinic were less anxious, more relaxed and more likely to investigate their surroundings when exposed to dog-appeasing pheromone (DAP) in the waiting room.

Pets differ as to whether they respond more calmly in the clinic in the owner's presence or absence, and this issue needs to be sensitively addressed by the practice staff. The owner's knowledge of their pet should be respected. If an owner says that their dog will feel less stressed being examined on the floor as opposed to the examination table then careful consideration needs to be given to examining the dog on the floor, with appropriate safety measures if necessary. If a cat might feel more comfortable sitting on its owners lap then the veterinarian can try to examine it there, as long as the owner acknowledges any risks. Unfortunately, almost every physical examination will involve potentially uncomfortable, if not painful, procedures – and this cannot be avoided. What can be changed, however, is how people approach and handle the animal. The aim is for the animal to be as comfortable as possible, to ensure maximum cooperation. Simply giving the animal time and space to acclimatise to its surroundings in the consultation room can help it to relax. Working slowly and being relaxed oneself can remove a lot of pressure from the animal and will in the end save everybody time and reduce the risk of injury to all.

In order to be perceived as minimally threatening, the person handling the animal must be familiar with the species and its normal means of communication, and must respond appropriately in light of this. Professional staff should try to adopt the following nonthreatening postures and techniques:

- Let the animal investigate the room and ideally let it initiate contact (as long as it is known not to be predisposed to aggressive behaviour). If approach must be initiated, do so indirectly and to the side.
- Avoid potentially threatening gestures such as direct eye contact, leaning or reaching over a dog or a cat.
- Avoid rushed, big, brusque or indecisive movements.
- Hold the animal only enough to secure it and not so much as to cause it to feel trapped.
- Give the owner clear instructions about what to expect and what they should do: whether they should be in our out of sight, touching or not touching the animal (depending on the individual) and so on.
- Let the animal know what is going to happen, by caressing it in the area first, for example, so as to make the next move predictable, and speaking in a soft, friendly voice.
- Recognise the different signs of the different forms of distress and respond appropriately to them (acknowledging the animal's signals through appropriate communication).
- Use pheromonatherapy to help minimise the negative effects of any uncertainty in the environment. This is discussed further later in this section in relation to its specific use in dogs and cats.

Döring *et al.* (2009) investigated the effect of DAP on dogs' behaviour in the consultation room. Dogs exposed to DAP were less anxious and tended to be less aroused, but a single exposure did not have an effect on their overt response to being handled. However, another study with a much larger sample size (105 dogs, with 52 exposed to DAP and 53 to placebo) concluded that dogs were calmer when having their ears and mouth checked, their abdomen palpated, their rectal temperature taken and receiving an injection. There was, however, no effect on their tendency to display aggressive behaviour, highlighting the importance of controlling this predisposition with other specific behaviour-modification techniques.

In conclusion, it seems that DAP is able to reduce the impact of less intense signs and forms of aversion but does not alter the style of response once the animal is aroused in a particular way (i.e. it is not sedative). However, anecdotal reports from a number of practices that use DAP regularly suggest a reduction in the risk of aggressive behaviour over time, perhaps as a result of animals not being so aroused in the first place. DAP is not a 'cure-all' or a substitute for good practice but rather is a complement to good practice. If animals are handled in a sensitive way and DAP is used, the risk to staff throughout the practice may be greatly reduced, the welfare of the animal may be significantly increased and the veterinarian should be more able to do their job.

In the case of cats, it has been reported that the use of the F4 facial fraction (Felifriend®) in the consultation room can significantly improve a cat's willingness to interact with the clinician and allow examination. It was found that cats in the F4 treated group typically approached the veterinarian in less than 2 minutes, whereas those in the placebo group took longer than 20 minutes on average to approach. Only 20% of the cats in the F4 group showed aggression, compared to nearly every cat in the placebo group. Clearly, pheromonatherapy has an important role to play in helping to reduce uncertainty in the veterinary clinic, but it must be accompanied by sensitive handling.

This is reinforced by anecdotal reports of an occasional, seemingly paradoxical increase in aggression by a cat exposed to F4 in this context. When we have looked into these cases the animal has had a long history of bad experiences at the veterinary clinic and it may well be that the contradictory signal causes the animal to more readily become aggressive. However, for animals new to the clinic, the use of F4 prior to handling in the consultation room may help. In conclusion, this form of pheromonatherapy is most effective when the encounter is new, rather than with an established history of problems; that is, F4 helps to minimise the aversion associated with an uncertain social encounter, while F3 may help an animal to perceive the physical environment as safe.

In order to maximise the potential of controlling chemical signals in the clinic setting it is very important to clean areas regularly (especially the examination table, which should be cleaned between patients) with an enzymatic cleaner in order to remove any alarm pheromones that may have been deposited and to minimise aerial contamination. Measures can also be taken to exert beneficial control over other sensory channels, such as auditory stressors. It is helpful to try to keep the waiting area and the consultation room as quiet as possible, furnishing them with sound-absorbing surfaces, avoiding loud talk and keeping the phone area as separate as possible from the patient area. The lighting can influence stress levels too: the flickering of a neon light might bother an animal more than it does a human, due to differences in critical flicker fusion frequencies in the eye. Visual decoration needs careful consideration too: the dog statue in the corner or animal silhouettes on the wall may be pleasant to owners but not their pets. Even if the reaction of the animal is just an increase in vigilance, this is another unnecessary stressor adding to the total load the patient has to cope with and therefore increasing the challenge of the situation.

## 12.3.2.2  *THE HOSPITAL KENNEL AND CATTERY AREA*

Many of the general management principles discussed in the previous section also apply to the back-room hospital areas: avoiding contact between cats and dogs and so on. Quite a lot of work has been done on the use of pheromonatherapy in rescue shelters, which may be of relevance. F4 seems to help cats cope with the transition into the shelter and the proximity of other cats, while DAP seems to help dogs adjust to the shelter, reducing the amount and average volume of barking, especially when someone walks by. There have also been a number of specific studies focused around the veterinary hospital. One study on the effects of DAP on perisurgical stress found that DAP reduced both behavioural signs of stress in dogs (they were more alert and visually explorative after surgery) and neuroendo-crinal responses (postoperative decreases in prolactin were smaller). Another reported that DAP reduced restlessness, elimination and excessive licking in the hospital kennel. F3 has been found to help calm cats during intravenous catheteri-sation, but like DAP in the consulting room it does not appear to have any sedative effect. In the hospital cage, F3 has been found to reduce time spent sleeping but increase lying, sitting and grooming activity, and most importantly increase interest in food and the amount eaten. Given the problems that often occur with appetite in hospitalised cats, this effect may literally be a life-saver. It is also important to provide cats with some form of hide when hospitalised, such as a cardboard box, in order to increase their perceived control over the situation.

We therefore recommend that DAP and F3 diffusers are routinely used in the hospital housing area and that the relevant product is also sprayed into the pen 20 minutes or so before a new patient uses it (it should first be thoroughly cleaned and rinsed, since remnants of an enzymatic cleaner may break down the phero-mone product). Hospitalised animals should also be provided with articles from home wherever possible. It is important to recognise that pheromonatherapy does not produce sedation, so if an animal is aroused into a given state it will express the chosen behaviour with the same intensity as normal. However, although aggression does not appear to be directly affected by the commercially available pheromone products, the reduction in stress-related behaviours seen with them does reduce the risk in the long term.

## 12.3.3  *POST-VISIT MANAGEMENT*

The learning experience from a vet visit does not end when leaving the veterinary practice: there is still the return home, where there might be other pets waiting. The trip back should be made as stress-free as possible, for example by using pheromonatherapy to aid transport. With cats, the carrier should be cleaned on return and left out again, with clean or familiar bedding. F3 may be applied again, to encourage continued use of the area. A trip to the vet's may also result in a change in the odour of the animal, and other pets in the household might not recognise them at first. This can lead to aggressive interactions. Although there are no published studies on this, pheromonatherapy may help here by encouraging animals to relax upon reintroduction, as if it were their first encounter (see Chapter 11). Owners should be informed of this risk and encouraged to gradually reintroduce the pet back into the household, while watching the responses of the other residents. If there is any tension, pheromonatherapy should be used on this and all future occasions.

In the unfortunate event of a significant adverse event occurring in the clinic, owners should be informed of this and encouraged to undertake remedial training to ensure the animal can relax there in future. This will focus around building pleasant associations with the clinic and staff, as discussed previously.

## 12.4  CONCLUSION

A visit to the vet's has the potential to be a very stressful event for a cat or dog, but this is not necessarily the case. Nor is it inevitable that some pets will learn not to like the vet. With an awareness of the risks and sensitive management, including the judicious use of pheromonatherapy, many problems can be averted. These measures need not take a lot of time, but only require a consistently implemented policy. Indeed, over time, they will almost inevitably mean not only that procedures run more smoothly, but also that they can be done more quickly and certainly more safely. As with the other scenarios discussed in Part II of this text, it is important to remember that pheromonatherapy is not a substitute for good management but rather an integral part of it. It is hoped that this text goes some way to helping those who care about animals to care for them a little bit better.

## REVIEW ACTIVITIES

- Create a list of the procedures and circumstances that might give rise to specific emotional responses within the clinic. What measures can be taken to prevent these from arising and what should be done at the early signs of their emergence?
- Develop a client handout concerning the things a caring owner can do to minimise the stress of going to the vet's.
- Develop a remedial training programme for pets who have had a significant adverse experience at the clinic.

## REFERENCES

Döring D, Roscher A, Scheipl F, Küchenhoff J, Erhard MH (2009) Fear-related behaviour of dogs in veterinary practice. The Veterinary Journal 182: 38–43.
FAB (2006) Creating a cat friendly practice. Available from http://www.fabcats.org/catfriendlypractice/catfriendly44pp.pdf. (See also http://www.wellcat.org/.)

Stanford TL (1982) Behavior of dogs entering a veterinary clinic. Applied Animal Ethology 7: 271–279.
Zulch H, Mills D (2012) Life Skills for Puppies: Laying the Foundation for a Loving, Lasting Relationship. Dorchester: Veloce Publishing Ltd.

## FURTHER READING

Bonnafous L, Lafont C, Gaultier E, Falawée C, Pageat P (2005) Interest in the use of a new galenic form of the feline allomarking pheromone (F4) analog (Felifriend) during medical examination. In: Mills D, Levine E, Landsberg G, Horwitz D, Duxbury M, Mertens P, Meyer K, Radosta Huntley L, Reich M, Willard J (eds) Current Issues and Research in Veterinary Behavioral Medicine. West Lafayette, IN: Purdue University Press. pp. 119–122.
Griffith CA, Steigerwald ES, Buffington CAT (2000) Effects of a synthetic facial pheromone on behavior of cats. Journal of the American Veterinary Medical Association 217: 1154–1156.
Mills DS, Ramos D, Gandia Estelles M, Hargrave C (2006) A triple blind placebo-controlled investigation into the assessment of the effect of Dog Appeasing Pheromone (DAP) on anxiety related behaviour of problem dogs in the veterinary clinic. Applied Animal Behaviour Science 98: 114–126.
Rodan I, Sundahl E, Carney H, Gagnon A-C, Heath S, Landsberg G, Seksel K, Yin S (2011) AAFP and ISFM feline-friendly handling guidelines. Journal of Feline Medicine and Surgery 13: 364–375.
Siracusa C, Manteca X, Cuenca R, del Mar Alcalá M, Alba A, Lavín S, Pastor J (2010) Effect of a synthetic appeasing pheromone on behavioural, neuroendocrine, immune, and acute-phase perioperative stress responses in dogs. Journal of the American Veterinary Medical Association 237: 673–681.
University of Lincoln. Cat behaviour described. http://catbehaviour.blogs.lincoln.ac.uk.
University of Lincoln Animal Behaviour Clinic. Muzzle training video. Available from http://www.lincoln.ac.uk/dbs/abc/Muzzle%20Video.htm.
Yin S (2009) Low Stress Handling, Restraint and Behaviour Modification of Dogs and Cats. Davis, CA: Cattle Dog Publishing.

# Appendix A

# EDED (Evaluation of a Dog's Emotional Disorder) Scale

This scale was developed in France and considers three domains: *centripetal behaviour*, *centrifugal behaviour* and *health*. Each behavioural element within these areas is given a score between 1 and 5, and these are combined with a score derived from the weighted sum of specific conditions within the third domain, health, to provide a quantifiable score of the animal's emotional state.

## CENTRIPETAL BEHAVIOUR

This is behaviour that alters an animal's physiology and may be either inhibited or excessive during 'emotional disorders'. It is suggested that self-centred activities tend to increase in 'emotional disorders'. Activity of interest relates to: eating, drinking, self-stimulation, elimination behaviour and sleep-related activity.

## CENTRIFUGAL BEHAVIOUR

This is more externally targeted behaviour that produces a modification of an animal's environment, and includes aspects of cognitive functioning.

*Stress and Pheromonatherapy in Small Animal Clinical Behaviour*, First Edition.
Daniel Mills, Maya Braem Dube and Helen Zulch.
© 2013 John Wiley & Sons, Ltd. Published 2013 by John Wiley & Sons, Ltd.

| Behaviour type | Specific behaviour | Score |
|---|---|---|
| Feeding | Normal appetite | 1 |
| | Hyperphagia | 3 |
| | Hyperphagia with regurgitation and reingestion | 3 |
| | Hyporexia/anorexia | 4 |
| | Dysorexia (moving between hyper and hypo) | 5 |
| Drinking | Normal drinking | 1 |
| | Ritualised manipulation of water bowl, e.g. carries empty bowl around | 2 |
| | Champing at water without much drinking | 3 |
| | Polydipsia | 5 |
| Auto-stimulation | Normal grooming | 1 |
| | Excessive licking/nibbling | 4 |
| | Stereotypical grooming, circling or other repetitive behaviour | 5 |
| Sleep | Normal (no change) | 1 |
| | Increased (>12–14 hours/day) | 2 |
| | Decreased (<6 hours/day) or frequently disturbed sleeping bouts | 3 |
| | Anxiety/restlessness prior to sleeping and failure to settle initially | 5 |
| Exploration | Normal | 1 |
| | Inhibited | 2 |
| | Frequent avoidance responses | 3 |
| | Increased and hypervigilant | 4 |
| | Oral tendencies | 5 |
| Aggressive behaviour | No problems or change | 1 |
| | Irritability/frustration | 3 |
| | Fear-related | 4 |
| | Fear-related and irritability | 5 |
| Learned social responses | Unchanged | 1 |
| | No self-control when playing or submissiveness | 2 |
| | Bites without growling | 4 |
| | Steals and will not surrender stolen items | 5 |
| Learning performance | Stable and normal for age | 1 |
| | Arbitrary responses | 3 |
| | Complete loss of certain learned behaviours | 5 |
| Health | Normal | 1 |
| | Bouts of tachycardia and/or tachypnoea | 2 |
| | Colic or diarrhoea | 2 |
| | Bloat, stomach rumbles, retching or drooling | 2 |
| | Frequent emotional urination | 3 |
| | Acral lick lesion or extensive hair loss from self-grooming | 4 |
| | Obesity | 4 |
| | Polydipsia and polyuria | 4 |

# Appendix B

# The Lincoln Sound-sensitivity Scale

Please describe your dog's normal response to firework noises *in the home* in terms of the frequency (how often it occurs relative to the number of times your dog is scared) and intensity of each of the following behaviours:

## 1. RUNNING AROUND
Frequency:

| 0 | 1 | 2 | 3 |
|---|---|---|---|
| Never | Rarely | Frequently | Every time |

Intensity:

| 1 | 2 | 3 | 4 | 5 |
|---|---|---|---|---|
| Small amount – occasional burst of activity | | | | Extensive amount – continuously running around |

## 2. DROOLING SALIVA
Frequency:

| 0 | 1 | 2 | 3 |
|---|---|---|---|
| Never | Rarely | Frequently | Every time |

Intensity:

| 1 | 2 | 3 | 4 | 5 |
|---|---|---|---|---|
| Small amount – damp around mouth | | | | Extensive amount – pools of saliva |

*Stress and Pheromonatherapy in Small Animal Clinical Behaviour*, First Edition.
Daniel Mills, Maya Braem Dube and Helen Zulch.
© 2013 John Wiley & Sons, Ltd. Published 2013 by John Wiley & Sons, Ltd.

## 3.  HIDING (e.g. under furniture, behind owner, etc.) –
## PLEASE INDICATE WHERE

Frequency:

| 0 | 1 | 2 | 3 |
|---|---|---|---|
| Never | Rarely | Frequently | Every time |

Intensity:

| 1 | 2 | 3 | 4 | 5 |
|---|---|---|---|---|
| Small amount – retreats | | | | Extensive amount – will not be removed from hiding area |

## 4.  DESTRUCTIVENESS (E.G. FURNITURE, DOORS, CARPETS, ETC.) –
## PLEASE INDICATE WHICH ITEMS TEND TO BE DAMAGED

Frequency:

| 0 | 1 | 2 | 3 |
|---|---|---|---|
| Never | Rarely | Frequently | Every time |

Intensity:

| 1 | 2 | 3 | 4 | 5 |
|---|---|---|---|---|
| Small amount – small items, e.g. pens | | | | Extensive amount – e.g. holes in the wall |

## 5.  COWERING (E.G. TUCKS TAIL FLATTENS EARS, ETC.)

Frequency:

| 0 | 1 | 2 | 3 |
|---|---|---|---|
| Never | Rarely | Frequently | Every time |

Intensity:

| 1 | 2 | 3 | 4 | 5 |
|---|---|---|---|---|
| Small amount – uneasy | | | | Extensive amount – petrified |

## 6.  RESTLESSNESS / PACING

Frequency:

| 0 | 1 | 2 | 3 |
|---|---|---|---|
| Never | Rarely | Frequently | Every time |

Intensity:

| 1 | 2 | 3 | 4 | 5 |
|---|---|---|---|---|
| Small amount | | | | Extensive amount – fixed route continuously traced |

## 7. AGGRESSIVE BEHAVIOUR (E.G. GROWLING, SNAPPING OR BITING)

Frequency:

| 0 | 1 | 2 | 3 |
|---|---|---|---|
| Never | Rarely | Frequently | Every time |

Intensity:

| 1 | 2 | 3 | 4 | 5 |
|---|---|---|---|---|
| Small amount – occasional growl | | | | Extensive amount – severe biting attempts made |

## 8. "FREEZING TO THE SPOT"

Frequency:

| 0 | 1 | 2 | 3 |
|---|---|---|---|
| Never | Rarely | Frequently | Every time |

Intensity:

| 1 | 2 | 3 | 4 | 5 |
|---|---|---|---|---|
| Occurs sporadically within an event | | | | Most of the time |

## 9. BARKING/WHINING/HOWLING – PLEASE INDICATE WHICH OF THESE BEHAVIOURS

Frequency:

| 0 | 1 | 2 | 3 |
|---|---|---|---|
| Never | Rarely | Frequently | Every time |

Intensity:

| 1 | 2 | 3 | 4 | 5 |
|---|---|---|---|---|
| Small amount | | | | Extensive amount |

## 10. PANTING

Frequency:

| 0 | 1 | 2 | 3 |
|---|---|---|---|
| Never | Rarely | Frequently | Every time |

Intensity:

| 1 | 2 | 3 | 4 | 5 |
|---|---|---|---|---|
| Occurs sporadically within an event | | | | Most of the time |

## 11. VOMITING, DEFECATING, URINATING AND/ OR DIARRHOEA – PLEASE INDICATE WHICH OF THESE BEHAVIOURS

Frequency:

| 0 | 1 | 2 | 3 |
|---|---|---|---|
| Never | Rarely | Frequently | Every time |

Intensity:

| 1 | 2 | 3 | 4 | 5 |
|---|---|---|---|---|
| Small amount | | | | Excessive amount |

## 12. OWNER-SEEKING BEHAVIOUR

Frequency:

| 0 | 1 | 2 | 3 |
|---|---|---|---|
| Never | Rarely | Frequently | Every time |

Intensity:

| 1 | 2 | 3 | 4 | 5 |
|---|---|---|---|---|
| Seeks out owner occasionally during the event | | | | Will not leave owner in any circumstance |

## 13. VIGILANCE/SCANNING OF THE ENVIRONMENT

Frequency:

| 0 | 1 | 2 | 3 |
|---|---|---|---|
| Never | Rarely | Frequently | Every time |

Intensity:

| 1 | 2 | 3 | 4 | 5 |
|---|---|---|---|---|
| Occurs sporadically within an event | | | | Most of the time |

## 14. BOLTS

Frequency:

| 0 | 1 | 2 | 3 |
|---|---|---|---|
| Never | Rarely | Frequently | Every time |

Intensity:

| 1 | 2 | 3 | 4 | 5 |
|---|---|---|---|---|
| Occurs occasionally, in response to certain noises | | | | Occurs always, in response to a wide range of sounds |

## 15.  EXAGGERATED RESPONSE WHEN STARTLED

Frequency:

| 0 | 1 | 2 | 3 |
|---|---|---|---|
| Never | Rarely | Frequently | Every time |

Intensity:

| 1 | 2 | 3 | 4 | 5 |
|---|---|---|---|---|
| Occurs occasionally, in response to certain noises | | | | Occurs always, in response to a wide range of sounds |

## 16.  SHAKING OR TREMBLING

Frequency:

| 0 | 1 | 2 | 3 |
|---|---|---|---|
| Never | Rarely | Frequently | Every time |

Intensity:

| 1 | 2 | 3 | 4 | 5 |
|---|---|---|---|---|
| Occurs occasionally, in response to certain noises | | | | Occurs always, in response to a wide range of sounds |

## 17.  SELF-HARM

Frequency:

| 0 | 1 | 2 | 3 |
|---|---|---|---|
| Never | Rarely | Frequently | Every time |

Intensity:

| 1 | 2 | 3 | 4 | 5 |
|---|---|---|---|---|
| Small amount – e.g. licking feet | | | | Extensive amount – e.g. broken teeth or nails |

## 18.  OTHERS:

**Please detail**

Frequency:

| 0 | 1 | 2 | 3 |
|---|---|---|---|
| Never | Rarely | Frequently | Every time |

Intensity:

| 1 | 2 | 3 | 4 | 5 |
|---|---|---|---|---|
| Small amount | | | | Extensive amount |

19.  **Considering both the frequency of signs and their intensity and duration, how would you rate your dog's fear of fireworks on a scale of 0–10, where 0 = quite mild and 10 = could not be worse?** _____

# Glossary

This brief glossary deals with some of the terminology used in this text which may be less familiar to the reader or whose definition may vary between authors. It is not intended to be an exhaustive list of all technical terms, but rather a reference list for the current text. For more extensive information and discussion of some of the points raised, readers are referred to: Mills D (2010) The Encyclopedia of Applied Animal Behaviour & Welfare. Wallingford: CABI.

## A

Adaptation phase
: One of two alternative third phases of Selye's general adaptation syndrome, in which the animal adapts to the new situation. If adaptation is not possible, it leads to exhaustion (see *Exhaustion phase*).

Alarm phase
: The first phase of Selye's general adaptation syndrome, with increases in epinephrine and norepinephrine.

Ambivalent behaviour
: Conflict behaviour, with the individual showing elements of at least two opposing behaviours, such as a mixture of approach and avoidance.

*Anxiety–fear* system
: A motivational–emotional system related to the subjective perception and organisation of individualised behaviour associated with the comfort provided by predictable access to essential resources. Arousal occurs within this system when access is threatened or lost.

Attachment
: An enduring and specific affiliative bond between two individuals, characterised by a need for social contact between the two and distress at separation.

## B

Behaviour problem
: A behaviour that poses a problem to the carer of an animal. This can be normal or pathological, but being a problem does not necessarily indicate the behaviour is a sign of poor welfare.

Behaviour therapy
: The management of an animal's behaviour through a focus on its underlying emotional regulation (see *Training*).

*Stress and Pheromonatherapy in Small Animal Clinical Behaviour*, First Edition.
Daniel Mills, Maya Braem Dube and Helen Zulch.
© 2013 John Wiley & Sons, Ltd. Published 2013 by John Wiley & Sons, Ltd.

| | |
|---|---|
| Bolt hole | Somewhere that an animal runs to in order to try to escape or monitor a situation. It does not necessarily provide the comfort necessary for relaxation (see *Safe haven*). |

**C**

| | |
|---|---|
| *Care* system | A motivational–emotional system related to the subjective perception and organisation of individualised behaviour associated with the support of significant others, such as parental care or nurturance of others. |
| Communication | The transfer of information from a sender to a receiver, where both sender and receiver map a signal to a particular meaning. |
| Counterconditioning | Eliciting a behaviour or emotional response which is not compatible with another that might be aroused in similar circumstances. |

**D**

| | |
|---|---|
| *Desire* system | A motivational–emotional system related to the subjective perception and organisation of individualised behaviour associated with the exploitation of incentives. This involves the subjective encoding of the personal significance of seeking and consummatory activity towards different types of physical resource which have their own specific behavioural motivational systems (e.g. foraging, object play). |
| Discrete signal | A binary signal that is either wholly present or absent, such as individual identity (see *Graded signal*). |
| Displacement behaviour | A simple behaviour shown by an individual in conflict situations which seems completely irrelevant to solving the problem, such as sniffing the ground upon seeing another dog. |
| Dog-appeasing pheromone (DAP) | A pheromonal semiochemical of the dog which is believed to induce a bias in favour of the perception of a sense of safety. |

**E**

| | |
|---|---|
| Eliciting contexts | Situations in which a behaviour has been known to occur. Monitoring of the proportion of eliciting contexts in which a behaviour occurs is often used to assess progress during management. This involves calculating the number of times the animal shows the behaviour in a specific context (e.g. destructive when left alone) divided by the number of times the context occurs (the number of times the animal is left alone). |
| Eustress | Arousing situations which an animal may find pleasurable, such as those associated with reproduction or play. |

| | |
|---|---|
| Evaluation of a Dog's Emotional Disorder (EDED) scale | A scale produced by French behaviour vets to evaluate and monitor a range of behaviour problems and associated emotional states. See Appendix A. |
| Exhaustion phase | One of two alternative third phases of Selye's general adaptation syndrome, resulting from an animal not being able to adapt to the stress load, which will ultimately lead to the development of pathological processes and potentially premature death (see *Adaptation phase*). |

**F**

| | |
|---|---|
| F3 | A pheromonal fraction of the feline facial secretions, which is thought to aid organisation of the core area and provide reassurance in the presence of a threat to resources (see *Feliway*®). |
| F4 | A pheromonal fraction of the feline facial secretions, which is thought to aid social familiarisation between cats (see *Felifriend*®). |
| Fear | A typically adaptive response, which helps to protect the animal in the face of unpleasant events (see *Anxiety–fear system, Phobia*). |
| Felifriend® | A commercial product based around feline facial fraction F4. |
| Feliway® | A commercial product based around feline facial fraction F3. |
| Flehmen | Behaviour expressed to aid the perception of phero-mones. This varies between species, but in all instances is associated with the opening of the vomeronasal organ and increased flow of air into this structure. |
| *Frustration* system | A motivational–emotional system related to the subjective perception and organisation of individualised behaviour associated with exploiting incentives that are being denied. The system integrates the personal significance of a failure to meet expectations relating to resource acquisition or control (including territorial integrity) with the consequences of bodily restraint, in order to determine resulting strategic priorities. |

**G**

| | |
|---|---|
| General adaptation syndrome (GAS) | Theory of Hans Selye, used to describe the most common form of arousal resulting from a range of stressors and consisting of three phases of response to a stressor (alarm phase, period of resistance, adaptation or exhaustion phase). |
| Graded signal | A signal that can vary in intensity, such as a threatening display (see *Discrete signal*). |

**H**

Habit

A general, consistent behavioural response that is shown repeatedly in similar situations, often with little emotional arousal (see *Trait*).

Habituation

Process in which an individual learns to ignore a specific stimulus because it is irrelevant and so stops responding to it both physiologically and behaviourally.

Hypothalamic–
pituitary–adrenal
(HPA) system

Interconnected system consisting of information flow between the hypothalamus, pituitary and adrenal glands, which can result in the secretion of corticosteroid hormones and an associated change in metabolic activity, including suppression of the immune system.

**I**

Intraspecific
communication

Communication between individuals of the same species.

Interspecific
communication

Communication between individuals belonging to different species.

**L**

Learned helplessness

State of emotional and behavioural depression in which an animal has learned that it has no control over the outcome of a significant aversive stimulus. Experimentally induced by the random delivery of electric shocks.

*Lust* system

A motivational–emotional system related to the subjective perception and organisation of individualised behaviour associated with the reproductive needs of the individual, ranging from the attraction or selection of a mate through courtship and any associated bond to mating with a sexual partner.

**M**

Maladaptive behaviour

The failure of a behaviour to fulfil its normal biological goal at either an appetitive (goal-seeking) or consummatory (goal-execution) level, resulting in suboptimal behaviour.

Malfunction behaviour

Disorganisation of the mechanisms underlying the regulation, execution or structure of a behaviour.

Management strategy

The broad conceptual mechanism underpinning the way in which a problem behaviour is brought under control. Management strategies can be divided into those that seek to prevent the behaviour, remove triggers, alter perception of triggers, alter expression of the motivation and encourage alternatives.

Management
technique

The method used to bring about a strategic change in problem behaviour. Management techniques can be

|  | broadly defined as chemical, environmental, physical or psychological interventions. |
|---|---|
| Mood | A particular emotional predisposition to behave in a certain way over a limited time span, which is not contingent on a specific stimulus for its creation or elimination. |
| Motivational–emotional systems | Different types of contextually contingent behavioural control systems which are significantly affected by subjective inputs. These systems integrate subjective perceptions related to the values of significant stimuli associated with particular needs in order to prioritise activity directed towards achieving an individual's personal priorities at any given time. |

**N**

| Negative reinforcement | Increased probability of a behaviour recurring in similar circumstances as a result of escape from a contingent aversive. |
|---|---|
| Negative punishment | Decreased probability of a behaviour recurring in similar circumstances as a result of the elimination of a contingent incentive. |

**O**

| OARS | **O**pen-ended questioning, **A**ffirmation, **R**eflective listening, **S**ummarising. |
|---|---|

**P**

| *Pain* system | A motivational–emotional system related to the subjective perception and organisation of individualised behaviour associated with the maintenance of body integrity and function. This system needs to be distinguished from the sensory system that which deals with processing the nociceptive element of a pain stimulus. |
|---|---|
| *Panic–grief* system | A motivational–emotional system related to the subjective perception and organisation of individualised behaviour associated with the protection provided by others and reflected in a need for social contact (attachment). |
| Period of resistance | The second phase of Selye's general adaptation syndrome, associated with high levels of adrenal hormones (epinepherine, norepinephrine and corticosteroids) and anabolic hormones. |
| Personality | Biologically based behavioural predispositions that contribute to the definition of a relative stable but individually distinct phenotype (see *Temperament*). |
| Pheromonatherapy | The use of chemical signals normally involved in intraspceific communication within a clinical context to manage the behaviour of animals. |

| | |
|---|---|
| Pheromone | Originally (from Karlson & Lüscher): a substance secreted to the outside by an individual and received by a second individual of the same species, in which it releases a specific reaction. In this text: chemical signals normally used in intraspecific communication that are typically detected through the vomeronasal organ and which appear to have an effect on the emotional processing of the receiver. |
| Phobia | An extreme (often maladaptive) fear response that is ungraded and interferes with the subject's normal functioning (see *Fear*). |
| Positive punishment | The decreased probability of a behaviour recurring in similar circumstances as a result of the application of a contingent aversive. |
| Positive reinforcement | The increased probability of a behaviour recurring in similar circumstances as a result of the contingent acquisition of an incentive. |
| Primer pheromone | Pheromone that triggers a developmental process in another individual of the same species (see *Releaser pheromone*). |
| Pseudofear | An apparently fearful response that is largely devoid of fearful arousal, such as an attention-seeking activity. |

**R**

| | |
|---|---|
| Redirected behaviour | A behaviour that is directed towards a stimulus other than the relevant target might help an animal to cope with the arousal associated with a given event. |
| Releaser pheromone | Pheromone that releases a specific behaviour in another individual of the same species (see *Primer pheromone*). |
| Risk | The product of the probability of an event occurring and the severity of its consequences. |
| RSPCA | Royal Society for the Prevention of Cruelty to Animals. |

**S**

| | |
|---|---|
| Safe haven | A predefined area that is associated with the reliable absence of harm and absence of signs of harm and in which an animal is in control of events. It thus generates a sense of safety (see *Bolt hole*). |
| Sensitisation | Process whereby the physiological and behavioural response to a particular stimulus or event becomes more intense with repeated exposure. |
| Sensitive phase | Developmental phase in the early life of an individual that is particularly relevant to learning certain types of association. |
| *Social-play* system | A motivational–emotional system related to the subjective perception and organisation of individualised behaviour |

|  | associated with learning about social relationships and interaction styles. |
|---|---|
| Stimulus–response association | The reliably defined relationship between a specific environmental event and its behavioural outcome within an individual. |
| Stress audit | A systematic evaluation of the daily management routines and environment of an animal, with regards to the demands being placed upon it and its potential to cope. |
| Stress-induced dishabituation | A phenomenon induced by a significant stress load (often chronic) in which an individual appears to forget previous habituation learning. |
| Stressor | Anything that moves an animal out of its normal optimal range. The trigger of a stress response. |
| Stress response | The physiological, behavioural and psychological response to a challenge to an individual's optimal state of well-being. |
| Sympathetico-adrenomedullary (SAM) system | Interconnected system consisting of information flow between the sympathetic nervous system and the hormones produced by the adrenal medulla (epinephrine and norepinephrine). It is mainly involved in making the adjustments necessary for response to an unexpected event, such as increased arousal, environmental attention and preparation for possible further action. |
| Systematic desensitisation | Raising the threshold of intensity at which an animal responds to a given stimulus in a controlled way. |

**T**

| Temperament | The affective style of an individual, which is typically shaped by the effects of both genetic predisposition and early experience on motivational–emotional systems (see *Personality*). |
|---|---|
| Training | Modification of the behaviour of an animal, with a focus on the behavioural output in response to certain stimuli (see *Behaviour therapy*). |
| Trait | A predisposition to react in a certain way in response to certain broad classes of stimuli (see *Habit*). |

**U**

| Unconditional stimulus | Signal that brings about a certain response without the need for prior learning. However, the response may be changed as a result of learning. |
|---|---|

# Index

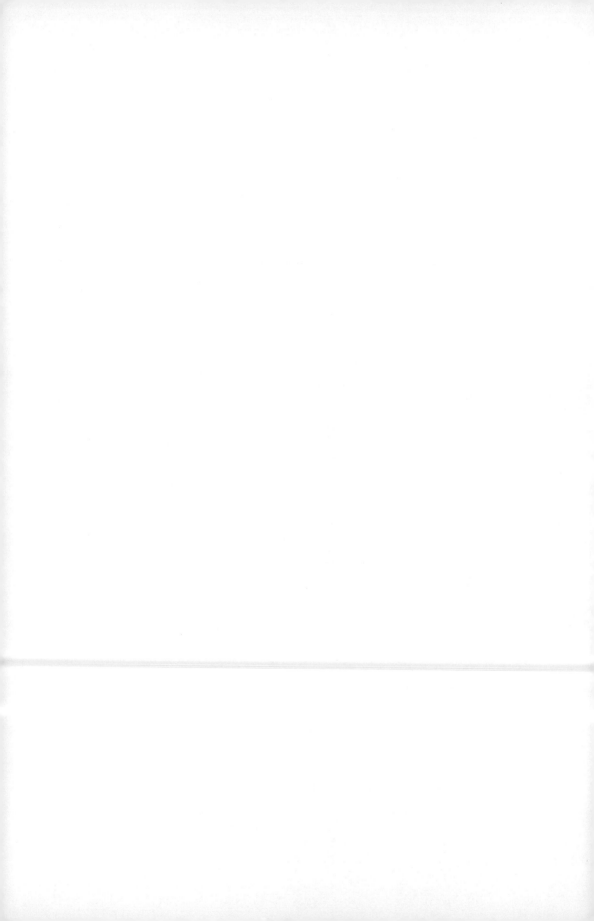

Printed and bound by CPI Group (UK) Ltd, Croydon, CR0 4YY

27/10/2024

14580288-0001